Proceedings in Life Sciences

Neural Transplantation and Regeneration

Edited by
Gopal D. Das and Robert B. Wallace

With Contributions by

M. Berry, A. Bignami, A. Björklund,
M.W. Brightman, P. Brundin, N.H. Chi, D. Dahl,
G.D. Das, F.F. Ebner, F.H. Gage, J.B. Gelderd,
S.A. Gilmore, J. Harnsberger, O. Isacson,
G.W. Kreutzberg, M.A. Matthews, L. Rees,
J.M. Rosenstein, D.T. Ross, J. Sievers, T.J. Sims,
L.M. Smith, R.B. Wallace

With 149 Figures

Springer-Verlag
New York Berlin Heidelberg Tokyo

Gopal D. Das
Department of Biological Sciences
Purdue University
West Lafayette, Indiana 47907
U.S.A.

Robert B. Wallace
Departments of Psychology and
  Biology
University of Hartford
West Hartford, Connecticut 06117
U.S.A.

On the front cover: A cluster of neurons in a neocortical transplant in the spinal
cord of a host animal. The neurons appear fully-differentiated, normal, and organized
in a cluster. Pyramidal and stellate cells can be identified in this cluster. (See
Chapter 1 for discussion.)

Library of Congress Cataloging-in-Publication Data
Main entry under title:
Neural transplantation and regeneration.
    (Proceedings in life sciences)
    Expanded version of material presented at a satellite
international symposium held in conjunction with the
13th Annual Meeting of the Society for Neuroscience
in Boston in 1983.
    Includes bibliographies and index.
    1. Nervous system—Regeneration—Congresses.
2. Nerve grafting—Congresses. I. Das, Gopal D.
II. Wallace, Robert B., 1937–   . III. Society for
Neuroscience. Meeting (13th : 1983 : Boston, Mass.)
IV. Series. [DNLM: 1. Nerve Regeneration—congresses.
2. Nerve Tissue—transplantation—congresses.
3. Neurosurgery—congresses. WL 368 N49394]
QP363.5.N47   1985   617′.48   85-17265

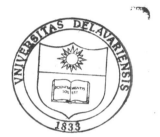

Typeset by Bi-Comp, Inc., York, Pennsylvania.
Printed and bound by H. Stürtz AG, Würzburg, Federal Republic of Germany.
Printed in the Federal Republic of Germany.

9 8 7 6 5 4 3 2 1

ISBN 0-387-96160-7 Springer-Verlag New York Berlin Heidelberg Tokyo
ISBN 3-540-96160-7 Springer-Verlag Berlin Heidelberg New York Tokyo

To those who will come after

Preface

Four years ago the first international symposium dealing with neural transplantation was organized as a satellite conference to the annual meeting of the Society for Neuroscience in Los Angeles, California. The expanded proceedings of that symposium were published by Springer-Verlag in 1983 in a volume entitled *Neural Tissue Transplantation Research*. We were sufficiently pleased with the results of that effort to organize a second satellite international symposium on Neural Transplantation and Regeneration in conjunction with the 13th Annual Meeting of the Society for Neuroscience in Boston in the fall of 1983.

Paralleling the growing body of research dealing with various aspects of neural transplantation, the scope of this second symposium was broadened to include not only transplantation but also regeneration. Additionally, topics of clinical interest were addressed as well as issues of basic research. The promise apparent in that first conference is still seen in the second as more and more investigators apply their talents in an attempt to understand this infant field of research. The present volume represents an expanded version of the material presented at the second symposium.

We wish to thank all of the contributors to the conference and to this volume for their insight and their assistance.

West Lafayette   Gopal D. Das
West Hartford   Robert B. Wallace

Acknowledgments

The editors wish to thank the Society for Neurosciences for help in the organization of this second satellite symposium on Transplantation and Regeneration. We also wish to thank Mrs. Claire Silverstein and Mrs. Shirley Siegel for their assistance in the preparation of this manuscript and in the organization of the symposium.

Contents

Contributors

The following is a list of contributors. The author's complete address is found on the first page of their contribution. Numbers in parentheses indicate the page on which the contribution begins.

M. Berry (63)
A. Bignami (229)
A. Björklund (103)
M.W. Brightman (277)
P. Brundin (103)
N.H. Chi (229)
D. Dahl (229)
G.D. Das (1, 181)

F.F. Ebner (81)
F.H. Gage (103)
J.B. Gelderd (149)
S.A. Gilmore (245)
J. Harnsberger (287)
O. Isacson (103)
G.W. Kreutzberg (271)
M.A. Matthews (125, 149)

L. Rees (63)
J.M. Rosenstein (277)
D.T. Ross (181)
J. Sievers (63)
T.J. Sims (245)
L.M. Smith (81)
R.B. Wallace (287)

Chapter 1

Neural Transplantation in Spinal Cord under Different Conditions of Lesions and Their Functional Significance

GOPAL D. DAS*

Introduction

Research on the problems of trauma and regeneration in the spinal cord has a long history. The importance of this research lies in the fact that trauma to this structure deprives the individual of voluntary control over the basic motor functions, such as movement of limbs involved in locomotion. The severity of trauma and the level of spinal cord where it is inflicted determine the nature and magnitude of loss of motor functions. Understanding the complexity of pathological events ensuing from the trauma, the nature and permanency of the functional loss, and the difficulties inherent in the restitution of the lost functions has been a concern for investigators in many fields. Pathologists, neurobiologists, neuroembryologists, and neurosurgeons, among others, have contributed to a considerable extent within their respective domains towards explaining why, following a serious trauma, there is no functional recovery, and have speculated variously on how to achieve it. At different periods, various investigators claimed recovery of lost locomotor functions following surgical or pharmacological treatments. But those claims could not be supported by other investigators working independently. Thus, despite the great progress made towards an understanding of the pathological events and the problems of limited or no regeneration of damaged fiber systems, the goal of achieving recovery of the lost motor functions has remained beyond our reach.

During the past decade or so, neural transplantation in the mammalian brain has emerged as an important field in neuroscience. Many basic issues related to survival, growth, differentiation, and integration of neural transplants have yet to be investigated systematically. But this field has generated some hope for the recovery of functions lost because of trauma to supraspinal structures. And, in the same vein, neural transplantation is seen to offer some promise for the conditions of spinal cord trauma.

* Department of Biological Sciences, Purdue University, West Lafayette, Indiana 47907 U.S.A.

The use of the spinal cord as a neural structure for the study of experimental trauma and neural transplantation poses many problems, among them: How to define a trauma that consistently yields paraplegic syndrome in a high percentage of preparations? What are the characteristics of paraplegic syndrome in experimental animals? What is the relationship between sparing of selected fiber tracts and spontaneous recovery from paraplegic syndrome within a few days following the trauma? What are the problems of survival and growth of neural transplants in a pathological milieu of a damaged spinal cord? Does neural transplantation aid in the recovery of the lost motor functions? If so, how much? And what precisely is the role of a neural transplant in such a recovery? Research in our laboratory over the last several years provides some information on these questions, which is presented in this chapter. It is essential to point out that these findings are based upon the use of the most common experimental animal, the rat, and that any extrapolation of these findings to human conditions must be done with great caution.

Models of Experimental Trauma to the Spinal Cord—Historical Background

A review of literature on the experimentally induced trauma to the spinal cord indicates that, broadly speaking, two types of traumas have been investigated extensively: impact injuries and severance injuries. The former involves injuries resulting from a violent blow to the vertebral column or the spinal cord that does not directly tear through the meningeal membranes or the spinal cord parenchyma. The latter, in contrast, involves direct tearing and damage to the meningeal membranes and the spinal cord parenchyma with a sharp and penetrating instrument. This classification is helpful not only in understanding different patterns of histopathological changes following the trauma but also in differentiating the conceptual basis for therapeutic procedures suggested by various investigators. Further, under both these conditions the trauma may vary in severity, leading to conditions whereby subthreshold trauma may not produce any symptoms at all and suprathreshold trauma may affect the very survival of the animal. Over the decades, these two models of experimental trauma have been modified and improved upon to satisfy the following requirements: Operationally, they should be as close to human conditions as possible; technically, the trauma should be highly reproducible; the syndrome produced by a trauma should be clearly observable and permanent; and the course of histopathological events should correspond to that in humans. These and other issues on the experimental production of spinal cord trauma have been discussed by Dohrmann (1972), Tator (1972), Osterholm (1974), Jellinger (1976), Collins and Kauer (1979), Windle (1980), and Bohlmann et al. (1982).

Windle (1980) has distinguished closed impact injuries from open impact injuries. The former include only those injuries that involve an impact by a blunt blow or a speeding missile on the vertebrae. As a result of this, the spinal cord suffers from concussion-type trauma. In a strict sense this may be considered as an indirect injury to the spinal cord (Jellinger 1976). This model of spinal cord injury has the closest bearing to the injuries in humans. But the work by Groat et al. (1945) and Brookhart et al. (1948) showed that the neurological deficit produced by this experimental approach was generally transient and difficult to reproduce with a high degree of consistency. It is possible that these limitations in this model made it less acceptable for continued investigations. The open impact injuries, in contrast, have been employed successfully by many investigators. Allen (1911, 1914) introduced a well-controlled, standardized, and quantifiable method for producing open impact injuries in experimental animals. According to this method, the anesthetized animals are surgically prepared for laminectomy, the spinal cord with its meningeal membranes intact is held in a fixed position, and a known weight from a predetermined height is dropped on the spinal cord. To the extent that the meningeal membranes are not torn apart and the spinal cord is not lacerated directly by the impact of the weight, this model is considered to yield contusion-type lesions. This model of producing spinal cord injury has many advantages. First, the injuries produced by this method are close to those encountered in human cases. Second, the trauma can be operationally defined and the force of impact quantified. This permits the varying of the severity of injury quantitatively, establishing threshold values for the impact force that yield a clearly observable syndrome and replication of experiments by independent investigators. Further, because with this method the meningeal membranes are left intact, there is no danger of loose connective tissue, interstitial fluid, or any other foreign agents penetrating into the traumatized region of the spinal cord. These aspects of open impact injury have proven very valuable to pathologists and neurosurgeons in their investigations on pathological events leading to paraplegia in the experimental animals.

The weight-dropping method, with all its advantages, suffers from some technical drawbacks. The major problem with this technique has been a high degree of variability in the severity of trauma and in the paraplegic syndrome, even when all the operational procedures are kept constant (Ducker and Hamit 1969, Campbell et al. 1973, Koozekanani et al. 1976, Koenig and Dohrmann 1977, Molt et al. 1979). The technical problems contributing to this variability seem to reside in the instability of the vertebral column and the spinal cord and lateral displacement of the cord at the time of impact. A lesion produced under these conditions is asymmetrical, with more sparing of fiber bundles on one side than on the other, and is inconsistent in size in different animals. For this reason, the experimental animals may or may not show any syndrome, and those that do may show paraplegic syndrome of different degrees of severity lasting for different durations after the injury. In order to overcome these artifacts of experimentation, various modifications have been introduced by different investigators (Yashon et al. 1973, de la Torre et al. 1975, Dohrmann et al. 1976, 1978, Gerber and Corrie 1979). Essentially all the improvements are aimed at holding the spinal cord firmly at the time of impact. With these modifications it is possible to obtain well-defined and reproducible lesions in the spinal cord. In his recent report, Ford (1983) has critically evaluated various modifications of the weight-dropping technique and has suggested further improvements that ensure the reproducibility of the injury and that help define the threshold lesion for paraplegic syndrome in cats.

A variation of the weight-dropping technique, successfully developed and employed by some investigators, is compression of the spinal cord. Tarlov et al (1953) developed balloons of different sizes and placed them in the extradural space of the spinal cord. By inflating them at different rates, lesions of different magnitude could be induced in the spinal cord. This technique, although simple and effective, did not yield uniform lesions. Tator (1971, 1973) introduced a modification that involved insertion of an inflatable silastic cuff extradurally surrounding the spinal cord in its entire transverse plane. With this, uniform compression lesions of spinal cord could be produced. These two methods and their variations have been used extensively to study pathological events and the effects of various pharmacological treatments on the pathological conditions (Richardson and Nakamura 1971, Beggs and Waggener 1973, Doppman et al. 1973, Hansebout et al. 1975, Anderson et al. 1976, Sandler and Tator 1976, Kobrine et al. 1978, Schramm et al. 1979, Means et al. 1981). Other attempts to produce a contusion-type lesion comparable to that in human patients have involved spinal cord distraction (Dolan et al. 1980, Hung et al. 1981, Cusick et al. 1982).

Studies on contusion-type trauma to the spinal cord have contributed significantly in three major directions: establishing a distinction between reversible and irreversible changes related to transient and permanent paraplegic syndrome (Assenmacher and Ducker 1971, Dohrmann et al. 1971), providing an analysis of the histopathological course of events that results in paraplegia (Tator 1972, Osterholm 1974, Ducker 1976, Bohlmann et al. 1982), and developing therapeutic measures to help retard and arrest, if not reverse, the course of pathological changes (Tator 1972, Osterholm 1974). An understanding of the reversible and irreversible changes following a trauma was of importance in that it pointed out the sources and dangers of artifacts of experimentation and observations on paraplegia, stressed the precise definition of threshold lesions for obtaining permanent paraplegia, and directed attention towards an analysis of pathological events underlying paraplegia. Findings made on the histopathological aspects of trauma, in addition to providing a wealth of data on pathophysiology of the spinal cord, have aided in the conceptualization of secondary injuries to the spinal cord. Although in the literature the primary injuries following a contusion-type trauma have not been precisely defined, one must assume that disruption of any cellular or tissue integrity constitutes the primary injury. Since hemorrhage at the site of trauma is the most striking event, it is safe to suggest that damage to the blood vessels may be the important primary injury. Other primary injuries may include damage to the cells and their membranes, axons, and myelin structure. Other pathological events, such as hemorrhage, edema, ischemia, and necrosis, that follow the trauma are considered as the secondary injuries or secondary traumatic changes. In other words, the contusion-type trauma, at least immediately following the injury, is more characterized by secondary pathological changes than by primary injuries. Allen

(1911, 1914) noticed the extensiveness of hemorrhage soon after the injury caused by the dropping of a weight on the spinal cord. But it was Freeman and his associates (Freeman and Wright 1953, Joyner and Freeman 1963) who emphasized the role of secondary injuries in determining the paraplegic syndrome. Since then various investigators have analyzed different aspects of secondary injuries in the spinal cord and their relative importance in leading to paraplegia. Extensive hemorrhage in the central gray of the spinal cord has been recognized as an important pathological event observable soon after the trauma (Goodkin and Campbell 1969, White et al. 1969, Assenmacher and Ducker 1971, Wagner et al. 1971). Ducker et al. (1971) demonstrated that the magnitude of hemorrhage was directly related to the severity of the trauma, thus emphasizing the importance of the concept of threshold lesions for producing irreversible or permanent paraplegia. Another important observation made by various investigators pertains to the increase in hemorrhage over a span of time following the lesion (Ducker et al. 1971, Osterholm 1974, Ducker 1976, Jellinger 1976, Balentine and Paris 1978a). These and other studies have shown that for some time after the trauma the zone of hemorrhage is seen to spread in both transverse and longitudinal planes until it achieves a stable value. At rostral and caudal levels it is seen to taper off. Thus, in the final analysis, the zone of hemorrhage is found to be much larger than the zone of direct trauma. Following closely these changes in the hemorrhage, edema is seen to set in and increase (Goodkin and Campbell 1969, Fairholm and Turnbull 1971, Yashon et al. 1973, Griffiths 1975). Generally, many investigators are of the opinion that both hemorrhage and edema are first set in the gray matter of the spinal cord and then spread peripherally into the white matter (Goodkin and Campbell 1969, White et al. 1969, Kelly et al. 1970, Dohrmann et al. 1971, Wagner et al. 1971, Green and Wagner 1973). This pattern of spread eventually results in a spindle-shaped region in the spinal cord defining the zone of hemorrhage and edema. Necrosis, or necrotic lesion, in the spinal cord, which is considered to be due to hemorrhagic conditions rather than the direct trauma, is seen to follow the same pattern and occupy the same territory as the hemorrhage and edema. More often than not, the necrotic lesion may extend beyond the zone of hemorrhage and edema, and this is attributed to obstructive consequences of vascular injury in the spinal cord parenchyma close to the zone of hemorrhage (Balentine and Paris 1978a). This sequence of pathological progression in experimental animals is seen to be completed within 24 hours (Osterholm 1974, Balentine and Paris 1978a); and, at the end, fragmented necrotic tissue, aggregates of erythrocytes and leucocytes, and macrophages are seen at the site of necrotic lesion. In addition to hemorrhage and edema, the pathological events related to secondary traumatic injuries, ischemia, and hypoxia in the traumatic zone of the spinal cord have been considered as factors contributing to tissue necrosis and paraplegia (Woodward and Freeman 1956, Kelly et al. 1970, Ducker and Perot 1971, Locke et al. 1971, Hukuda and Wilson 1972, Rawe et al. 1978, Seuter and Venes 1979). Of equal importance were the findings by Osterholm and Mathews (1972a,b) that in the region of trauma there was a significant increase in norepinephrine. This could cause vasoconstriction of uninjured blood vessels, thus resulting in ischemia and hypoxia in and near the region of trauma in the spinal cord. However, Bingham et al. (1975) in their studies found an increase in the level of dopamine, but not in that of nor-epinephrine, not only at the site of trauma but also at rostral and caudal levels to it. Although these biogenic amines have an influence on the blood vessels, it is very likely that their high levels may also have profound effects on the necrotic mass and the viable neural parenchyma of the spinal cord. But these effects are not known. The phase of pathological changes is followed by phago-cytic activity, clearing of necrotic debris, emergence of cysts, repair and regen-eration of damaged blood vessels, delimitation of the region of necrosis from viable neural parenchyma, and glial reaction. These changes contribute to sta-bilization and containment of pathological reaction, preservation of axons that may have still remained viable, and provide a milieu conducive for any possible regenerative processes. The glial reaction, which ultimately results in the de-velopment of glial scar formation, may have an important role to play in delim-iting viable spinal cord tissue from the necrotic mass.

Many investigators employing contusion-type trauma to the spinal cord have emphasized secondary injuries as the main cause of necrosis and of paraplegia, but this does not mean that neurons and axons subjected to such a trauma are not affected at all. Groat et al. (1945), Gelfan and Tarlov (1956), Tarlov (1957, 1972), and Fairholm and Turnbull (1970, 1971) observed histopathological changes in the gray as well as the white matter of the spinal cord. Soon after trauma, neurons as well as glia cells show pathological reactions. Astroglial elements, in particular, show swelling in a striking manner (Dohrmann et al. 1971, 1973). Kobrine et al. (1975), Bresnahan et al. (1976), Bresnahan (1978), and Balentine and Paris (1978b) have shown that axons in various ascending as well as descending fiber tracts are directly damaged by the mechanical force of the trauma. The early changes observed include fragmentation of myelin, axonal swelling, axonal fragmentation, and abnormal accumulation of various organelles in the axons. Such pathological changes are observed to be lasting and progressive in nature (Wakefield and Eidelberg 1975). Bresnahan (1978) found that under these traumatic conditions small fibers degenerate first and large-caliber fibers later. However, Blight (1983a) has observed that it is the large-caliber axons that are more readily subjected to degenerative changes following the trauma. He has shown, further, that owing to the injury there is a severe reduction in the number of axons with sustained loss of myelin over a prolonged period of time, and the surviving axons, if any, tend to be located along the periphery, subpially. The surviving axons are seen to be distributed in the form of a rim equally in the posterior, lateral, and anterior funiculi. The finding on the sparing and survival of axons following a trauma is of importance in understanding the nature of factors underlying reversible or transient para-plegia.

When the above studies are viewed comprehensively it is found that the weight-dropping model for spinal cord trauma has contributed significantly towards the understanding of the histopathological nature of paraplegia. In essence, there seem to be three different, but overlapping, events that determine the development of paraplegic syndrome: primary trauma, secondary traumatic changes, and progressive degenerative changes. Obviously, all these three events must be of suprathreshold value to yield permanent paraplegia, but thus far major emphasis has been placed upon the secondary traumatic changes. In the studies described in this presentation an attempt is made to define the role of progressive degenerative changes in the development of paraplegia.

Experimental studies employing severance injuries to the spinal cord have always involved the severing of fiber tracts and gray matter with a surgical blade. Such lesions, whether complete or partial, are straight-line and clean lesions, with minimal amount of bleeding at the site of trauma. Investigators employing these lesions in their studies generally make use of various chemo- and electro-cauterizing agents to control and stop bleeding. These experimental conditions, although far removed from human conditions of spinal trauma, assure clean lesions with very little, if any, ensuing secondary traumatic changes. Therefore, the paraplegic syndrome obtained with this model of trauma is directly attributable to the primary trauma of the severance of axons and the gray matter and, more precisely, to the absence of anatomical and physiological continuity and connectivity between the segments rostral and caudal to the lesion. These considerations have led investigators to postulate that if the severed axons could regenerate, there would be a recovery from the paraplegic syndrome. This line of reasoning seems to be the underlying force that has determined the types of questions posed, the nature of experimental designs followed, and the nature of observations made by investigators in this field of neurobiology. Thus, for the researchers employing this model of spinal cord trauma, the regeneration of axons, or lack thereof, and paraplegia are the two most intimately related issues. Investigations on the regeneration of axons in the central nervous system, no doubt, are of importance in their own right, but it remains questionable how far they are related to the actual conditions of spinal cord trauma and ensuing paraplegic syndrome in human cases. Review articles by Lee (1929), Windle (1956), Clemente (1964), Guth and Windle (1970), Puchala and Windle (1977), and Kiernan (1979) and a conference report by Veraa and Grafstein (1981) provide an extensive literature survey on various aspects of regeneration. Without going into historical details some major issues will be considered here.

Ramon y Cajal (1928), Brown and McCouch (1947), Lampert and Cressman (1964), and various other investigators have observed that regeneration shown by the axons of the central nervous system is, at best, abortive in nature. Their observations indicated that the regenerative process may begin after some days following the lesion, but eventually the axonal sprouts die back. The lack of sustained and elongated regrowth of severed axons has been observed under various other conditions of trauma. However, of interest were the reports by Sugar and Gerard (1940) and Freeman (1952, 1954, 1962) who found that following complete transection of the spinal cord the animals showed paraplegic syndrome and that, subsequently, they showed recovery from the syndrome that was related to regeneration of the severed axons. Their reports indicate that regeneration was observed only in a small number of axons. Since then a number of investigators, who have performed complete transection of the spinal cord under well-defined conditions, have not been able to support their claims on regeneration in the spinal cord (Brown and McCouch 1974, Davidoff and Ransohoff 1948, Barnard and Carpenter 1950, Feigin et al. 1951, Stelzner et al. 1975, Cummings et al. 1981). The functional recovery from paraplegic syndrome, observed by early investigators, is generally considered to be due to sparing of a small number of axons while making lesions in the spinal cord (Windle et al. 1958, Barker and Eayrs 1967, Feringa et al. 1976, Eidelberg et al. 1977, Vahlsing and Feringa 1980). In other words, what was considered as complete transection in all likelihood was incomplete severance of the spinal cord. The spared axons, although small in number, probably recovered from the spinal shock after some time and, thus, recovered from the paraplegic syndrome. Since then, reports on total transection of spinal cord and claims on recovery from paraplegia following such lesions are treated with a great degree of skepticism. Guth et al. (1980a), in an attempt to establish some rigor in this research, have formulated some essential criteria for the evaluation of spinal cord lesions and regeneration of severed axons.

The sparing of a small number of axons in the ventral funiculi has been found to be associated with transient paraplegia, which is considered to indicate recovery from paraplegic syndrome (Windle et al. 1958). On the basis of this observation, it is often concluded that, following complete transection of the spinal cord, even if a small number of axons were to show regeneration there would be sufficient grounds to expect some degree of functional recovery. This seems to be the basic assumption underlying various researches on regeneration in the spinal cord. This line of thinking overlooks one important difference, and it is that when a small number of axons are spared from the lesion they are the adult and fully differentiated axons, and that they are left intact, still maintaining their original full length with original fields of axonal collaterals and terminations. These axons have gone through a protracted and complex developmental history during their growth and differentiation. A small number of regenerating axons, even if they were to show more than abortive regeneration, need not necessarily grow back to regain their original length and original fields of axonal collaterals and terminations. They may, at best, show random growth immediately within a short distance from the lesion site. No matter how profuse and permanent this random growth may be, it is unlikely that it would lead to any functional recovery. This is supported by observations made in those studies, described below, where attempts have been made to reduce glial scar formation, or where various agents have been used to enhance regeneration of the severed axons.

Various studies on regeneration have contributed to the universally accepted fact that glial scar formation at the site of lesion is a major barrier in the path of the regenerating axons (Brown and McCouch 1947, Davidoff and Ransohoff 1948, Windle and Chambers 1950, Windle et al. 1952a, 1958, Clemente and Windle 1954, Guth et al. 1978, Gearhart et al. 1979, Barrett et al. 1981). It has often been suggested that if the glial scar formation were eliminated, or at least reduced, the severed axons would regenerate and functional recovery would be achieved. Towards this goal various different approaches have been made. One of the early approaches involved the use of bacterial pyrogen, more specifically, pyrogenic bacterial polysaccharides, to induce regeneration in the damaged axons (Windle and Chambers 1950, Windle et al. 1952b, Clemente and Windle 1954). It was found that the animals receiving pyrogens intravenously or intramuscularly following lesions showed a reduction in glial scar formation and some regeneration of axons. The regenerating axons appeared organized in the form of minute fascicles penetrating through the persisting glial scar formation to reach the other side of the lesion. Scott and Clemente (1955) were able to observe physiological activity related to these regenerating fibers. After reviewing an extensive amount of anatomical and physiological work, Windle (1956) noted that the animals following this treatment did not show functional recovery from the paraplegic syndrome. Various other investigators, including Lance (1954), Arteta (1956), and O'Callaghan and Speakman (1963), did not find any positive effects of pyrogens on the regeneration of axons. Along similar lines Magenis et al. (1952) and Freeman et al. (1960) employed trypsin to reduce the development of glial scar formation at the site of the lesion following hemisectioning of the spinal cord. They observed functional recovery and a reduction in the glial scar formation that led to the conclusion that, indeed, regeneration of severed axons had taken place. However, recently Guth et al. (1980b) and Pettegrew (1980) were not able to support these claims. Fertig et al. (1971) and Heinicke (1977) observed that following a lesion most of the severed axons undergo degenerative changes. It is only a small number of axons that may show abortive or true regeneration.

Glial reaction at the site of the lesion is a histopathological reaction to the traumatic conditions and culminates in a glial scar formation along the borders of the cavity left by the lesion after a considerable interval. It is seen to follow a developmental history. In brief, a glial scar formation does not appear immediately after the lesion. It appears after a considerable lag of time as the secondary traumatic changes develop and subside (Ducker 1976, Jellinger 1976). Further, when the spinal cord is severed partially, the glial scar formation is present only in the regions where the axons are traumatized and not where they are spared from the direct trauma. These and similar observations on the histopathology of the spinal cord following a trauma induced by the weight-dropping method strongly suggest that the glial scar formation in actuality is a protective mechanism. It is possible that in a nonpathological environment the severed axons may show considerable regeneration, but it is close to impossible to provide such an ideal environment to the damaged axons following a lesion. Owing to pathological conditions the severed axons may remain dormant and may not show regeneration for some time, but the pathological processes follow their own independent progressive course. In order to contain it, the glial cells proliferate and give rise to a glial scar formation. Thus, perhaps, it is the absence of *adequate and timely* regeneration of severed axons that influences the development of glial scar formation, which covers the exposed surface of the tissue containing severed and degenerating axonal endings. The glial scar formation, from this viewpoint, appears to protect the spinal neural tissue from protracted and extensive progressive degeneration. If, by some means, glial scar formation could be completely eliminated, most of the atrophying axons still might not show regeneration, and the spinal cord would be continuously invaded by loose connective tissue and other foreign materials and organisms while undergoing a protracted degeneration. Glial scar formation very likely serves to prevent such progressive degenerative changes. Histopathological observations on the spinal cord following a trauma by the weight-dropping method show that immediately after the trauma many axons are apparently left intact but do not show any regeneration even weeks after the trauma; they simply degenerate over a span of time (Wakefield and Eidelberg 1975, Bresnahan et al. 1976, Bresnahan 1978, Ford 1983). These observations, when viewed comprehensively, suggest that the nature and severity of trauma may have a very important bearing on the regeneration or lack of regeneration of the axons, that regeneration or lack of regeneration of damaged axons, at least during early stages following the trauma, may be independent of glial scar formation, and that glial scar formation develops only in those regions where the damaged axons fail to regenerate. These observations are supported by recent findings on neural transplantation in the traumatized spinal cord (Das 1983a,c).

Transplantation of peripheral and central nervous tissues in the traumatized spinal cord, as another approach to aid in the regeneration of severed axons, has been attempted by many investigators. Generally, the main objective in most of these investigations has been to provide some conducive morphological substratum for the severed axons to grow and reach the other end of the severed spinal cord. The earliest report available is by Shirres (1905). He transplanted a segment of spinal cord obtained from a dog in an adult patient who had been paraplegic for about 11 months at the time of surgery. Although there was no evidence of any functional recovery, he observed a limited regeneration of axons in the spinal cord. The transplant had served as a bridge for the regenerating axons. Since then various investigators have transplanted fragments of peripheral nerves in the traumatized spinal cord to provide a substratum for the regenerating axons (Sugar and Gerard 1940, Turbes and Freeman 1958, Campbell et al. 1960, Jakoby et al. 1960, Freeman and Turbes 1961, Cseuz and Speakman 1963, Perkins et al. 1964, Kao 1974, Kao et al., 1977a). From an overall viewpoint, these studies showed that the transplanted nerve fragments degenerated, that they provided a substratum for the growth of the regenerating axons, and that the number of regenerating axons was rather small. Conceptually, since at the time of surgery these nerve fragments were inserted through the necrotic tissue at both ends of the severed spinal cord, they served as bridges for the regenerating axons. However, in these studies it was not established how far these regenerated axons grew into the other end of the spinal cord and how conclusively the animals showed functional recovery from the paraplegic syndrome. It is important to note that Brown and McCouch (1947), Barnard and Carpenter (1950), and Feigin et al. (1951) did not observe any regeneration following implantation of peripheral nerve segments. Transplantation of central nervous tissue has also been used to inhibit the growth of the glial scar formation. Aihara (1970) and Kao et al. (1970) transplanted cultured cerebellar tissue and noncultured neocortical tissues from adult donors into the spinal cord of adult dogs. The transplants soon became necrotic and degenerated, but the presence of neural transplants at the site of lesion appeared to arrest or retard the growth of the scar formation. Under these conditions, regeneration of axons was found to be facilitated. Shimizu (1983), employing the same experimental approach, not only confirmed their observations but also has shown functional recovery from paraplegia in dogs. It must be stressed that all these investigations were not addressed to the problems of transplantability of neural tissue. The neural transplants, which invariably degenerated after transplantation, were simply a means to achieve regeneration of the severed axons.

During the last decade there has been a renewed interest in neural transplantation in the central nervous system. This field of research has a long history, and it has been reviewed in earlier publications (Das 1974, 1983b). Various investigators have helped establish the fact that embryonic neural tissues can be successfully transplanted, and that these tissues following transplantation grow, differentiate, and become integrated with the host brain tissue (Das 1974, 1975, 1983a,b,c, 1984, Lund and Hauschka 1976, Stenevi et al. 1976, Das and Altman 1971, 1972, Das and Hallas 1978, Das et al. 1979, 1980, 1983, Bjorklund et al. 1979, Hallas et al. 1980a, Jaeger and Lund 1980, Kromer et al. 1983, Albert and Das 1984). These investigators have employed different types of neural tissues from embryos of various developmental stages as transplants and have successfully transplanted them in different sites of host brain such as cerebellum, tectum, neocortex, and hippocampus of neonatal as well as adult host animals. The neural transplants that are anatomically integrated with the host brain show afferent and efferent connectivity with it (Jaeger and Lund 1979, Hallas et al. 1980b, Oblinger et al. 1980, Harvey and Lund 1981, Kromer et al. 1981, Lund and Harvey 1981, Oblinger and Das 1982, 1983). During this period various techniques of transplantation and techniques of freezing neural tissues for storage and subsequent transplantation have also been worked out (Das 1974, 1983a,b, Stenevi et al. 1976, Das et al. 1979, 1983b, Houle and Das 1980a,b, Das and Ross 1982). These studies, from a comprehensive viewpoint, have been addressed to the problems of transplantability of neural tissues and developmental and anatomical characteristics of successful neural transplantation. With this background it is now possible to pose questions related to neural transplantation under various conditions of trauma to the host central nervous system.

The spinal cord, as a site for neural transplantation, has been found to be a rather difficult structure (Nygren et al. 1977, Das 1981, 1983a). When neural tissues are transplanted in an intact spinal cord, the transplants are ejected out. Since they are not retained within the host brain parenchyma, they become extraparenchymal transplants and eventually become atrophied and degenerated (Das 1982). Owing to these technical limitations, generally investigators make a surgical cavity prior to transplanting a neural tissue, and this is seen to aid in the retention of the transplants (Das 1981, 1983a,c, 1984, Nornes et al.

1983, Patel and Bernstein 1983). These studies on neural transplantation in the spinal cord have shown that embryonic neural tissues no doubt survive and grow, but they do so in a pathological environment. The conditions of introducing a lesion in order to make a surgical cavity provide extensive traumatic conditions to the host spinal cord tissue. When viewed from this perspective, neural transplantation in the spinal cord actually provides a model for transplantation in a traumatized spinal cord. With this it is possible to study not only growth and differentiation of neural transplants but also interaction between the pathological conditions and the growing transplants.

In the following, various studies on surgically induced trauma to the spinal cord of adult rats and neural transplantation are presented. The main focus of attention is on the laceration-type lesions, for they appeared to provide conditions close to those in human cases and also to those seen in the studies employing the weight-dropping model. Studies on knife-lesions are included because they appeared to serve as control studies and also provided an insight into the observations made by other investigators using this model of lesion. A comparative evaluation of these two models reveals how two different experimental approaches have influenced the perspective of and observations made by the investigators and how they have directed the search for findings in two different directions as if there were nothing common between them.

Experimental Studies

Comments on Various Technical Aspects

The experiments described below were conducted on laboratory-bred Long-Evans hooded rats. The animals were 3–6 months old. In these experiments, lesions were made in the spinal cord at thoracic level by surgical means. This method of making lesions was preferred over that employing weight dropping because it permitted a relatively accurate method of defining lesions in anatomical terms at the time of inducing trauma. With this it was possible to analyze histopathological changes in the spinal cord from the initial point of trauma to the stage when the animals were sacrificed. The developmental approach, as employed in the following studies, provided an insight into the differential contributions of primary trauma, secondary traumatic changes, and progressive degenerative changes in the emergence of permanent paraplegic syndrome. Further, in the experimental animals that received neural transplants following lesions, this approach of analysis permitted an insight into the survival, growth, and integration of neural transplants with the spinal cord tissue.

In these experiments different lesions with varying degrees of severity were made in the thoracic spinal cord. They were at the level of T8–T9 or T9–T10. The choice of this level of spinal cord for making lesions was determined by the following facts. First, lesions of various degrees of severity could be induced consistently with a very small degree of variability. Second, paraplegic syndrome under different conditions of lesions could be produced consistently. The lesions that resulted in paraplegic syndrome were such that they yielded the syndrome in a very high percentage of control as well as experimental animals. This was an essential requirement, in particular for the experimental animals that showed functional recovery following neural transplantation. Third, the survival rate of animals, particularly those receiving total transections, was high, thus permitting a full analysis of animals with such extensive lesions. When such lesions were made in the cervical or lumbar regions of the spinal cord, the survival rate of animals was very low. Fourth, this is the preferred site employed by many investigators using surgical lesions or weight-dropping methods to induce trauma. Furthermore, in these studies lesions were made under a surgical microscope, and they were defined in terms of both rostro-caudal axis and dorso-ventral or transverse plane. After exposing the spinal cord, lesions were made bilaterally. They were made from the dorsal aspect, and in all the preparations the dorsal funiculi were always completely severed. The ventrally located structures, depending upon the severity of lesion required, were severed differentially. The techniques of creating such lesions in the thoracic spinal cord have been described earlier in other publications (Das 1983a,c).

The lesions described in these studies fell into two categories: knife lesions and laceration-type lesions. The knife lesions were made by a fine surgical blade (Figure 1-1). They were straight-line lesions, and no neural tissue from the spinal cord was removed. Different groups of animals received lesions of different degrees of severity. This means that the spinal cord in different animals was severed to different degrees of depth in its transverse plane. Following such lesions the two cut ends of the spinal cord remained apposed to each other. In other words, these lesions simply severed the fiber tracts and the gray

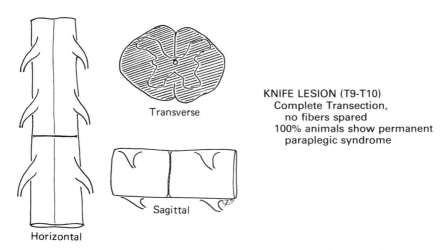

Transverse

Horizontal

Sagittal

KNIFE LESION (T9-T10)
Complete Transection,
no fibers spared
100% animals show permanent
paraplegic syndrome

Figure 1-1. Schematic drawing showing complete transection of spinal cord with knife lesion.

matter of the spinal cord. In control animals the lesions were made and no neural tissues were transplanted. In experimental animals following such lesions, depending upon the nature of the experimental requirements, either the spinal cord tissue or neocortical tissue obtained from embryos of various ages were transplanted. The knife lesions were employed for two reasons: to serve as a control for the laceration-type lesions, and to replicate studies conducted by other investigators employing this model of making lesions. In all the preparations following lesion, there was bleeding and it was controlled with the help of a piece of Gelfoam soaked in lactated Ringer's solution. No other method of controlling or stopping bleeding was employed. After bleeding was stopped, the incision was sutured, and the animals were placed back in their respective cages.

The laceration-type lesions, in contrast, were extensive and involved not only cutting of the spinal cord but also removal of neural tissue from the site of lesion (Figure 1-2). Such lesions were seen to be far more traumatic than the knife lesions. After exposing the spinal cord at lower thoracic levels two transverse cuts were made, one rostral and other caudal, extending for at least one segment. These lesions varied in depth in different groups of animals. In some groups of animals the spinal cord was severed completely and in others partially. Following such lesions the spinal cord tissue between the two cut ends was further cut using iris scissors and was removed with the aid of microforceps. These lesions resulted in creation of large surgical cavities extending 4–5 mm in rostro-caudal axis. The laceration-type lesions were chosen for these studies because they seemed to provide traumatic conditions close to those in human cases. It is very rare that human patients are seen to have clean, straight-line knife lesions. Although it is possible to create laceration-type lesions by other means, the surgical approach, as employed in these studies, was

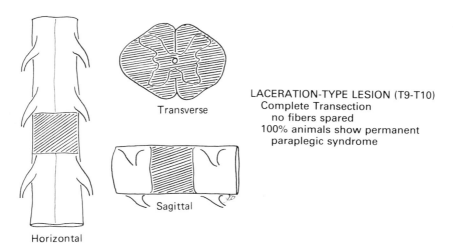

LACERATION-TYPE LESION (T9-T10)
Complete Transection
no fibers spared
100% animals show permanent
paraplegic syndrome

Transverse

Sagittal

Horizontal

Figure 1-2. Schematic drawing showing complete transection of spinal cord with laceration-type lesion.

found valuable because it permitted direct visualization and determination of the extent of lesions. With this method it was possible to determine whether the lesions were complete or incomplete. In the case of incomplete lesions, it was possible to establish the degree of partial sectioning of the spinal cord. In control animals after the laceration-type lesions were made, bleeding was controlled with the aid of a piece of Gelfoam soaked in lactated Ringer's solution, and the incision was sutured. The experimental animals, following such lesions and identical treatment for controlling bleeding, received neural transplants of spinal cord tissue or neocortical tissue depending upon the experimental conditions. It is important to stress that in no animal was any foreign material, such as Gelfoam or silicon-coated Dacron (Dura Film), left at the site of lesion or on top of the transplant.

Transplantation of neural tissues in the animals in experimental groups was done intraparenchymally (Das 1983a,b, Das et al. 1979). The tissues were injected into the spinal cord in such a fashion that some amount of tissue remained within the parenchyma and some in the space between the two cut ends. In the case of knife lesions, the transplants were small and filled the space immediately. But in the case of laceration-type lesions, where the cavities were large, large amounts of neural tissue, as much as 10 mm^3, were injected to fill the cavity to achieve satisfactory transplantation. It must be stressed that in no case were the neural tissues simply left or deposited in the lesion site or the cavity without injecting inside the spinal cord parenchyma. The experimental animals, after receiving neural transplants, were left undisturbed for some time, and the transplants were checked repeatedly to make sure that they were retained at the lesion site. Observations from previous studies have shown that retainability of neural transplants is a major problem and that failure to observe various precautions, more often than not, leads to loss of neural tissues and their settling in the subdural space. Such displaced neural transplants, even when they survive, are extraparenchymal and are not actually integrated with the host spinal cord. Such technically faulty preparations can lead to unwarranted and erroneous conclusions on the beneficial effects, or lack of them, of transplants in the recovery from neurological deficits or abnormalities. At the end of the surgery the incision was sutured, and the animals were placed back undisturbed in their cages (Das 1983a,c, 1984).

All the control and experimental animals, under various conditions of lesions and transplantations, were kept alive for 6–8 months after the surgery, and observations on paraplegic syndrome and autonomic dysfunctions were made every day. For observations on paraplegic syndrome, particularly on the loss of locomotor and supportive functions, elevated metal grids were used. All the animals were attended to regularly for cleaning, feeding, and medications required to alleviate discomfort. At the end of the study, the animals were sacrificed and the spinal cord segments containing lesions and transplants were removed and processed for histology. Material stained with Nissl stain, H&E stain, and Bodian's Protargol stain provided data on the survival and integration of the transplants and histological appearance of cellular elements of the transplants. Further, connectivity of transplants was investigated by employing

Fink-Heimer staining technique. Prior to sacrificing these animals, under appropriate surgical conditions, knife lesions either at lower cervical level or at lumbar level were made to induce degeneration in the descending and ascending afferents to the transplants. Five days after these lesions, animals were sacrificed and segments of spinal cord containing lesions and transplants were processed for Fink-Heimer staining. All this material was studied in serial sections in order to comprehend topographic changes in the transplant, its interface with the spinal cord, and changes in the pattern of connectivity from one level of the transplant to the other.

In addition to the above described preparations for the analysis of long-term characteristics of lesions and neural transplants, other studies were conducted that provided developmental information on histopathological changes leading to cavitation in the control animals and on histopathology of cavitation and growth of transplants in the experimental animals. In essence, in different conditions, control as well as experimental animals were sacrificed at various intervals such as 1, 2, 3, 4, 6, 10, 15, 20, 30, and 60 days after the surgery, and segments of spinal cord containing lesions and transplants were processed for histology. This material was found valuable in providing an insight into the problems of primary trauma and secondary traumatic changes in the spinal cord and the nature of interaction between the developmental histopathological changes in the spinal cord and the growing neural transplants.

Characteristics of Neural Transplants

In various pilot studies in the past, attempts were made in this laboratory to transplant embryonic neural tissues obtained from different regions of neuraxis of embryos of various developmental stages in the spinal cord. It was found that in order to achieve intraparenchymal and well-integrated transplants, it was essential to use neural tissues that were characterized by a high growth potential. Of all the tissues investigated, it was found that the neocortical tissues obtained from 15- or 16-day embryos, which contained predominantly neuroepithelial cells, were the most suitable tissues. These neural tissues, by virtue of the fact that they contained neuroepithelial cells, showed a very high rate of survival, extensive growth, and a high capability of penetrating through the degenerating mass of the spinal cord at the site of lesion and achieving an anatomical integration with it. In contrast to this, neural tissues obtained from the spinal cord of 14-, 15-, or 16-day embryos that contained neuroblasts in various degrees of differentiation showed a low growth. Such neural transplants, no matter how carefully they were transplanted, generally remained extraparenchymal, were unable to fill the surgical lesion cavity, and remained anatomically unintegrated with the spinal cord. Some of these transplants did survive, but they were in small fragments, showed a thin umbilical-type attachment with the spinal cord, and survived for variable periods of a few weeks or months but eventually became necrotic and degenerated. Histologically, at no stage of their survival did they appear as healthy and viable as those obtained from the neocortical tissues. Transplants of other neural tissues, such as those from brain stem, that showed moderate or low growth potential presented similar problems in their growth and integration in a pathological environment of the spinal cord with lesions. Like other extraparenchymal transplants in other studies, they all were seen to undergo different phases of degeneration (Das 1982). Furthermore, anatomically as well as functionally, transplants of spinal cord did not contribute to positive findings and therefore are not presented in this study. With these considerations, the findings presented here are focused exclusively on the neocortical transplants in the spinal cord.

Spinal Cord Lesions and Paraplegia

At this point it is important to clarify the nature of the paraplegic syndrome under different conditions of lesions, the distinction between transient and permanent paraplegic syndrome, and the criteria employed in arriving at this distinction. These characteristics were best observed in control animals that received lesions only. The lesions described below varied in degree of severity, and this was generally related to the nature and severity of the syndrome.

The animals receiving complete transection of spinal cord were permanently paraplegic (Figures 1-1 and 1-2). Their hindlimbs were flaccid, and they were not used for either locomotion or supporting the body. These animals moved about in their cages with their forelimbs, dragging their hindlimbs flaccidly. They rested their bodies on one side of the floor of the cage. The hindlimbs were not used for lifting and supporting their bodies above the cage floor. If the paws of the hindlimbs of these animals were pinched, they showed fast and jerky withdrawal reflexes of the whole limbs. These reflexes could not be elicited by tactile stimulation. In addition to these severe motor deficits, these animals showed a variety of autonomic dysfunctions, which included loss of control of bladder, loss of body-temperature regulation often resulting in hypothermia, loss of appetite as reflected by reduction in food and water intake, and irregular and abnormal pattern of breathing. Total transection of spinal cord was seen to yield a very low survival rate of the animals (Table 1-1). Most of the animals that failed to survive the trauma died within 24–48 hours after the surgery. They were hypothermic and could not regain their normal body temperature. Even when they were kept warm they could not maintain their body temperature satisfactorily. Hypothermia was the major cause of death in these and other animals with extensive subtotal lesions that died within a day or two after the surgery. Another equally important cause of death in these animals was the abnormal pattern of breathing. Even a slight stimulus, such as a noise in the room or holding them for cleaning, disturbed their breathing pattern seriously. In some cases, uncontrollably rapid breathing led to a sudden arrest in breathing. The movement of the diaphragm in these animals was arrested, and it was held abnormally taut; it showed no signs of release even some minutes after their death. The animals that survived these initial complications showed some recovery of autonomic functions in about 8–12 days after sur-

Table 1-1. Percentage of Animals Surviving Surgical Trauma of Lesion and Neural Transplantation in Spinal Cord for More Than 2 Weeks

	Knife lesion	Laceration-type lesion
Total transection		
Control: lesion only	28 (4/14)[a]	21 (4/19)
Experimental: lesion-		
transplantation	24 (5/21)	19 (15/78)
Partial transection-		
extensive lesion:		
Control: lesion only	75 (9/12)	66 (8/12)
Experimental: lesion-		
transplantation	78 (15/19)	74 (20/27)
Partial transection-		
restricted lesion:		
Control: lesion only	—	85 (12/14)
Experimental: lesion		
transplantation	—	75 (21/28)

[a] Numbers in parenthesis: denominator = number of animals subjected to surgery, numerator = number of animals survived.

gery, but they remained permanently paraplegic. The paraplegic syndrome in these animals was defined in terms of *loss of voluntary movement in hindlimbs related to locomotion in coordination with the forelimbs and loss of supporting of body by the hindlimbs*. These two characteristics served as the main criteria for establishing permanent paraplegic syndrome.

The animals receiving subtotal or partial transection of the spinal cord showed various degrees of somatic and autonomic functional abnormalities, and they were generally related to the degree of severity of the trauma. From an overall viewpoint, most of the animals, under various conditions of partial transection, did not show true paraplegic syndrome. They did show flaccidity of hindlimbs, lack of movement in them as related to locomotion, and lack of ability to support the body by hindlimbs only for a few days after the surgery, but they soon showed a rapid recovery of the somatic functions. Similarly, they showed autonomic dysfunctions only for a few days, followed by rapid recovery. Generally, the animals receiving lesions less than 85% in the transverse plane showed no paraplegic syndrome whatsoever. This was true of the animals receiving knife as well as laceration-type lesions. From an anatomical viewpoint these lesions included sectioning of dorsal and lateral funiculi completely, gray matter completely, and ventral funiculi partially (Figure 1-3). Fibers in the ventral region of the ventral funiculi were spared from the lesion. Animals receiving these lesions were able to use their hindlimbs and move about within 24 hours after the surgery. Under the conditions of knife lesion, even as large a lesion as that extending for 90% of the spinal cord in the transverse plane did not produce any paraplegic syndrome (Figure 1-3). The animals with this extensive lesion were able to move about in 4–5 days after the surgery. It must be indicated that although these animals did not satisfy the

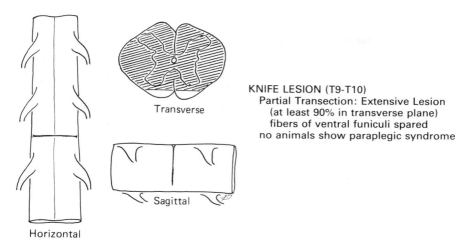

Transverse

KNIFE LESION (T9-T10)
Partial Transection: Extensive Lesion
(at least 90% in transverse plane)
fibers of ventral funiculi spared
no animals show paraplegic syndrome

Sagittal

Horizontal

Figure 1-3. Schematic drawing showing partial transection-extensive lesion with knife lesion.

criteria used for true paraplegic syndrome, their walking was not normal. Their gait was affected, and they moved about in a waddling fashion. They could not walk for a sustained period of 2–5 minutes without falling on their sides. They did not show any serious autonomic dysfunctions.

Under the conditions of laceration-type lesions, where the trauma caused to the spinal cord was far more extensive, lesions extending for 85% or more in the transverse plane did show paraplegic syndrome. However, in these preparations not all the animals were paraplegic. When the lesions extended to 85–90% in the transverse plane, about 70% of animals showed permanent paraplegic syndrome and 30% showed a slow recovery within a few days after the surgery (Figure 1-4). If the severity of lesion was increased to such an extent that it extended to 95% in the transverse plane, about 95% of animals showed paraplegic syndrome and only 5% showed recovery within a few days following the trauma (Figure 1-5). However, if the lesions extended further, involving 100% severance of the spinal cord in the transverse plane, all the animals showed paraplegic syndrome. Thus, it was found that by increasing the severity of trauma, the percentage of animals becoming paraplegic increased and at the same time the survival rate of the animals following such a surgery decreased (Table 1-1). In other words, animals receiving less severe trauma showed a better survival rate than those receiving very severe trauma. It is possible to conceive of a lesion of such severity that on the average 50% of animals would show permanent paraplegia and the remaining 50% would not show such a syndrome. Such a lesion would certainly be less than 85% in transverse extent and would yield a high survival rate of the animals. No attempt was made to determine this lesion and use it in these studies because variability in the number of animals showing paraplegia from one set of preparations to the other would have been very high, and the findings on functional

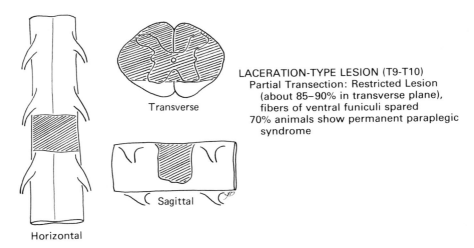

Transverse

LACERATION-TYPE LESION (T9-T10)
Partial Transection: Restricted Lesion
(about 85–90% in transverse plane),
fibers of ventral funiculi spared
70% animals show permanent paraplegic
syndrome

Sagittal

Horizontal

Figure 1-4. Schematic drawing showing partial transection-restricted lesion with laceration-type lesion.

recovery, following neural transplantation in experimental animals, would not have been clear-cut and unequivocal.

It is important to comment on the nature of recovery in the animals that did not show permanent paraplegic syndrome following partial transection of the spinal cord. The animals showing any recovery of locomotor and supportive functions were seen to recover slowly and gradually. They were able to use their hindlimbs for these two functions in about 10–12 days after the surgery. The recovery in these animals was never complete. They walked in an abnor-

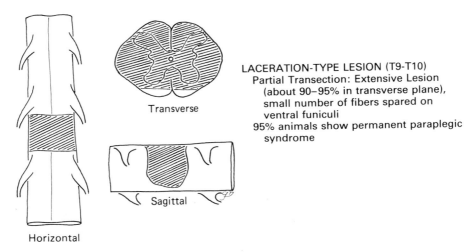

Transverse

LACERATION-TYPE LESION (T9-T10)
Partial Transection: Extensive Lesion
(about 90–95% in transverse plane),
small number of fibers spared on
ventral funiculi
95% animals show permanent paraplegic
syndrome

Sagittal

Horizontal

Figure 1-5. Schematic drawing showing partial transection-extensive lesion with laceration-type lesion.

mal fashion, and their gait was affected. They could not walk in a sustained fashion for more than 2–3 minutes. They fell on their sides repeatedly. Those animals that were paraplegic for 10–12 days after surgery remained permanently paraplegic without ever showing any recovery of locomotor or supportive functions. In other words, in control animals if there was any spontaneous recovery of any degree from paraplegic syndrome, it was always within 2 weeks after the surgery, and if there was no recovery within this period, the animals remained permanently paraplegic. These observations helped establish a distinction between the transient and permanent paraplegia. *The animals showing recovery of locomotor and supportive functions to any degree within 2 weeks were considered to show transient paraplegic syndrome, and the animals that remained paraplegic for 2 weeks or longer were permanently paraplegic animals.* Although it was difficult to establish in anatomical terms the slight differences in lesions that caused transient paraplegia in some animals and permanent paraplegic syndrome in others, these observations suggested that, very likely, the differences may have been in the severity of secondary traumatic conditions and of the progressive degenerative changes in the two cases that contributed to transient paraplegia in one and permanent paraplegia in the other. As a matter of fact, the time factor distinguishing transient and permanent paraplegia in control animals was also helpful in understanding the nature of recovery, or lack of it, from paraplegic syndrome in experimental animals that received neural transplants following lesions in the spinal cord. If these animals showed any recovery in locomotor or supportive functions in less than 2 weeks after the surgery, it was not attributed to the neural transplants. It was considered as spontaneous recovery owing to inadequate nature of the lesion. Those experimental animals that showed recovery from paraplegia within 2–3 weeks after the surgery were considered to show improvement attributable to neural transplants. And the experimental animals that showed no recovery, even after receiving neural transplants, were evaluated as failures of transplantation. Variability in the incidence of permanent paraplegic syndrome in the animals receiving subtotal lesions has always been a problem of major consideration by investigators using weight-dropping methods or knife-lesion techniques. However, if attention is paid to the distinction between transient and permanent paraplegia and to the percentage of animals showing permanent paraplegic syndrome following lesions produced by different methods, it is possible to achieve a better understanding of subtotal lesions resulting in paraplegia and the anatomical and histopathological conditions underlying it.

In addition to the above-described lesions, various other kinds of laceration-type lesions were also investigated. Of them, two appear of important consideration. In one type, the laceration-type lesions were bilateral and extensive, but instead of sparing fibers in the ventral funiculi only a small portion of fibers of the lateral funiculi were spared (Figure 1-6). All other fibers in the dorsal, lateral, and ventral funiculi and the gray matter were severed. With this type of lesion not even a single animal showed any paraplegic syndrome. These observations strongly supported the findings made by Eidelberg et al. (1981). The animals were able to use their hindlimbs for locomotor as well as supportive

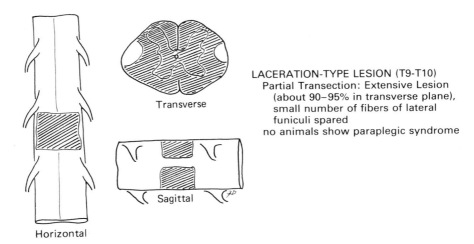

Transverse

LACERATION-TYPE LESION (T9-T10)
Partial Transection: Extensive Lesion
(about 90–95% in transverse plane),
small number of fibers of lateral
funiculi spared
no animals show paraplegic syndrome

Sagittal

Horizontal

Figure 1-6. Schematic drawing showing partial transection-extensive lesion with laceration-type lesion sparing some fibers in the lateral funiculi.

functions within 24–48 hours after the surgery. They did not even show the transient paraplegia observed in other lesion conditions. Their walking pattern was, at first, abnormal, but that also progressively improved for about 8–12 days after the surgery. In another set of animals, sparing of small numbers of fibers in the lateral funiculi was unilateral instead of bilateral. These animals showed a closely normal control on their hindlimb ipsilateral to where the fibers were spared. However, contralaterally, where the fibers of the lateral funiculi were completely severed, the hindlimb showed flaccid-type paralysis. They showed considerable recovery even in this limb within 10–12 days after the surgery. On the basis of these findings, it is possible to reconstruct and suggest that in various other studies where recovery from paraplegia followed total transection of the spinal cord has been attributed to the regeneration of damaged axons or regeneration of axons induced by various chemicals and pharmaceutical agents, this recovery may have been, in actuality, due to nothing more than recovery from the transient paraplegic syndrome because of the sparing of fibers in the lateral funiculi. Lesions producing total transection in the spinal cord are always associated with extensive bleeding at the site of lesion, and it is possible to leave, inadvertantly, some fibers of the lateral funiculi intact, thus creating conditions of subtotal lesions yielding a transient paraplegic condition. Perhaps because of these artifacts of techniques and observation, the studies claiming recovery from paraplegic syndrome following total transection of spinal cord have not been replicated by other independent investigators.

In the other type of lesion, extensive hemorrhagic conditions were created at the site of lesion. The lesion involved severance of dorsal funiculi, parts of lateral and ventral funiculi, and an extensive damage to the gray matter. Large portions of lateral and ventral funiculi along the outer regions were spared from direct trauma of severance of axons (Figure 1-7). Bleeding at the site of lesion

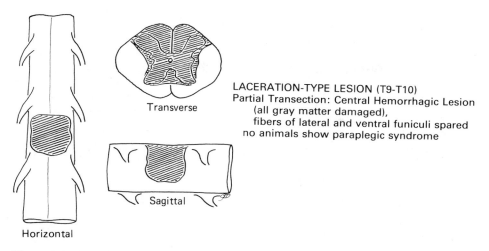

Transverse

LACERATION-TYPE LESION (T9-T10)
Partial Transection: Central Hemorrhagic Lesion
(all gray matter damaged),
fibers of lateral and ventral funiculi spared
no animals show paraplegic syndrome

Sagittal

Horizontal

Figure 1-7. Schematic drawing showing partial transection-central hemorrhagic lesion with laceration-type lesion. Many fibers of lateral and ventral funiculi are left intact.

was extensive, and it was not controlled as meticulously and completely as in other lesion conditions. In other words, bleeding was allowed to continue to contribute to central hemorrhagic conditions. The main advantages of making such surgical lesions over lesions by weight-dropping were that extensive hemorrhagic conditions were directly visualized, and at the same time the spared fibers in the lateral and ventral funiculi were not subjected to primary trauma. With this type of lesion, not even a single animal showed any paraplegic syndrome. All the animals were able to use their hindlimbs for locomotor and supportive functions within 24–48 hours after the surgery. As a matter of fact, observations made in other lesion conditions would have logically led to a prediction of this outcome. Histological observations of these preparations after the surgery did confirm extensive hemorrhage and necrosis in the gray matter extending for more than one segment, as well as sparing of the majority of axons in the lateral and ventral funiculi from the direct surgical trauma. Observations made on this type of lesion suggested that, contrary to the suggestions made in the studies employing the weight-dropping model, central hemorrhage in the gray matter of the spinal cord is not the primary factor resulting in paraplegia. Central hemorrhage in the gray matter of the spinal cord following a trauma by weight-dropping technique is the most readily and immediately observable pathological change. But it does not necessarily mean that it is the primary cause leading to paraplegic syndrome. There may be other changes such as direct as well as indirect primary trauma to, and gradual progressive degeneration of, the apparently intact axons, which are not readily observable immediately after the trauma, but in actuality may progressively lead to a paraplegic syndrome, and, therefore, may be the primary factor responsible for paraplegic conditions in these experimental animals. Studies by Wakefield and Eidelberg (1975), Bresnahan et al. (1976), Bresnahan (1978),

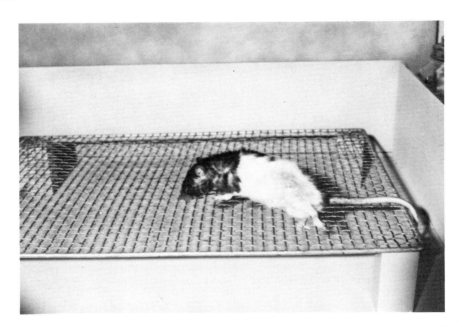

Figure 1-8. Knife lesion and complete transection of spinal cord at T_9-T_{10}. This animal was operated on when 2 months old, and received neocortical tissue from 16-day embryo as the transplant. It was allowed to survive for 6 months after the surgery. It remained permanently paraplegic for this duration. Note that this animal is on its side and is dragging its himdlimbs as it attempts to move about.

Balentine and Paris (1978b), and Blight (1983a) indicate that with the weight-dropping method the threshold trauma resulting in paraplegia does indeed cause an extensive amount of direct trauma to the axons of the spinal cord.

Complete Transection and Transplantation

Under both knife and laceration-type lesions there were animals in control groups that were subjected to complete or total transection of the spinal cord and animals in the experimental groups that received total transection of the spinal cord followed by neocortical transplantation. In every animal the lesion was examined repeatedly at the time of surgery as well as at the end of the study. As described above, the survival rate of animals with this lesion was very low. The presence of neural transplants in the experimental animals neither improved nor worsened the survival rate of the animals. In both control and experimental groups the animals that survived showed recovery from various autonomic dysfunctions within 2 weeks after the surgery. The recovery was generally very slow, but in some cases it was rather fast. The somatic functions of these animals, namely, locomotor and supportive functions by hindlimbs, remained lost as long as they lived. When these animals were tested

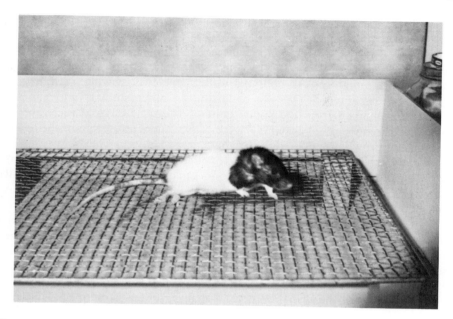

Figure 1-9. Laceration-type lesion and complete transection of spinal cord at T_9-T_{10}. This animal received lesion and transplant when it was 2 months old. The transplant was obtained from neocortex of 16-day embryo. It was allowed to survive for 6 months following the surgery. During this interval it remained permanently paraplegic. This animal also is seen on its side, unable to use its hindlimbs either for locomotion or supporting its body.

on elevated metal grids, the paraplegic syndrome became clearly evident (Figures 1-8 and 1-9). They moved about only with their forelimbs, dragging their hindlimbs flaccidly. These animals were permanently paraplegic. In this testing situation, if the hindlimbs slipped through the grids, they were unable to lift their hindlimbs up and move about. The hindlimbs of some animals remained dangling for a long duration of 10–15 minutes until they were removed from the testing situation. No animal under these conditions of lesion showed transient paraplegia, and no experimental animal with a neocortical transplant showed any recovery from the paraplegic syndrome. However, animals in both groups showed reflexive kicking of hindlimbs when a nociceptive stimulus was applied. They also showed spastic extension of hindlimbs without any relevance to locomotor or supportive functions. Thus, total transection of spinal cord, whether neural transplants were present or not, resulted in permanent paraplegia.

Histological analysis of spinal cords from these animals showed that in the case of control animals the lesion site had enlarged considerably, and the two cut ends of the spinal cord had further retracted leaving behind a large cavity. The phenomenon of cavitation following such lesions has been described by other investigators (Kao 1980, Kao and Chang 1977, Kao et al. 1977b). In the case of experimental animals, too, cavitation at the site of lesion was observed. The neocortical transplants had filled the cavity between the two cut ends and were found anatomically integrated with the spinal cord along the regions of its gray matter (Figures 1-10 and 1-11). This indicated that neocortical transplants endowed with a high growth potential were capable of growing and filling the cavity as it expanded at the site of lesion. In other studies, where neural transplants obtained from the spinal cord of 14- or 15-day-old rat embryos, which show a low growth potential, were transplanted at the site of the lesion, they did not grow large enough to fill the enlarged cavity. They were small in size, remained isolated, and were surrounded and enwrapped by the dense matrix of meningeal membranes and connective tissue. They were generally extraparenchymal, and in those few instances where they appeared integrated with the host spinal cord, the integration was minimal.

The neocortical transplants, although large and integrated with the spinal cord, were integrated only with the gray matter. But at the regions where they were apposed to the cut surfaces of white matter of the spinal cord, they were unintegrated. At these regions of apposition, there was an extensive glial scar formation that stood as a barrier between the transplants and the cut axons of the white matter of the spinal cord. These observations confirmed those presented in our earlier publications (Das 1983a,c). In Fink-Heimer preparations, it was observed that the neocortical transplants did receive both ascending and descending afferents from the spinal cord through the interface with the gray matter. Although efferents of transplants extending into the spinal cord were not investigated by experimental means, an analysis of serial sections in Bodian's Protargol preparations indicated that they did provide efferents into the spinal cord. It may be reiterated that despite the fact that the neocortical transplants had grown and filled the cavity, had differentiated into normal-looking neural tissue, and had connectivity with the host spinal cord, the experimental animals did not show any recovery from the paraplegic syndrome (Table 1-2).

An analysis of material obtained from animals sacrificed in a developmental sequence showed that in the control animals following lesion there was extensive hemorrhage, edema, and necrosis of tissue in the spinal cord extending from its cut ends into the parenchyma (Figures 1-12A,B,C and 1-13A,B,C). The lesion site was filled with erythrocytes and leucocytes. In this region of degenerative changes a large number of highly distended capillaries were seen indicating their proliferation following a trauma. Although this necrotic region at first was diffuse, in a few days it appeared delineated. The transition between the necrotic region and normal-looking tissue of the spinal cord became well defined. The degenerative changes appeared contained and did not appear to extend deep into the spinal cord. Over a period of time, the necrotic tissue was cleared, edema had subsided, and the hematogenous elements were gradually removed. This process of clearing the degenerating mass resulted in the development of a cavity or a cyst at the site of the lesion. In other words, although with knife lesions no real cavity was created at the time of lesion, the ensuing degenerative changes in the tissue and clearing of the necrotic mass contributed

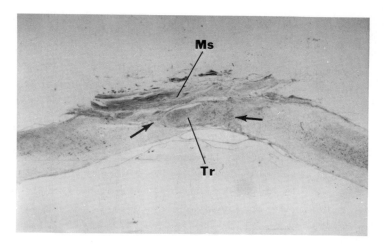

Figure 1-10. Spinal cord from the animal shown in Figure 1-8. This animal had received knife lesion and complete transection, and 16-day embryonic neocortical tissue as the transplant. The lesion site has become enlarged as a result of cavitation in the spinal cord due to degenerative changes. The transplant (Tr) has survived and is integrated with the gray matter of the host spinal cord (arrows). Thin band of loose connective tissue and dense muscular tissue (Ms) are seen to cover the top surface of the transplant. 6 months survival; Cresyl-violet stain; ×8.

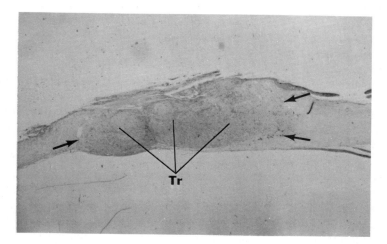

Figure 1-11. Spinal cord from the animal shown in Figure 1-9. This animal had received laceration-type lesion and complete transection of the spinal cord, followed by transplantation of neocortical tissue from 16-day donor embryo. The transplant (Tr) has survived, grown, and filled the cavity left by the lesion. It is integrated with the host spinal cord, mainly with its gray matter (arrows). In this as well as other cases note that the lesion has enlarged, due to cavitation of the spinal cord. 6 months survival; Cresyl-violet stain; ×8.

Table 1-2. Percentage of Animals Showing Loss of Locomotor and Supportive Functions of Both Hindlimbs (Paraplegia) and Those Showing Recovery from This Following Transplantation of Neocortical Tissue in the Spinal Cord

	Animals showing paraplegia (loss of locomotor and supportive functions)	Animals showing recovery of locomotor function only	Animals showing recovery of locomotor and supportive functions
Total transection-			
Knife lesion			
Control: lesion only	100	—	—
Experimental: lesion-transplantation	100	0	0
Laceration-type lesion			
Control: lesion only	100	—	—
Experimental: lesion-transplantation	100	0	0
Partial transection-extensive lesion			
Knife lesion			
Control: lesion only	0	0	100
Experimental: lesion-transplantation	0	0	100
Laceration-type lesion			
Control: lesion only	95	—	—
Experimental: lesion-transplantation	95	70	0
Partial transection-restricted lesion			
Laceration-type lesion			
Control: lesion only	70	—	—
Experimental: lesion-transplantation	75	0	80

KNIFE LESION: COMPLETE TRANSECTION

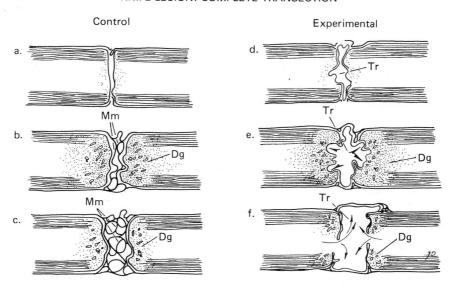

Control   Experimental

Figure 1-12. Schematic drawings to show developmental events in control and experimental animals following complete transection with knife lesion. Control: (a) Lesion within spinal cord. (b) Lesion after 5–7 days. There is considerable degeneration (Dg) in the spinal cord at both the cut ends. In the space between them, meningeal membranes (Mm) and connective tissue penetrate. (c) Lesion after about 1 month. The cavity has enlarged, and degeneration (Dg) in the spinal cord is seen to persist. Meningeal membranes (Mm) and connective tissue form a dense matrix in the cavity. Experimental: (d) Lesion is made in the spinal cord and neocortical tissue (Tr) is transplanted to fill the lesion site. (e) About 5–7 days after the lesion there is degeneration (Dg) in the spinal cord and the growing transplant (Tr) is seen to penetrate through it. Arrowheads indicate the outward-growing regions of the transplant. (f) About 1 month after the surgery, the transplant (Tr) is seen fully grown and integrated with the gray matter. In the regions of white matter the transplant is not integrated, and there is some persisting degeneration (Dg) in the spinal cord.

to the development of cavities in the spinal cord (Figure 1-12A,B,C). Similarly, with laceration-type lesions, there was a region at each cut end of the spinal cord that showed degenerative changes including hemorrhage, edema, and tissue necrosis. As this necrotic mass was cleared away, the cavity made at the time of lesion was considerably enlarged (Figure 1-13A,B,C). It was important to observe that of the various pathological conditions at the lesion site, the degree of hemorrhage, at the time of lesion, seemed to determine how large the cavity would be. If there was extensive bleeding at the time of making the lesion, the final size of the cavity was large. And if there was small amount of bleeding at the time of surgery, the cavities were small. Of course it is possible that in some cases even when bleeding at the time of surgery was controlled, some amount of bleeding may have continued after the incision was closed and sutured and may have contributed to an increase in the size of the cavity.

LACERATION-TYPE LESION: COMPLETE TRANSECTION

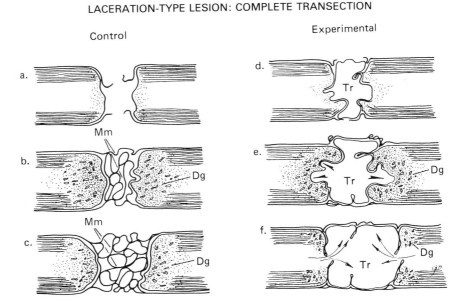

Figure 1-13. Schematic drawings to show developmental events in control and experimental animals following complete transection with laceration-type lesion. Control: (a) Lesion in the spinal cord. The lesion appears large because considerable amount of neural tissue has been removed after making lesion. (b) Lesion after 5–7 days. There is a large amount of degeneration (Dg) in the spinal cord at both the cut ends. In the space between them meningeal membranes (Mm) and connective tissue penetrate to form a matrix. (c) Lesion after about 1 month. The cavity has enlarged, and degeneration (Dg) in the spinal cord is still seen to persist. Meningeal membranes (Mm) and connective tissue fill the cavity completely. Experimental: (d) Lesion is made in the spinal cord, and neocortical transplant (Tr) is injected intraparenchymally to fill the lesion site. (e) About 5–7 days after the surgery, the degeneration (Dg) is seen in the spinal cord. The growing transplant (Tr) penetrates through the degenerating mass. The forward-growing regions of transplant are shown by arrowheads. (f) About 1 month after the surgery, the transplant (Tr) is seen fully grown and integrated with the gray matter. In the white matter regions of spinal cord some degree of degeneration (Dg) is still seen to persist. The transplant is not integrated at these regions.

The development of a cavity at the site of lesion was closely associated with the proliferation of meningeal membranes and the connective tissue that penetrated into the cavity. At first the proliferating meningeal membranes and connective tissue seemed diffuse and unorganized. But as the necrotic tissue was cleared away and the surface of the viable spinal cord tissue was delineated from the necrotic tissue, the proliferating meningeal membranes were seen to penetrate and provide a membranous sheet covering the viable spinal cord. Eventually, the surface of the spared spinal cord was fully covered by the meningeal membranes. Adjacent to this covering, in the spinal cord parenchyma, there was an evidence of glial proliferation, glial hypertrophy, and dense accumulation of glial cells. They contributed to the development of glial scar formation. These sequelae following pathological reaction in the spinal cord appeared as protective mechanisms for preserving the viable and normal neural tissue of the spinal cord. Outside the spinal cord the meningeal membranes not only covered the surface of the spinal cord at the two cut ends but also formed a lining in the cavity. The cavity itself was filled largely with the loose connective tissue and the disorganized meningeal membranes. The two cut ends of the spinal cord were held together by a loose matrix of meningeal membranes and connective tissue. The severed axons at both the cut ends showed no regenerative growth, but a number of large- and small-caliber blood vessels were seen to proliferate and penetrate into this connective tissue matrix. These blood vessels were seen to penetrate into the spinal cord through the glial scar formation and through the remaining degenerating mass into the normal spinal cord. The regenerating blood vessels were not inhibited or restricted from penetrating into the spinal cord by the presence of glial scar formation or loose matrix of meningeal membranes and connective tissue. It may be added that the developmental histopathological changes observed in these control animals were also seen in other control animals with partial transection lesions.

In the experimental animals, which received knife and laceration-type lesions followed by neocortical transplants, various developmental histopathological processes related to the development of degenerative changes, gradual clearance of necrotic tissue, and the development of a cavity were similar to those described above. Transplantation of neocortical tissues in these animals provided a situation of an interaction between the degenerative changes in the fully differentiated adult spinal cord and the growth, differentiation, and integration of undifferentiated embryonic neural tissues (Figures 1-12D,E,F and 1-13D,E,F). At first, most of the transplant was within the cavity between the two cut ends of the spinal cord with some portions in the spinal cord parenchyma. During development, the growing transplant was seen to penetrate into the degenerating mass in the spinal cord and displace the necrotic tissue. With this process the compact necrotic tissue was broken down, and fragmented, and pushed away from the viable spinal cord tissue. It is possible that this course of events contributed to a faster removal of the necrotic tissue, parenchymal attachment of the growing transplant with the viable spinal cord tissue, and prevention of any further development of necrosis in the spinal cord. Within 4 weeks, the transplant had grown large, had occupied the entire region of the cavity, and had established an interface with the spinal cord at the region of the gray matter. It had not established any type of neural interface with the white matter of the spinal cord. The white matter at the two cut ends was composed of swollen axonal endings, thin and atrophying axons, fragmentation of myelin, and extensive vacuolation. The meningeal membranes had penetrated in between the cut axons and the transplants and contributed to a barrier between them. In the spinal cord at the cut ends of white matter, there was an increase in the number of glial cells, very likely most of them being astrocytes and some oligodendroglial cells, contributing to the glial scar formation. Thus, the glial scar formation was confined to the regions of apposition between the white matter of the spinal cord and the transplant but not between the gray matter of the spinal cord and the transplant. The gray matter of the spinal cord seemed more conducive and receptive to providing neural milieu for the development of an interface with the growing transplant than the white matter composed of damaged and frayed axons and damaged myelin. Further, necrotic reaction in the spinal cord of the control animals with lesions was extensive and persisted for a long time, lasting for 2–3 months after the surgery. But in the experimental animals that had received neural transplants following the lesions, the necrotic mass had receded and subsided within 4–6 weeks after transplantation. There was little evidence of persistence of necrotic reaction in the spinal cord. These observations suggested that very likely the presence of a viable and growing neural transplant had prevented the spared spinal cord from undergoing excessive degenerative changes over a protracted period of time. From an overall viewpoint, the histopathological changes and interactions between pathological conditions and growing neural transplants observed in these preparations were also seen in the experimental animals receiving only partial transection lesions of the spinal cord.

The above-described observations on complete transection of the spinal cord showed that these lesions involved a complex course of various pathological changes. In light of the literature on the weight-dropping model, it may be suggested that these lesions also involved a primary trauma followed by secondary traumatic conditions. The primary trauma or primary traumatic condition pertained to the direct severance of the spinal cord tissue by surgical means. With this complete severance of the neural tissue the anatomical continuity between the segments, rostral and caudal to the lesion, was lost. The secondary traumatic condition, also known as secondary traumatic reaction, involved damage to the vascular system resulting in hemorrhage and ischemia, followed by edema and subsequent necrosis of tissue at the site of lesion. In the literature on weight-dropping experiments, the secondary traumatic conditions are considered to be the main, if not the sole, factors contributing to paraplegia. In the present studies, described above, the secondary traumatic changes were associated with extensive degeneration of the spinal cord tissue at and near the site of lesion. These degenerative changes in the tissue and clearing of the necrotic mass were found to be the major factors contributing to the development of cavities. Furthermore, it was observed that the secondary traumatic conditions and degeneration of spinal cord tissue were of short duration. The former, in general, subsided within 8–12 days after the surgery and the latter in about 2–3 weeks. In addition to these, other degenerative changes were found to persist even 6–8 months after the surgery. These persisting degenerative changes included gradual degeneration of axons, demyelination of axons, and atrophic reaction in the neurons in the spinal cord as well as other neural structures far removed from the site of the lesion. These were considered as progressive degenerative changes. In all likelihood, these changes were due to a complex course of pathological events including effects of the secondary traumatic changes, retrograde degenerative reaction in the neurons whose axons were severed, and anterograde degeneration of axons that were severed from their somata. The role played by progressive degenerative changes under the conditions of total transection of the spinal cord in contributing to permanent paraplegia was masked by the complete severance of all the ascending and descending axons by the lesion. But their role in the development of paraplegia under the conditions of partial transection of spinal cord is seen to be of great importance.

Partial Transection and Transplantation

Partial transection of the spinal cord was performed under both conditions of knife and laceration-type lesions. The lesions were at T8–T9 or T9–T10, the level of thoracic spinal cord also employed for total transection of the spinal cord. These lesions varied in depth in dorso-ventral plane, thus providing lesions of different degrees of severity. The results obtained with knife lesions were different from those with laceration-type lesions, and therefore they are treated separately.

Knife Lesions

The surgical approach for making partial transections of the spinal cord at lower thoracic levels was identical to that followed for making total transections of the spinal cord except that with these lesions ventral funiculi were partially spared from sectioning. The lesions studied in this investigation extended for at least 90% of the spinal cord in its transverse plane (Figure 1-3). With this, the dorsal and lateral funiculi and the gray matter of the spinal cord were completely severed. The ventral funiculi were partially severed, leaving some portions of white matter spared. Such lesions represented a condition of partial transection-extensive lesion. The control as well as experimental animals with these lesions did not show any permanent paraplegia (Table 1-2). They showed transient paraplegic syndrome lasting only for 4–5 days, and after this they regained most of the control over locomotor and supportive functions of their hindlimbs. When these animals were placed on elevated metal grids, they showed variable degrees of abnormality in their gait, but from an overall viewpoint neither locomotor not supportive functions were seriously affected by such lesions. Since there were no differences in control and experimental animals, the rapid recovery from the transient paraplegic syndrome in animals in both groups could be attributed to sparing of some fibers in the ventral funiculi. In the experimental animals, the neocortical transplants had grown and become anatomically integrated with the gray matter of the spinal cord. Despite this the neural transplants could not be attributed with any ameliorative properties for the following two reasons: First, since in the control animals sparing of fibers in the ventral funiculi was related to spontaneous recovery from the transient paraplegic syndrome, it was safe to conclude that in the experimental animals, too, sparing of fibers in the ventral funiculi was the primary cause of spontaneous recovery from the paraplegic syndrome. Second, the spontaneous recovery was observed within 4–5 days after the surgery, and it was highly unlikely that an undifferentiated and unintegrated mass of embryonic neural tissue undergoing the initial phases of necrosis and recovery would have established connections with the host spinal cord to provide for this fast recovery. Even under the most ideal conditions of transplantation, a neural tissue takes 2–3 weeks to grow, differentiate, and become anatomically integrated with the host brain tissue. If neural transplants had any beneficial effects on the functional recovery, these effects would not appear for at least 2–3 weeks after the surgery, but by then the animals had already recovered from the transient paraplegic syndrome attributable to the spared fibers in the ventral funiculi.

An anatomical analysis of neocortical transplants in the experimental animals, in summary, showed that the transplants had grown and filled the enlarged lesion site. They contained fully differentiated neurons and had become integrated with the gray matter of the host spinal cord. They were separated from the apposing white matter that was severed by the lesion by an intervening glial scar formation. In other words, even in these preparations the severed axons of dorsal and lateral funiculi showed no regenerative growth into the transplants. The afferents to these transplants, both ascending and descending, as established in Fink-Heimer preparations, were seen to come mainly through the interface with the gray matter of the spinal cord. Although the exact source of these afferents could not be established, very likely they represented the axonal collaterals from the gray matter and also, to some extent, from the spared axons in the ventral funiculi. It is of importance to observe that in both control and experimental animals the lesions at the time of surgery did result in a considerable amount of hemorrhage and ischemia, but the spared axons in the ventral funiculi had survived the indirect trauma from the act of lesion and the hemorrhagic and ischemic conditions. This observation was found valuable when knife lesions were compared with the laceration-type lesions.

Other knife lesions that were less than 90% in transverse extent of the spinal cord did not result in any obviously detectable somatic abnormalities. When the lesions were less than 90% in the transverse extent, the animals were able to support their bodies and move about using their hindlimbs in 24–48 hours after the surgery. Partial lesions extending more than 90% in the transverse plane did not yield consistent and reliable results. The majority of animals with lesions larger than 90% in transverse extent were found to have become like animals with total transection of the spinal cord. This change was due to progressive degeneration of the few spared, and probably traumatized, axonal fibers. They were permanently paraplegic. Thus, knife lesions involving partial transection of the spinal cord were found to be of little value in understanding the problem of paraplegia and the effectiveness of neural transplants in relation to paraplegic syndrome.

Laceration-Type Lesions

These lesions, from an overall viewpoint, were similar to those made under the total transection conditions, except that they involved only partial transection of the spinal cord in its transverse plane. They extended for a segment or more in rostro-caudal axis. The very nature of laceration-type lesions was such that under this condition an extensive amount of damage was caused to the spinal cord, and this was associated with two immediate pathological events: an extensive amount of hemorrhage at the site of lesion, and some indirect trauma to the spared axons in the spinal cord. Extensive hemorrhage presaged and initiated the complex secondary traumatic changes, thus aggravating the effects of the primary trauma, and indirect trauma to the spared axons, which, depending upon the degree of its severity and other conditions, contributed to various degrees of progressive degeneration. These pathological events were always present in the condition of laceration-type lesions but were not seen to this degree with the knife lesion. Although under the condition of laceration-type lesions various different degrees of severity of lesions were investigated, two appeared very important: partial transection-extensive lesions and partial transection-restricted lesions.

Partial transection-extensive lesions involved making very deep lesions. Dorsal and lateral funiculi and gray matter were completely severed and ventral funiculi were severed in such a manner that less than half of the fibers were spared. Such lesions covered 90–95% of the spinal cord in its transverse extent (Figure 1-5). With this lesion about 95% of animals in the control group showed permanent paraplegia (Table 1-2). They were unable to use their hindlimbs for locomotor and supportive functions. During the first 2 weeks after surgery, they showed a variety of autonomic dysfunctions, but after this they were able to recover gradually. Although they were permanently paraplegic they did show some reflexive activity in their hindlimbs. The reflexes observed were withdrawal reflexes and vigorous kicking responses to a nociceptive stimulus. At the end of the experiment histological preparations showed that in the spinal cord of these paraplegic animals the lesions had enlarged into large cavities, and there were only a few thin atrophying axons left in the ventral funiculi. The spared axons in the control animals were undergoing degenerative changes. The myelin in this region appeared fragmented (Figure 1-16A,B,C).

The experimental animals that received extensive lesions, very similar to those in the control animals, but with neocortical transplants showed similar autonomic dysfunctions as the control animals. They were completely paraplegic for 2–3 weeks after the surgery. After this period, during which time they had recovered from autonomic dysfunctions, they showed a slow and gradual recovery in the use of their hindlimbs for locomotion (Table 1-2). This recovery progressed for about 2 months at a very slow rate. This was only a partial recovery, for they did not show any recovery in the supportive functions. When these animals were placed on the elevated metal grids, their bellies rested on the grid. They were unable to support their bodies on the hindlimbs, although they were able to move their hindlimbs in a paddling fashion that was coordinated with the movements in the forelimbs during locomotion (Figure 1-14). From an overall viewpoint, the movements observed in the hindlimbs were not random. They were well-integrated, although in a primitive fashion, with those in the forelimbs and were used for locomotor function. They were able to flex their hindlimbs, place them against the bars of the metal grid, grasp the

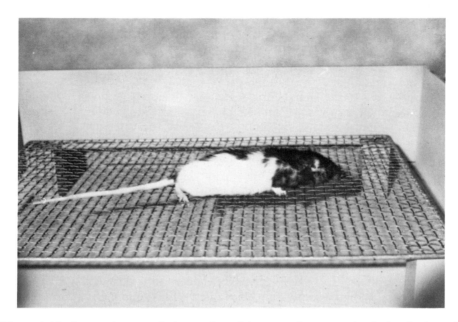

Figure 1-14. Laceration-type lesion and partial transection-extensive lesion in the spinal cord at T_9-T_{10}. This animal was operated on when 3 months old, and received neocortical tissue as the transplant from a 16-day donor embryo. It survived for 8 months after the surgery. It was able to recover some functions in its hindlimbs and use them for locomotion. But it was unable to use them for supporting its body. While resting or moving its belly always rested on the floor of the cage. Here its right hindlimb is flexed and has grasped the grid, and will extend it in coordination with other limbs in locomotion.

bars, extend the hindlimbs, and propel their bodies forward. In essence, this was the pattern of the locomotor function. Further, their hindlimbs moved in alternation during this sequence of movements, and the movements were fully coordinated with those in the forelimbs. It must be emphasized that although the hindlimbs did show a recovery of voluntary control over their movements, as related to locomotor function, they were not as smooth and well-regulated as those seen in a normal animal. These movements were at best rudimentary and primitive. Further, these animals could not show this locomotor function for a sustained period of more than 2–3 minutes at a time. This indicated only an incomplete recovery in the locomotor function, but it was permanent. These animals showed this primitive locomotor function as long as they lived without relapsing to the paraplegic syndrome. Thus, the experimental animals with extensive lesions showed only a partial recovery from paraplegic syndrome, in that it was a recovery of locomotor function and not of supportive function. And it was an incomplete recovery of locomotor function, in that it was rudimentary and primitive and not normal.

Histological analysis of these spinal cords with transplants showed that the neocortical transplants had grown large and filled the cavity (Figure 1-15). They

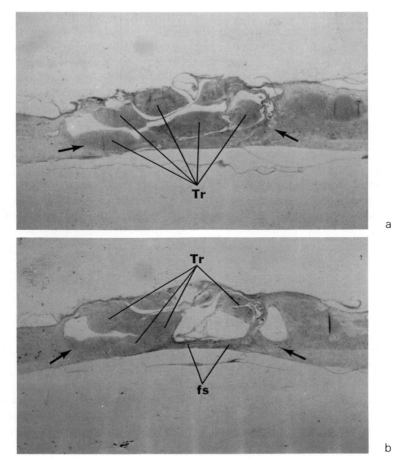

Figure 1-15. Spinal cord from the animal shown in Figure 1-14. It has received laceration-type lesion and partial transection and extensive lesion, followed by transplantation of neocortical tissue from a 16-day donor embryo. The neocortical transplant (Tr) has survived, grown, and become differentiated. It is integrated with the gray matter of the spinal cord (arrows). Although the transplant appears fragmented, in actuality these fragments are interconnected and continuous. In serial sections the transplant is seen to be one single mass with a tortuous cavity in its center. It is an intraparenchymal transplant. (a) The transplant is seen to fill the whole cavity with little evidence of spared fibers. But after a distance of a few sections (b), the spared fibers in the ventral funiculi (fs) are seen preserved. These small number of fibers are closely related to the transplant and have not undergone degeneration. 8 months survival; Cresyl-violet stain; ×8.

were anatomically integrated with the gray matter of the spinal cord through which they received both ascending and descending afferents. The glial scar formation between the apposing white matter of the spinal cord and the transplant was extensive, often extending partially into the region of apposition between the gray matter and the transplants. Despite this, the transplants looked well differentiated and well integrated with the host spinal cord tissue.

Of importance was the observation that the few axonal fibers spared in the ventral funiculi did not degenerate. They remained normal and viable. In this region there was no indication of degeneration of myelin. Some axonal collaterals were seen to emerge from these spared fibers and penetrate into the transplants. These observations indicated that the few fibers that were spared from the lesion, instead of degenerating, were preserved in the presence of a growing neural transplant. These preserved axons seemed to have provided axonal collaterals into the transplants indicating their regenerative expression.

It is important to comment on the fact that only 70% of animals in the experimental group showed this partial and rudimentary recovery from the paraplegic syndrome (Table 1-2). In the remaining 30% of animals, generally the neocortical transplants had survived but they were not integrated with the host spinal cord. They were extraparenchymal and had no connections with the spinal cord. A dense glial scar formation intervened between them and the host spinal cord along the entire surface of the cavity. There was extensive degeneration in the spinal cord, and the few fibers spared in the ventral funiculi at the time of surgery appeared degenerated. Except for the presence of extraparenchymally located transplants, these preparations were histologically similar to those of the control animals.

An analysis of developmental material showed a pattern of histopathological reaction similar to that observed in animals with complete transection of the spinal cord. In brief, in control animals, there was a considerable amount of hemorrhage along with edema and necrosis immediately after the surgery (Figure 1-16A,B,C). As these secondary traumatic changes in the spinal cord increased, the necrotic or degenerating mass in the spinal cord also increased. Over a period of time, it was cleared away and a large cavity was formed. This cavity was lined by the meningeal membranes and filled with loose connective tissue. The indirect traumatic effects on the spared axons in the ventral funiculi induced at the time of surgery, and the secondary traumatic conditions ensuing them, very likely contributed to atrophy and gradual degeneration of the spared axons. Although the secondary traumatic changes subsided within a few days, the degenerative changes in the spinal cord continued to progress. It is these progressive degenerative changes that resulted in the loss of the few spared axonal fibers in the ventral funiculi.

In the experimental animals, too, a similar pattern of secondary traumatic changes followed by degenerative changes in the spinal cord was observed (Figure 1-16D,E,F), but the growing transplants after having pushed aside the necrotic mass and having established parenchymal attachment with the viable spinal cord seemed to restrict the degenerative changes from progressing too far. The degenerative changes in the spinal cord slowed down considerably, and most important of all, the spared axons in the ventral funiculi were preserved from any progressive degeneration. It is possible that, of the spared axons at the time of surgery, not all were preserved. Some may have degenerated even as the transplant was growing, but the remaining were preserved from progressive degeneration. If the indirect traumatic changes associated with the primary trauma of severance of axons and neural tissue and the pres-

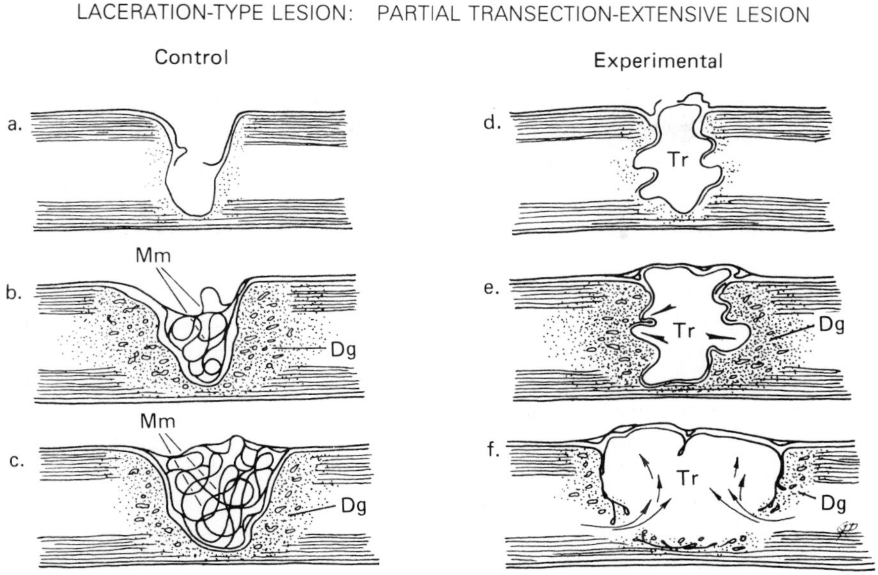

LACERATION-TYPE LESION: PARTIAL TRANSECTION-EXTENSIVE LESION

Control   Experimental

Figure 1-16. Schematic drawings to show developmental events in control and experimental animals following partial transection-extensive lesion with laceration-type lesion. Control: (a) Lesion in the spinal cord. It extends for 90–95% of spinal cord in transverse plane. Only a few fibers of ventral funiculi are spared. (b) Lesion after 5–7 days. The cavity has enlarged. There is a large amount of degeneration (Dg) in the spinal cord; and meningeal membranes (Mm) and connective tissue have penetrated into the cavity. (c) Lesion after about 1 month. The cavity has further enlarged. The degeneration (Dg) in the spinal cord still persists considerably. The few spared axons in the ventral funiculi are found atrophied and degenerating. The cavity is filled with a dense matrix of meningeal membranes (Mm) and loose connective tissue. Experimental: (d) Lesion is made in the spinal cord, and neocortical tissue (Tr) is transplanted intraparenchymally to fill the cavity. (e) About 5–7 days after the surgery, the degeneration is seen in the spinal cord. The transplant (Tr) is growing, and its regions of active growth (arrowheads) are seen to penetrate through the degenerating mass. (f) About 1 month after the surgery, the transplant (Tr) is fully grown and is integrated with the gray matter along its basal aspects. Degeneration (Dg) in the white matter is still seen to persist. The spared fibers in the ventral funiculi are preserved. They are intact and provide some afferents (arrows) to the transplant.

ence of secondary traumatic changes could be considered to contribute to trauma to the spared axons of the ventral funiculi, the degenerating axons were subjected to suprathreshold indirect trauma and the preserved axons to a subthreshold indirect trauma. The spared axons subjected to subthreshold trauma in the presence of growing neural transplants were able to survive and show some degree of regeneration in the form of axonal collaterals to the transplants.

A partial transection of the spinal cord, somewhat less severe than that described above, involved sectioning of the spinal cord in such a fashion that the entire dorsal and lateral funiculi and the gray matter were severed. In the ventral funiculi only some fibers were severed and the rest were spared. Such lesions extended for 85–90% in the transverse plane, and they were designated as partial transection-restricted lesions (Figure 1-4). Under this condition, 70% of control animals showed permanent paraplegic syndrome (Table 1-2). They were unable to use their hindlimbs for locomotor as well as supportive functions. These animals also underwent the initial autonomic disturbances from which they recovered gradually. The course of functional abnormalities that they underwent was similar to that described earlier for animals in other control groups. The remaining 30% of control animals showed transient paraplegia. They were able to use their hindlimbs for locomotor and supportive functions in less than 8–12 days after the surgery. The permanently paraplegic animals, in this case too, showed the presence of reflexes, as described earlier, when subjected to nociceptive stimulation.

Histological evaluation of the spinal cord in these animals showed that, in these preparations also, primary trauma was followed by extensive secondary traumatic changes, including loss of spinal cord tissue along the two sides of the cavity. Other pathological changes related to progressive degenerative changes, such as atrophy and degeneration of the spared axons in the ventral funiculi, were also observed (Figure 1-17A,B,C). The degenerating axons in the ventral funiculi were found in different stages of degeneration, which probably was determined by the degree of proximity to the lesion. In other words, axons close to the lesion were in a far more advanced stage of degeneration than those far away from it.

The animals in the experimental group that had received similar laceration-type lesions followed by neocortical transplants also showed various autonomic dysfunctions and paraplegic syndrome. But after 2–3 weeks they showed a gradual recovery from paraplegia. At first, the movements of hindlimbs related to locomotion appeared. They were rudimentary and primitive, similar to those observed in the experimental animals with partial transection-extensive lesion. When placed on an elevated metal grid, they were able to use their hindlimbs in grasping the metal bars and in propelling their bodies forward in coordination with the movements of the forelimbs. Overlapping this recovery, they showed a slow and gradual recovery in their supportive function (Figure 1-18). They were able to flex their hindlimbs and slowly extend them and support their bodies. At first the supportive function by the hindlimbs was seen only when the animals were stationary, but gradually they were able to integrate both locomotor and supportive functions and move about with their bellies lifted above the metal grid (Table 1-2). This recovery was permanent. In other words, the animals that showed this functional recovery did not show any relapse of paraplegic syndrome.

Histological evaluation of material from these animals showed that the degenerative changes in the spinal cord following lesions were very similar to those observed in the control animals, but they were not as extensive (Figure 1-17D,E,F). In this case, too, the growing transplants had penetrated through the degenerating mass, pushed it aside, established parenchymal attachment

LACERATION-TYPE LESION:
PARTIAL TRANSECTION-RESTRICTED LESION

Control   Experimental

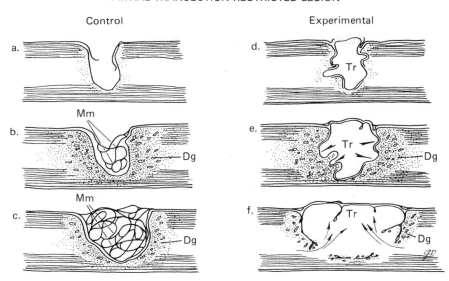

Figure 1-17. Schematic drawings to show developmental events in control and experimental animals following partial transection-restricted lesion with laceration-type lesion. Control: (a) Lesion in the spinal cord. It extends for 85–90% of spinal cord in its transverse plane. Many fibers in the ventral funiculi are spared from the lesion. (b) Lesion after about 5–7 days. The cavity has become larger. There is a large amount of degeneration (Dg) in the spinal cord. Meningeal membranes (Mm) and loose connective tissue have filled the cavity. (c) Lesion after about 1 month. The cavity has further enlarged. Degeneration (Dg) in the spinal cord is still seen to persist. Meningeal membranes (Mm) and connective tissues have filled the cavity. Many spared fibers in the ventral funiculi are found atrophied and degenerating. Experimental: (d) Lesion is made in the spinal cord, and transplant (Tr) is injected intraparenchymally to fill the cavity. (e) About 5–7 days after the surgery, degeneration (Dg) in the spinal cord is present. The transplant (Tr) is seen growing, with its active regions of growth (arrowheads) penetrating into the degenerating mass. (f) About 1 month after the surgery, the transplant (Tr) is fully grown, and it is integrated with the gray matter of the spinal cord along its basal aspects. Degeneration (Dg) in the white matter is still seen to persist. The spared fibers of ventral funiculi are found preserved. They do not show any degeneration. Some of them seem to provide afferents (arrows) to the transplant.

with the host spinal cord, and, above all, had contributed to the preservation of the spared axons in the ventral funiculi (Figure 1-19). Since under this condition of lesion more fibers in the ventral funiculi were spared at the time of surgery, the number of axonal fibers preserved also was high. The neural transplants, as they grew and became integrated with the spinal cord, aided in the preservation of a large number of spared fibers in the ventral funiculi. In these preparations it was possible to see a very large number of axonal collaterals penetrating into the spinal cord as the afferent fibers.

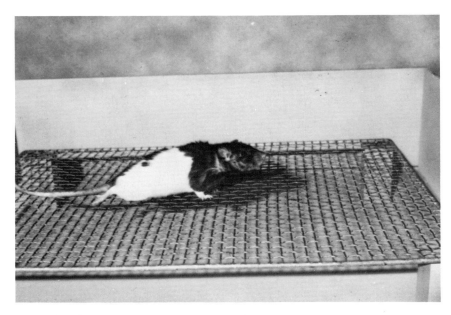

Figure 1-18. Laceration-type lesion and partial transection-restricted lesion in the spinal cord at T_9-T_{10}. This animal was operated on when 3 months old, and received neocortical transplant from a 16-day donor embryo. It survived for 8 months after the surgery, and was able to recover both locomotor and supportive functions in hindlimbs. While resting, this animal generally lay on its side. But when it moved about, it was able to lift its belly above the floor of the cage. Here its right hindlimb is in extension position for locomotion, and its belly is clearly above the grid.

In this condition of lesion, about 80% of experimental animals showed recovery, and the remaining 20% that did not show a recovery were found to remain permanently paraplegic (Table 1-2). Histological analysis of the spinal cord from the 20% of animals that did not show recovery from paraplegia showed that the transplants in these animals had become necrotic. They contained highly shrunken and atrophied neurons. These transplants were isolated from the host spinal cord and were extraparenchymally located. In a few cases, where the transplants were large, they too were extraparenchymal and were unintegrated with the host spinal cord tissue. In all these preparations, where the transplants did not become integrated with the spinal cord, there was an extensive amount of glial scar formation intervening between the two. The spared axons in the ventral funiculi in these animals appeared thin, and they appeared to be undergoing progressive degeneration. In these preparations, there was no evidence of any axonal collaterals penetrating into the extraparenchymally located transplants.

In summary, partial transection of the spinal cord under the conditions of knife lesions was of little value in producing paraplegic syndrome in a consistent and systematic manner. Therefore, in such preparations, which were at

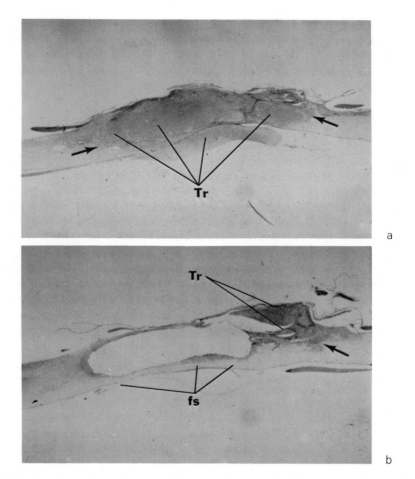

a

b

Figure 1-19. Spinal cord from the animal shown in Figure 1-18. It had received laceration-type lesion and partial transection, followed by transplantation of neocortical tissue from a 16-day donor embryo. The transplant (Tr) has survived, grown, and filled most of the cavity created by the lesion. It is integrated with the gray matter of the spinal cord (arrows). (a) The transplant has fully occupied the cavity, and has also grown ventrally outside the spinal cord. But a few sections away (b), there is a cyst in the transplant, and a large bundle of fibers (fs) in the ventral funiculi is seen preserved. These fibers were spared from the lesion, and are closely related to the transplant. They have not undergone progressive degeneration. 8 months survival; Cresyl-violet stain; ×8.

best characterized by transient paraplegia, the presence or absence of neural transplants had no significance. In the case of partial transection, under the conditions of laceration-type lesions, the following general observations could be made. First, partial transections extending for 85% or more in the transverse plane yielded permanent paraplegic syndrome, which was investigated in control as well as experimental animals. Second, in control animals, partial transections of this type resulted in progressive degeneration of the spared axons, and owing to these pathological events partial transections developed into total transections of the spinal cord. Third, in the experimental animals that received neocortical transplants following laceration-type lesions, the transplants had survived, grown, and become integrated with the host spinal cord. The spared axons, at least most of them if not all, did not undergo progressive degeneration in the presence of viable and integrated neural transplants. They appeared healthy and normal and showed some degree of regeneration in the form of collateral sprouting that served as afferents to the transplants. Fourth, the majority of animals in the experimental groups showed some degree of recovery from the paraplegic syndrome. The degree of recovery was related to the severity of the lesion. Animals with extensive lesions showed a recovery of rudimentary and primitive locomotor functions in the hindlimbs, but those with restricted lesions showed a recovery of both locomotor and supportive functions by the hindlimbs. The recovery of rudimentary locomotor functions in one case and that of locomotor and supportive functions in the other was never complete. Although recovery of these functions did not lead to normal locomotor and supportive functions by the hindlimbs, the recovery was permanent. Fifth, anatomically the neural transplants appeared to establish interfaces readily with the traumatized gray matter of the spinal cord but not with the severed axons of the white matter. The glial scar formation was a ubiquitous phenomenon between the white matter and the neural transplants.

Interpretation and Discussion

The findings submitted above provide information on many issues of spinal cord trauma and paraplegia, but here attention will be focused on the following three major issues: paraplegic syndrome under different conditions of lesions, the role of primary and secondary traumatic conditions and progressive degeneration in the development of paraplegia, and the role of neural transplants in the recovery from paraplegia. Before discussing these three different aspects of the findings it is important to define the conceptual framework within which these findings may be interpreted comprehensively. It is based upon the work of other investigators and that submitted in this presentation (Allen 1911, 1914, Freeman and Wright 1953, Joyner and Freeman 1963, Goodkin and Campbell 1969, White et al. 1969, Assenmacher and Ducker 1971, Ducker et al. 1971, Wagner et al. 1971, Osterholm and Mathews 1972a,b, Osterholm 1974, Jellinger 1976, Ducker 1976, Balentine and Paris 1978a).

Conceptually, it is important to distinguish primary trauma, secondary traumatic changes, and progressive degenerative changes. Primary trauma refers to the trauma caused to the spinal cord tissue directly by the surgical knife while making lesions. It involves the severance of axons and the gray matter. A primary trauma may vary in its degree of severity, and it is generally determined by whether the spinal cord is severed completely or partially. When the spinal cord is severed completely, all the neural tissues in the path of the knife are directly affected by the primary trauma. Therefore, the functional loss can be completely attributed to the primary trauma. But when the spinal cord is severed partially, it becomes very difficult to establish the role of primary trauma in determining the functional deficit or loss unequivocally. In such preparations it cannot be claimed that the spared axons are completely unaffected by the primary trauma. They may not be directly affected, but it is very likely that they may be indirectly affected during the surgery. The nature of the indirect primary trauma may be in the form of pulling, pressing, or stretching the spared axons while making lesions or cleaning up the lesion site. The indirect primary trauma on the spared spinal cord tissue may not be severe by itself, but in the presence of other pathological conditions it may have some important bearing on the development of the paraplegic syndrome. The effects of direct primary trauma are known to be irreversible, whereas those of indirect primary trauma, depending upon the degree of severity, may be reversible or irreversible. Immediately following primary trauma are the secondary traumatic conditions, which refer to various pathological changes, and they include hemorrhage, ischemia, and edema. Depending upon the nature and severity of the primary trauma, they may be extensive or restricted. Generally, under the experimental conditions involving laceration-type lesions, as employed in these studies, the secondary traumatic conditions are extensive. As the secondary traumatic conditions develop, there is evidence of necrosis in the spinal cord tissue that may extend for variable distances in the spinal cord and last for considerable duration. As a matter of fact, necrosis of tissue also is considered as a secondary traumatic change. The secondary traumatic conditions generally are contained and subside after variable intervals following the lesion. Hemorrhage, ischemia, and edema subside within 8 days, but the necrotic changes in the spinal cord tissue may linger for a long time. The clearing of necrotic mass depends upon the phagocytic activity in the region. Eventually these changes also subside leaving behind a cavity in the spinal cord. Although primary and secondary traumatic conditions are the most strikingly observable events during and after the surgery, there are other pathological changes too that may not be as readily detectable. Nonetheless, they play an important role in the lingering pathological condition of the spinal cord for a long time. They are subsumed under progressive degenerative changes. The progressive degenerative changes, for this presentation, pertain to a slow and gradual degeneration of spared as well as severed axons, fragmentation of myelin, and degeneration of neurons far removed from the site of lesions whose axons are affected by the lesion. Close to the site of lesion, in both rostral and caudal segments of the spinal cord, it is possible to see degenerating changes in the neuropil in the form of vacuolations. These changes are characterized by the fact that they become manifest after the secondary traumatic changes have subsided, and they may persist for months or as long as the animals live. They may be initiated by the direct as well as indirect effects of the primary trauma and accentuated by the secondary traumatic changes. It is possible that under minimal primary trauma and minimal secondary traumatic conditions, such as clean partial sectioning of the spinal cord by knife, the progressive degenerative changes may be so restricted that they may go unnoticed and may not lead to any functional loss or deficit. But when the primary and secondary traumatic conditions are severe, such as those seen under the conditions of laceration-type lesions involving partial transection of the spinal cord, the progressive degenerative changes are extensive and are seen to be closely related to the development of a permanent paraplegic syndrome. Various investigators employing the weight-dropping technique to induce trauma have observed and described the nature of progressive degenerative changes in the spinal cord and have stressed their bearing on the functional loss (Kobrine et al. 1975, Wakefield and Eidelberg 1975, Bresnahan et al. 1976, Balentine and Paris, 1978b, Bresnahan 1978, Blight, 1983a). It is important to observe that the researchers using knife lesions have not reported any findings on the progressive degenerative changes in the spinal cord following lesions. Very likely, this may be due to the fact that their focus of attention is directed towards nothing but regeneration, or lack of it, in the severed axons at the site of lesion.

Different types of traumas of appropriate degree of severity are capable of producing paraplegic syndrome. Total transection of the spinal cord, whether under the conditions of knife lesions or laceration-type lesions, yields paraplegia unfailingly. In this case, it is the total severance of all the fiber tracts and of the gray matter, the direct primary trauma, that is the cause of the syndrome. Following such a severe trauma there are various secondary traumatic changes, including hemorrhage, ischemia, edema, and necrosis of tissue and subsequent progressive degenerative changes, which include degeneration of the severed axons and their myelin and neuronal elements projecting through the site of the lesion. Because of the severity of the primary trauma, these pathological changes also are of severe degree. Even if these pathological changes were controlled or reduced, they would serve very little in reversing the effects of the primary trauma. Therefore, paraplegic syndrome induced directly by primary trauma in these conditions is seen to be permanent. Even in those preparations of experimental animals where the neocortical transplants had grown and become integrated with the gray matter of the spinal cord, there was no recovery from paraplegia (Figure 1-20). The lasting and irreversible effects of total transection of the spinal cord could not be in any way altered by even the most successful neural transplantation. In the studies employing the dropping of a weight on the spinal cord, where the impact is of suprathreshold value resulting in permanent paraplegic syndrome, very likely all the axons and the gray matter are directly damaged by the impact. They may not appear cleanly severed immediately after the lesion, but they may be severely and irreversibly damaged to such an extent that irrespective of the ensuing secondary traumatic changes they would start to degenerate (Bresnahan et al. 1976, Bresnahan 1978, Blight 1983a, Ford 1983). The secondary traumatic changes being inevitable with such a severe trauma, it is possible that they may accentuate the pathological conditions of the spinal cord, leading to large segments of spinal cord undergoing necrotic reaction.

Lesions involving partial transection of the spinal cord are of importance in understanding the contribution of various pathological changes in the emer-

NEOCORTICAL TRANSPLANTS IN THREE
DIFFERENT LACERATION-TYPE LESIONS

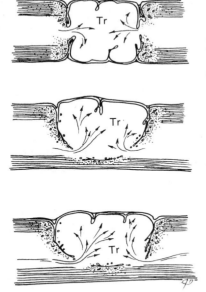

Complete Transection:
    transplant integrated with
gray matter of spinal cord; no
evidence of regeneration of
funicular fibers
    no recovery from paraplegic
syndrome

Partial Transection: Extensive
Lesion
    transplant integrated with
gray matter of spinal cord;
some fibers spared in ventral
funiculi preserved from degeneration
    70% animals show recovery
of locomotor function only

Partial Transection: Restricted
Lesion
    transplant integrated with
gray matter of the spinal cord;
most of the fibers spared in
ventral funiculi preserved from
degeneration
    80% animals show recovery
of both locomotor and supportive functions

Figure 1-20. Schematic drawings summarizing the final picture of neural transplantation under three different degrees of lesion with laceration-type lesions. Top: Complete transection of spinal cord and transplantation. Middle: Partial transection-extensive lesion of spinal cord and transplantation. Bottom: Partial transection-restricted lesion and transplantation. Nature and degree of recovery from paraplegia and percentage of animals showing such a recovery are given for each case.

gence of paraplegic syndrome. The partial transection lesion by knife, extending for as much as 90% of the spinal cord in its transverse plane, did not yield permanent paraplegia. The transient paraplegic syndrome in these animals, and also that observed in animals with other types of lesions, may be attributed to the spinal shock. In these animals most, if not all, of the spared axons in the ventral funiculi were possibly subjected to a subthreshold indirect primary trauma. Therefore, even though there were other pathological changes associated with the secondary traumatic changes at the site of lesion, they did not contribute to progressive degenerative changes in the spared axons. They remained intact and viable and therefore were able to recover their function as the animals recovered from the shock. In actuality, there may have been some axons at the transition between the severed and the spared axons that, because of threshold indirect primary trauma, may have degenerated, but the remaining spared axons were preserved from the progressive degenerative changes, and, hence, the animals did not develop permanent paraplegic syndrome. If the partial lesions were less extensive, that is, less than 90% in the transverse plane, the animals did not even show transient paraplegia. This, in all likelihood, was due to sparing of a large number of axons from the direct primary trauma and most of them being subjected to a subthreshold indirect primary trauma. In these animals, secondary traumatic changes of hemorrhage, ischemia, and edema did not even contribute to transient paraplegic syndrome.

The laceration-type partial transection lesions, involving far more damage to the spinal cord than the knife lesions, were characterized not only by extensive damage to the spinal cord tissue, but also extensive secondary traumatic changes at the site of the lesion. These lesions, whether they extended for 90–95% in the transverse plane (extensive lesions) or 85–90% in the transverse plane (restricted lesions) resulted in permanent paraplegia in a large number of animals. The damage caused to the spinal cord and other ensuing pathological changes with these lesions were far more extensive than those caused by the knife lesions. The direct primary trauma involving severance of axons and gray matter and the ensuing secondary traumatic changes were extensive. The surgical procedures involved in making these lesions were such that the spared axons in the ventral funiculi, although spared from the direct lesion, were in actuality subjected to an extensive amount of indirect primary trauma. They were left in such a threshold state that any additional pathological condition surrounding them would precipitate degenerative processes in them. Thus, in the control animals after a few months, these spared axons were found atrophied and degenerating. They were undergoing progressive degenerative changes. It is possible that the degenerating processes of these axons may have been dormant for a few days after the surgery but, in the presence of extensive secondary traumatic changes, may have been accentuated and become manifest after a week or two. This means that these animals at first were in a state of transient paraplegia, but with the progress of secondary traumatic changes and the threshold traumatic condition of the spared axons, the degenerative processes were set in in the spared axons. As these axons degenerated, the condition of the spinal cord at the site of lesion gradually came close to that of total transection. It is this course of events, i.e., threshold condition of the indirect primary trauma to the spared axons and aggravating extensive secondary traumatic changes leading to progressive degeneration of these axons, that seemed to be the cause of permanent paraplegia. These pathological conditions, to such a high degree of severity, were not present in the conditions of partial transection with knife lesions, and therefore the animals did not develop paraplegia.

Various other laceration-type lesions, particularly those involving subthreshold lesions extending for less than 85% in the transverse plane (Figure 1-3 and 1-4), and those involving hemorrhage to the gray matter (Figure 1-7), and sparing of axons in the lateral and ventral funiculi (Figure 1-6), did not yield paraplegic syndrome. As a matter of fact, many animals with these preparations did not even show transient paraplegia. This was due to the sparing of a large number of axons, and many of them, at best, were subjected to subthreshold indirect primary trauma. In these preparations, although the secondary traumatic conditions including hemorrhage, ischemia, and edema were extensive in the gray matter and were found to spread into the white matter containing spared axons, they by themselves did not induce paraplegic syndrome. The spared axons, at least most of them, were not in a state to undergo progressive degeneration. In the studies employing the weight-dropping model, subthreshold trauma, although accompanied by secondary traumatic changes, also does not yield paraplegia. In this case, too, the absence of progressive degeneration in the spared axons seems to be the important factor in preventing the animals from developing paraplegic syndrome.

The above observations on partial transections of the spinal cord bring out an important fact. In the case of total transection of spinal cord, the paraplegic syndrome sets in at the time of inflicting direct primary trauma, whereas in the case of partial transections of threshold value, various pathological changes following the direct primary trauma contribute to the development of paraplegia. In the latter, permanent paraplegia does not set in at one instant but is a result of developmental pathological events. If the developmental events in the latter could be arrested or retarded at appropriate stages, it is possible to conceive of arresting the transient paraplegic syndrome from developing into the permanent paraplegia.

Findings on the experimental animals that received lesions followed by neural transplantation showed that the animals receiving total transection of the spinal cord did not show any recovery from the paraplegic syndrome. This was true for the animals receiving knife as well as laceration-type lesions. In these animals the neocortical transplants had grown and become anatomically integrated with the gray matter of the host spinal cord but not with the severed axons in the white matter of the dorsal, lateral, and ventral funiculi. The transplants did receive afferents from the rostral and caudal segments of the spinal cord, but they did not seem to course through the transplants to reach the other end. They terminated within the transplants. To this extent, the transplants did not in reality serve as a bridge between the two cut ends of the spinal cord. Further, the neocortical transplants contained stellate and pyramidal neurons found in neocortex and showed a loose cytoarchitectural organization resembling neither the neocortex nor the spinal cord. Conceptually, therefore, the neocortical transplants could not be considered to contribute to reconstruction of the damaged spinal cord. The neocortical transplants were simply transplants with unique cellular and cytoarchitectural characteristics that were anatomically integrated with the cut ends of the spinal cord. Although these findings provide a different perspective for viewing the issues of glial scar formation, regeneration or lack of regeneration of severed axons, inhibitory influences of neural transplants on the glial scar formation, and inductive influences of neural transplants on regeneration, suffice it to say that none of them can be viewed in isolation. These events happen together at the same time in appropriate sequential order. Therefore, they must be viewed comprehensively in the perspective of developmental pathological changes in order to comprehend fully not only the development of paraplegic syndrome, but also the interaction between developmental pathological changes in the spinal cord and the development of neocortical transplants at the site of the lesion. For this presentation suffice it to say that the neocortical transplants in the totally transected spinal cord, although integrated with the gray matter of the spinal cord, had no influence whatsoever on the recovery from paraplegic syndrome; and, from a functional viewpoint, the spinal cord remained completely severed.

In the case of laceration-type lesions involving partial transections of the spinal cord, some recovery was observed in the experimental animals. Those having extensive lesions, which involved sectioning of spinal cord 90–95% in the transverse plane, showed only a slight recovery related to locomotor functions. This was rudimentary and primitive. The animals that received restricted lesions, which entailed sectioning of the spinal cord for 85–90% in the transverse plane, the recovery from paraplegia was somewhat better. These animals were able to use their hindlimbs for locomotor as well as supportive functions. In both these conditions, the recovery was never complete, and the animals could not perform these functions in a sustained manner for more than a few minutes at any given time. But the fact remains that they did show some degree of recovery and that they did regain some voluntary control on their hindlimbs. In the spinal cord of these animals, the transplants had grown and were integrated with the gray matter but were separated from the severed axons of the dorsal and lateral funiculi by an intervening glial scar formation. The transplants received ascending and descending afferents from the gray matter of the spinal cord. These characteristics were similar to those seen in the experimental animals with total transection and neocortical transplantation. What made them different was the preservation of the spared axons in the ventral funiculi that crossed through the spinal cord without any interruption. The anatomical integrity of the spinal cord, even to a very small extent, was preserved and maintained. It is very likely that these axons were physiologically viable and provided a rudimentary control from the higher centers to the lumbar segments of the spinal cord. The animals were able to have some degree of voluntary control on their hindlimbs, although their performance in locomotor and supportive functions was far from normal. It was important to note that the two groups of experimental animals showed different degrees of preservation of the spared axons. In the animals with extensive lesions the spared axons were relatively small in number and recovery was restricted to rudimentary locomotor functions. In the animals with restricted lesions the number of spared axons was relatively large, and, associated with it, the recovery from paraplegic syndrome included a higher degree of locomotor as well as supportive functions. Thus, the degree of recovery from paraplegic syndrome was related to the number of spared axons preserved from undergoing degenerative changes (Das, 1984).

The interesting question emerging from these observations is: Why were the spared axons preserved in the experimental animals receiving neocortical transplants and not in the control animals that had no transplants? In order to understand this issue it is important to comment on the findings by Blight (1983b), who has shown that following suprathreshold trauma to the spinal cord by the weight-dropping method, many axons are seen to degenerate and only a small number appear to remain morphologically intact. The latter, when tested for their physiological properties, showed abnormal conduction properties. In the present studies, in the control animals with laceration-type lesions, the spared axons, although apparently morphologically intact, had become physiologically nonviable. They could not recover their physiological viability and, therefore, gradually became morphologically atrophied and degenerated. In essence, lack of recovery from physiological nonviability led to their morphological death. In the experimental animals, the spared axons were preserved from progressive degenerative changes only in those cases where the neocortical transplants were parenchymally integrated with the host spinal cord, whereas in those cases where the transplants failed to become anatomically integrated with the host spinal cord and were extraparenchymal, the spared axons had degenerated. In such conditions the spared axons, although in the close vicinity of the growing transplants, did not show any preservation. The extraparenchymal transplants, containing a mixture of normal-looking and atrophied neurons, did not have any diffusable trophic substances crossing the glial scar formation to aid in the recovery of physiological viability and, thus, the morphological viability of the axons. This suggested that it was not the mere presence of a neural transplant but the presence of a normal-looking and an anatomically integrated transplant that was important for the preservation of the spared axons. The anatomical integration of transplants also involved receiving axonal collaterals from the spared axons. These facts suggested that a neural transplant with a high growth potential, such as a neocortical transplant from a 15- or 16-day embryo, achieves preservation of the spared axons from progressive degeneration first by pushing out the necrotic tissue from the site of trauma and then by establishing parenchymal attachment with the spinal cord, thus providing a normal neural milieu, with developing characteristics, in the region of the spared axons and the gray matter. A change from pathological to normal neural milieu meant elimination of secondary traumatic conditions at a fast rate. This was perhaps sufficient, and necessary too, to aid the spared axons in recovering their physiological viability and, thus, their morphological viability. The phase of recovery from threshold and subthreshold trauma, very likely, also was characterized by a growth of *de novo* axonal collaterals that penetrated into the gray matter of the spinal cord as well as the transplants through their interface. The axonal collaterals in these preparations may also have functioned as anchors to sustain the spared axons permanently. These axons, in addition to maintaining their original connections with the lumbar region of the spinal cord, may also have given rise to *de novo* axonal collaterals in that part of the spinal cord. These spared axons with their newly acquired collaterals were the physiological and morphological substratum for the partial recovery from paraplegic syndrome following neural transplantation (Das, 1984).

In summary, the neural transplants neither served as bridges for the regenerating axons nor as agents for the reconstruction of the damaged spinal cord. They simply aided in providing normal neural milieu for the preservation of the spared axons. The functional recovery from paraplegia, therefore, was primarily due to the preservation of the spared axons and only secondarily to the presence of normal-looking and integrated neural transplants. From this viewpoint, any neural transplant that can grow large at a fast rate and become integrated with the damaged spinal cord very likely can achieve these ameliorative effects. Neocortical transplants, with a high growth potential, and not the spinal cord or brain stem transplants showing low growth potential, seem to fit this role effectively.

Concluding Comments

Total transection of the spinal cord, irrespective of the type of lesion, results in permanent paraplegia. Neocortical transplants that have grown and become integrated with the two cut ends of the spinal cord do not aid in any way in the recovery from the paraplegic syndrome.

Partial transections with knife lesions, even when they are extensive, do not result in paraplegia. A small number of fibers, spared in the ventral funiculi, are found preserved and intact, and they seem to provide physiological and anatomical continuity between the two segments of the spinal cord. This preservation of original continuity, although very small, appears to be of critical importance in preventing development of permanent paraplegia.

Partial transections of the spinal cord with laceration-type lesions present a different picture. These lesions, when they are large, covering at least 85–90% of spinal cord in transverse plane, result in permanent paraplegia in a large number of animals. The few spared axons in the ventral funiculi are found degenerating. This is due to progressive degenerative changes closely following the secondary traumatic changes. In experimental animals that have received embryonic neocortical transplants at the site of the lesion, the spared axons are not found degenerating. The neural transplants seem to provide a normal neural milieu to the spared axons, and this seems to prevent their progressive degeneration. These axons are preserved morphologically and physiologically. They, as a matter of fact, show some degree of regeneration in the form of *de novo* collateral sproutings, which penetrate as afferents into the transplants. With these spared axons preserved, the animals show some degree of recovery from the paraplegic syndrome.

The neocortical transplants that show a high growth potential achieve anatomical integration with the gray matter of the spinal cord but not with the white matter containing severed endings of the axons of the dorsal and lateral funiculi. In the region of apposition between transplants and the severed axons there is always a glial scar formation. Although the consideration that glial scar formation is a barrier to the regeneration of axons has acquired the qualities of a truism and a dogma, the possibility that the glial scar formation develops because of the lack of adequate and timely regeneration of axons cannot be readily ruled out. From this viewpoint, development of a glial scar formation at the site of lesion, in actuality, is a protective mechanism that protects the spinal cord from protracted progressive degeneration. Glial scar formation keeps pathological changes from penetrating into the spinal cord.

Recovery from paraplegia is primarily attributable to the preservation of the few spared axons in the spinal cord and only secondarily to the neural transplantation. Neural transplants aid in the rapid elimination of pathological conditions and in providing a normal neural milieu to the spared axons.

Acknowledgments. Research supported by NIH Research Grant NS-88. The assistance of Kunda Das and Jane Brasko in various phases of this research is gratefully acknowledged.

References

Aihara, H. (1970). Autotransplantation of the cultured cerebellar cortex for spinal cord reconstruction (in Japanese). Brain and Nerve 22, 769–784.

Albert, E.N., Das, G.D. (1984). Neocortical transplants in the rat brain: An ultrastructural study. Experientia 40, 294–298.

Allen, A.R. (1911). Surgery of experimental lesions of spinal cord equivalent to crush injury of fracture dislocation of spinal column. A preliminary report. J. Am. Med. Assoc. 57, 878–880.

Allen, A.R. (1914). Remarks on the histopathological changes in the spinal cord due to impact. An experimental study. J. Nerv. Ment. Dis. 41, 141–147.

Anderson, D.K., Prockop, L.D., Means, E.D., Hartley, L.E. (1976). Cerebrospinal fluid lactate and electrolyte levels following experimental spinal cord injury. J. Neurosurg. 44, 715–722.

Arteta, J.L. (1956). Research on the regeneration of the spinal cord in the cat submitted to the action of pyrogenous substances (50R3895) of bacterial origin. J. Comp. Neurol. 105, 171–184.

Assenmacher, D.R., Ducker, T.B. (1971). Experimental traumatic paraplegia: The vascular and pathologic changes seen in reversible and irreversible spinal cord lesions. J. Bone Jt. Surg. 53, 671–680.

Balentine, J.D., Paris, D.U. (1978a). Pathology of experimental spinal cord trauma. I. The necrotic lesion as a function of vascular injury. Lab. Invest. 39, 236–253.

Balentine, J.D., Paris, D.U. (1978b). Pathology of experimental spinal cord trauma. II. Ultrastructure of axons and myelin. Lab. Invest. 39, 254–266.

Barker, B.M., Eayrs, J.T. (1967). Recovery mechanisms following lesions to the central nervous system. J. Physiol. 191, 25–26.

Barnard, J.W., Carpenter, W. (1950). Lack of regeneration in spinal cord of rat. J. Neurophysiol. 13, 223–228.

Barrett, C.P., Guth, L., Donati, E.J., Krikorian, J.G. (1981). Astroglial reaction in the gray matter of lumbar segments after mid thoracic transection of the adult rat spinal cord. Exp. Neurol. 73, 365–377.

Beggs, J.L., Waggener, J.D. (1973). The compression model: Its application in determining post-traumatic vascular leakage routes. Proc. 19th V.A. Spinal Cord Injury Conf. 101–105.

Bingham, W.J., Ruffolo, R., Friedman, S.J. (1975). Catecholamine levels in the injured spinal cord of monkeys. J. Neurosurg. 42, 174–178.

Björklund, A., Segal, M., Stenevi, U. (1979). Functional reinnervation of the rat hippocampus by locus coeruleus implants. Brain Res. 170, 409–426.

Blight, A.R. (1983a). Cellular morphology of chronic spinal cord injury in the cat:
Analysis of myelinated axons by line-sampling. Neuroscience 10, 521–543.

Blight, A.R. (1983b). Axonal physiology of chronic spinal cord injury in the cat: Intracellular recording in vitro. Neuroscience 10, 1471–1486.

Bohlmann, H.H., Ducker, T.B., Lucas, J.T. (1982). Spine and spinal cord injuries. In:
The Spine, Vol. II. Rothman, R.H., Simeone, F.A. (eds.). Philadelphia: W.B.
Saunders Co., pp. 661–756.

Bresnahan, J.C. (1978). An electron-microscopic analysis of axonal alterations following blunt contusion of the spinal cord of the rhesus monkey (*Macaca mulatta*). J.
Neurol. Sci. 37, 59–82.

Bresnahan, J.C., King, J.S., Martin, G.F., Yashon, D. (1976). A neuroanatomical analysis of spinal cord injury in the rhesus monkey (*Macaca mulatta*). J. Neurol. Sci.
28, 521–542.

Brookhart, J.M., Groat, R.W., Windle, W.F. (1948). A study of the mechanics of
gunshot injury to the spinal cord of the cat. Milit. Surg. 102, 386–395.

Brown, J.D., McCouch, G.P. (1947). Abortive regeneration of the transected spinal
cord. J. Comp. Neurol. 87, 131–137.

Campbell, J.B., Bassett, C.A.L., Thulin, C.A., Feringa, E.R. (1960). The use of nerve
grafts to orient axonal regeneration in transected spinal cords. Anat. Rec. 136, 174.

Campbell, J.B., DeCriscito, V., Tomasula, J.J., Demopoulos, H.B., Flamm, E.S.,
Ransohoff, J. (1973). Experimental treatment of spinal cord contusion in the cat.
Surg. Neurol. 1, 102–106.

Clemente, C.D. (1964). Regeneration in the vertebrate central nervous system. In:
International Review of Neurobiology, Vol. 6. Pfeiffer, C.C., Smythies, I.R. (eds.).
New York/London: Academic Press, pp. 257–301.

Clemente, C.D., Windle, W.F. (1954). Regeneration of severed nerve fibers in the spinal
cord of the adult cat. J. Comp. Neurol. 101, 691–731.

Collins, W.F., Kauer, J.S. (1979). The past and future of animal models used for spinal
cord trauma. In: Neural Trauma. Popp, A.J., Bourke, R.S., Nelson, L.R., Ki-
melberg, H.K. (eds.). New York: Raven Press, pp. 273–279.

Cseuz, K.A.J., Speakman, T.J. (1963). Peripheral nerve implantation in experimental
paraplegia. J. Neurosurg. 20, 557–563.

Cummings, J.P., Bernstein, D.R., Stelzner, D.J. (1981). Further evidence that sparing
of function after spinal cord transection in the neonatal rat is not due to axonal
generation or regeneration. Exp. Neurol. 74, 615–620.

Cusick, J.F., Myklebust, J., Zyvoloski, M., Sances, A., Houterman, C., Larson, C.J.
(1982). Effects of vertebral column distraction in the monkey. J. Neurosurg. 57,
651–659.

Das, G.D. (1974). Transplantation of embryonic neural tissue in the mammalian brain. I.
Growth and differentiation of neuroblasts from various regions of the embryonic
brain in the cerebellum of neonate rats. TIT J. Life Sci. 4, 93–124.

Das, G.D. (1975). Differentiation of dendrites in the transplanted neuroblasts in the
mammalian brain. In: Advances in Neurobiology: Physiology and Pathology of
Dendrites, Vol. 12. Kreutzberg, G.W. (ed.). New York: Raven Press, pp. 181–199.

Das, G.D. (1981). Neural transplants in the spinal cord of the adult rats. Anat. Rec.
199, 64A.

Das, G.D. (1982). Extraparenchymal neural transplants: Their cytology and survivability. Brain Res. 241, 182–186.

Das, G.D. (1983a). Neural transplantation in the spinal cord of the adult mammals. In: Reconstruction of the Spinal Cord. Kao, C.C., Bunge, R.P., Reier, P.J. (eds.). New York: Raven Press, pp. 367–396.

Das, G.D. (1983b). Neural transplantation in mammalian brain: Some conceptual and technical considerations. In: Neural Tissue Transplantation Research. Wallace, R.B., Das, G.D. (eds.). New York/Heidelberg/Berlin/Tokyo: Springer-Verlag, pp. 1–64.

Das, G.D. (1983c). Neural transplantation in the spinal cord of the adult rats: Conditions, survival, cytology and connectivity of the transplants. J. Neurol. Sci. 62, 191–210.

Das, G.D. (1984). Neural transplantation in the spinal cord and its functional significance. In: Paraplegia and Tetraplegia. Rossier, A., Radaelli, E., Redaelli, T. (eds.), Milan, Italy: Libreria Scientifica gia GHEDINI s.r.l., pp. 23–54.

Das, G.D., Altman, J. (1971). The fate of transplanted precursors of nerve cells in the cerebellum of young rats. Science 173, 637–638.

Das, G.D., Altman, J. (1972). Studies of the transplantation of developing neural tissue in the mammalian brain. I. Transplantation of cerebellar slabs into the cerebellum of neonate rats. Brain Res. 38, 233–249.

Das, G.D., Das, K.G., Brasko, J., Aleman-Gomez, J. (1983a). Neural transplants: Volumetric analysis of their growth and histopathological changes. Neuroscience Lett. 41, 73–79.

Das, G.D., Hallas, B.H. (1978). Transplantation of brain tissue in the brain of adult rat. Experientia 34, 1304–1306.

Das, G.D., Hallas, B.H., Das, K.G. (1979). Transplantation of neural tissues in the brains of laboratory mammals: Technical details and comments. Experientia 35, 143–153.

Das, G.D., Hallas, B.H., Das, K.G. (1980). Transplantation of brain tissue in the brain of rats. I. Growth characteristics of neocortical transplants from embryos of different ages. Am. J. Anat. 158, 135–145.

Das, G.D., Houlé, J.D., Brasko, J., Das, K.G. (1983b). Freezing of neural tissues and their transplantation in the brain of the rat: Technical details and histological observations. J. Neurosci. Meth. 8, 1–15.

Das, G.D., Ross, D.T. (1982). Stereotaxic technique for transplantation of neural tissues in the brain of adult rats. Experientia 38, 848–851.

Davidoff, L.M., Ransohoff, J. (1948). Absence of spinal cord regeneration in the cat. J. Neurophysiol. 11, 9–11.

de la Torre, J.C., Johnson, C.M., Goode, D.J., Mullen, S. (1975). Pharmacological treatment and evaluation of permanent experimental spinal cord trauma. Neurology 25, 508–514.

Dohrmann, G.J. (1972). Experimental spinal cord trauma. A historical review. Arch. Neurol. (Chicago) 27, 468–473.

Dohrmann, G.J., Panjabi, M.M., Banks, D. (1978). Biomechanics of experimental spinal cord trauma. J. Neurosurg. 48, 993–1001.

Dohrmann, G.J., Panjabi, M.M., Wagner, F.C., Jr. (1976). An apparatus for quantitating experimental spinal cord trauma. Surg. Neurol. 5, 315–318.

Dohrmann, G.J., Wagner, F.C., Jr., Bucy, P.C. (1971). The microvasculature in transitory traumatic paraplegia. An electron microscopic study in the monkey. J. Neurosurg. 35, 263–271.

Dohrmann, G.J., Wick, K.M., Bucy, P.C. (1973). Spinal cord blood flow patterns in experimental traumatic paraplegia. J. Neurosurg. 38, 52–58.

Dolan, E.J., Transfeldt, E.E., Tator, C.H., Simmons, E.H., Hughes, K.F. (1980). The effect of spinal distraction on regional spinal cord blood flow in cats. J. Neurosurg. 53, 756–764,

Doppman, J.L., Ramsey, R., Theis, R.J. (1973). A precutaneous technique for producing intra-spinal mass lesions in experimental animals. J. Neurosurg. 38, 438–447.

Ducker, T.B. (1976). Experimental injury of the spinal cord. In: Handbook of Clinical Neurology. Injuries of the Spine and Spinal Cord, Part I, Vol. 25. Vinken, P.J., Bruyn, G.W. (eds.) Amsterdam: North-Holland Publishing Co., pp. 9–26.

Ducker, T.B., Hamit, H.F. (1969). Experimental treatments of acute spinal cord injury. J. Neurosurg. 30, 693–697.

Ducker, T.B., Kindt, G.W., Kempe, G.L. (1971). Pathological findings in acute experimental spinal cord trauma. J. Neurosurg. 35, 700–708.

Ducker, T.B., Perot, P.L., Jr. (1971). Spinal cord oxygen and blood flow in trauma. Surg. Forum. 22, 413–415.

Eidelberg, E., Story, J.L., Walden, J.G., Meyer, B.L. (1981). Anatomical correlates of return of locomotor function after partial spinal cord lesions in cats. Exp. Brain Res. 42, 81–88.

Eidelberg, E., Straehley, R., Erspamer, R., Watkins, C.J. (1977). Relationship between residual hindlimb-assisted locomotion and surviving axons after incomplete spinal cord injuries. Exp. Neurol. 56, 312–322.

Fairholm, D.J., Turnbull, I.M. (1970). Microangiographic study of experimental spinal injuries in dogs and rabbits. Surg. Forum 21, 453–455.

Fairholm, D.J., Turnbull, I.M. (1971). Microangiographic study of experimental spinal cord injuries. J. Neurosurg. 35, 277–286.

Feigin, I., Geller, E.H., Wolf, A. (1951). Absence of regeneration in the spinal cord of the young rat. J. Neuropath. Exp. Neurol. 10, 420–425.

Feringa, E.R., Kinning, W.K., Britten, A.G., Vahlsing, H.L. (1976). Recovery in rats after spinal cord injury. Neurology 26, 839–843.

Fertig, A., Kiernan, J.A., Seyan, S.S.A.S. (1971). Enhancement of axonal regeneration in the brain of the rat by corticotrophin and triiodothyronine. Exp. Neurol. 33, 372–385.

Ford, R.W.J. (1983). A reproducible spinal cord injury model in the cat. J. Neurosurg. 59, 268–275.

Freeman, L.W. (1952). Return of function after complete transection of the spinal cord of the rat, cat and dog. Ann. Surg. 136, 193–205.

Freeman, L.W. (1954). Return of spinal cord function in mammals after transection lesions. Ann. N.Y. Acad. Sci. 58, 564–569.

Freeman, L.W. (1962). Experimental observations upon axonal regeneration in the transected spinal cord of mammals. Clin. Neurosurg. 8, 294–316.

Freeman, L.W., MacDougall, J., Turbes, C.C., Bowman, D.E. (1960). The treatment of experimental lesions of the spinal cord of dogs with trypsin. J. Neurosurg. 17, 259–265.

Freeman, L.W., Turbes, C. C. (1961). Influence upon reflex activity of viable nerve implants into the distal segment of the divided spinal cord of paraplegic animals. Exp. Med. Surg. 19, 270–277.

Freeman, L.W., Wright, T.W. (1953). Experimental observations of concussion and contusion of the spinal cord. Ann. Surg. 137, 433–443.

Gearhart, J., Oster-Granite, M.L., Guth, L. (1979). Histological changes after transection of the spinal cord of fetal and neonatal mice. Exp. Neurol. 66, 1–15.

Gelfan, S., Tarlov, I.M. (1956). Physiology of spinal cord, nerve root and peripheral nerve compression. Am. J. Physiol. 185, 217–229.

Gerber, A.M., Corrie, W.S. (1979). Effect of impounder contact area on experimental spinal cord injury. J. Neurosurg. 51, 539–542.

Goodkin, R., Campbell, J.B. (1969). Sequential pathologic changes in spinal cord injury: A preliminary report. Surg. Forum 20, 430–432.

Green, B.A., Wagner, F.C. (1973). Evolution of edema in the acutely injured spinal cord: A fluorescence microscopy study. Surg. Neurol. 1, 98–101.

Griffiths, I.R. (1975). Vasogenic edema following acute and chronic spinal cord compression in the dog. J. Neurosurg. 42, 155–165.

Groat, R.W., Rambach, W.A., Windle, W.F. (1945). Concussion of the spinal cord. Surg. Gynecol. Obstetr. 81, 63–74.

Guth, L., Albuquerque, E.X., Deshpande, S.S., Barrett, C.P., Donati, E.J., Warnick, J.E. (1980b). Ineffectiveness of enzyme therapy on regeneration in the transected spinal cord of the rat. J. Neurosurg. 52, 73–86.

Guth, L., Brewer, C.R., Collins, W.F., Jr., Goldberger, M.E., Perl, E.R. (1980a). Criteria for evaluating spinal cord regeneration experiments. Exp. Neurol. 69, 1–3.

Guth, L., Bright, D., Donati, E.J. (1978). Functional deficits and anatomical alterations after high cervical spinal hemisection in the rat. Exp. Neurol. 58, 511–520.

Guth, L., Windle, W.F. (1970). The enigma of central nervous regeneration. Exp. Neurol. 28, Suppl. 5, 1–43.

Hallas, B.H., Das, G.D., Das, K.G. (1980a). Transplantation of brain tissue in the brain of rat. II. Growth characteristics of neocortical transplants in hosts of different ages. Am. J. Anat. 158, 147–159.

Hallas, B.H., Oblinger, M.M., Das, G.D. (1980b). Heterotopic neural transplants in the cerebellum of the rat: Their afferents. Brain Res. 196, 242–246.

Hansebout, R.R., Kuchner, E.F., Romero-Sierra, C. (1975). Effects of local hypothermia and of steroids upon recovery from experimental spinal cord compression injury. Surg. Neurol. 4, 531–536.

Harvey, A.R., Lund, R.D. (1981). Transplantation of tectal tissue in rats. II. Distribution of host neurons which project to transplants. J. Comp. Neurol. 202, 505–520.

Heinicke, E.A. (1977). Influence of exogenous triiodothyronine on axonal regeneration and wound healing in the brain of the rat. J. Neurol. Sci. 31, 293–305.

Houlé, J.D., Das, G.D. (1980a). Freezing of embryonic neural tissue and its transplantation in the rat brain. Brain Res. 192, 570–574.

Houlé, J.D., Das, G.D. (1980b). Freezing and transplantation of brain tissue in rats. Experientia 36, 1114–1115.

Hukuda, S., Wilson, C.B. (1972). Experimental cervical myelopathy: Effects of compression and ischemia on the canine cervical cord. J. Neurosurg. 37, 631–652.

Hung, T.K., Chang, G.L., Chang, J.L., Albin, M. (1981). Stress-strain relationship and neurological sequelae of uniaxial elongation of the spinal cord of cats. Surg. Neurol. 15, 471–476.

Jaeger, C.B., Lund, R.D. (1979). Efferent fibers from transplanted cerebral cortex of rats. Brain Res. 165, 338–342.

Jaeger, C.B., Lund, R.D. (1980). Transplantation of embryonic occipital cortex to the tectal region of newborn rats: A light microscopic study of organization and connectivity of the transplants. J. Comp. Neurol. 194, 571–597.

Jakoby, R.K., Turbes, C.C., Freeman, L.W. (1960). The problem of neuronal regeneration in the central nervous system. I. The insertion of centrally connected peripheral nerve stumps into the spinal cord. J. Neurosurg. 17, 385–393.

Jellinger, K. (1976). Neuropathology of cord injuries. In: Handbook of Clinical Neurology. Injuries of the Spine and Spinal Cord, Part I, Vol. 25. Vinken, P.J., Bruyn, G.W. (eds.). Amsterdam: North-Holland Publishing Co., pp. 43–121.

Joyner, F., Freeman, L.W. (1963). Urea and spinal cord trauma. Neurology (Minneapolis) 13, 69–72.

Kao, C.C. (1974). Comparison of healing process in transected spinal cords grafted with autogenous brain tissue, sciatic nerve, and nodose ganglion. Exp. Neurol. 44, 424–439.

Kao, C.C. (1980). Spinal cord cavitation after injury. In: The Spinal Cord and Its Relation to Traumatic Injury. Windle, W.F. (ed.). New York/Basel: Marcel Dekker, pp. 249–270.

Kao, C.C., Chang, L.W. (1977). The mechanism of spinal cord cavitation following spinal cord transection. Part I. A correlated histochemical study. J. Neurosurg. 46, 197–209.

Kao, C.C., Chang, L.W., Bloodworth, J.M.B., Jr. (1977a). Axonal regeneration across transected mammalian spinal cords: An electron microscopic study of delayed nerve grafting. Exp. Neurol. 54, 591–615.

Kao, C.C., Chang, L.W., Bloodworth, J.M.B., Jr., (1977b). The mechanism of spinal cord cavitation following spinal cord transection. Part II. Electron microscopic observations. J. Neurosurg. 46, 745–756.

Kao, C.C., Shimizu, Y., Perkins, L.C., Freeman, L.W. (1970). Experimental use of cultured cerebellar cortical tissue to inhibit the collagenous scar following spinal cord transection. J. Neurosurg. 33(2), 127–139.

Kelly, D.L., Lassiter, K.R.L., Calogero, J.A. (1970). Effects of local hypothermia and tissue oxygen studies in experimental paraplegia. J. Neurosurg. 33, 554–563.

Kiernan, J.A. (1979). Hypotheses concerned with axonal regeneration in the mammalian nervous system. Biol. Rev. 54, 155–197.

Kobrine, A.I., Doyle, T.F., Martins, A.N. (1975). Local spinal cord blood flow in experimental traumatic myelopathy. J. Neurosurg. 42, 144–149.

Kobrine, A.I., Evans, D.E., Rizzoli, H. (1978). Correlation of spinal cord blood flow and function in experimental compression. Surg. Neurol. 10, 54–59.

Koenig, G., Dohrmann, G.J. (1977). Histopathological variability in "standardised" spinal cord trauma. J. Neurol. Neurosurg. Psychiat, 40, 1203–1210.

Koozekanani, S.H., Vise, W.M., Hashemi, R.M., McGhee, R.B. (1976). Possible mechanisms for observed patho-physiological variability in experimental spinal cord injury by the method of Allen. J. Neurosurg. 44, 429–434.

Kromer, L.F., Björklund, A., Stenevi, U. (1981). Innervation of embryonic hippocampal implants by regenerating axons of cholinergic septal neurons in the adult rat. Brain Res. 210, 153–171.

Kromer, L.F., Björklund, A., Stenevi, U. (1983). Intracephalic embryonic neural implants in the adult rat brain. I. Growth and mature organization of brain stem, cerebellar, and hippocampal implants. J. Comp. Neurol. 218, 433–459.

Lampert, P., Cressman, M. (1964). Axonal regeneration in the dorsal columns of the spinal cord of adult rats. Lab. Invest. 13, 825–839.

Lance, J.W. (1954). Behavior of pyramidal axons following section. Brain 77, 314–324.

Lee, F.C. (1929). The regeneration of nervous tissue. Physiol. Rev. 9, 575–623.

Locke, G.E., Yashon, D., Feldman, R.A., Hunt, W.E. (1971). Ischemia in primate spinal cord injury. J. Neurosurg. 34, 614–617.

Lund, R.D., Harvey, A.R. (1981). Transplantation of tectal tissue in rats. I. Organization of transplants and pattern of distribution of host afferents within them. J. Comp. Neurol. 201, 191–209.

Lund, R.D., Hauschka, S.D. (1976). Transplanted neural tissue develops connections with host rat brain. Science 193, 582–584.

Magenis, T.P., Freeman, L.W., Bowman, D.E. (1952). Functional recovery following spinal cord hemisection and intrathecal use of hypochlorite treated trypsin. Fed. Proc. 11, 99.

Means, E.D., Anderson, D.K., Waters, T.R., Kalaf, L. (1981). Effect of methylprednisolone in compression trauma to the feline spinal cord. J. Neurosurg. 55, 200–208.

Molt, J.T., Nelson, L.R., Poulos, D.A., Bourke, R.S. (1979). Analysis and measurement of some sources of variability in experimental spinal cord trauma. J. Neurosurg. 50, 784–791.

Nornes, H.O., Björklund, A., Stenevi, U. (1983). Reinnervation of the denervated adult spinal cord of rats by intraspinal transplants of embryonic brain stem neurons. Cell Tiss. Res. 230, 15–35.

Nygren, L.G., Olson, L., Seiger, A. (1977). Monoaminergic reinnervation of the transected spinal cord by homologous fetal brain grafts. Brain Res. 129, 227–235.

Oblinger, M.M., Das, G.D. (1982). Connectivity of neural transplants in adult rats: Analysis of afferents and efferents of neocortical transplants in the cerebellar hemisphere. Brain Res. 249, 31–49.

Oblinger, M.M., Das, G.D. (1983). Connectivity of neural transplants in the cerebellum: A model of developmental differences in neuroplasticity. In: Neural Tissue Transplantation Research. Wallace, R.B., Das, G.D. (eds.). New York/Heidelberg/Berlin/Tokyo: Springer-Verlag, pp. 105–134.

Oblinger, M.M., Hallas, B.H., Das, G.D. (1980). Neocortical transplants in the cerebellum of the rat: Their afferents and efferents. Brain Res. 189, 228–232.

O'Callaghan, S.S., Speakman, T.J. (1963). Axon regeneration in the rat spinal cord. Surg. Forum 14, 410–411.

Osterholm, J.L. (1974). The pathophysiological response to spinal cord injury. The current status of related research. J. Neurosurg. 40, 5–33.

Osterholm, J.L., Mathews, G.J. (1972a). Altered norepinephrine metabolism following experimental spinal cord injury. I. Relationship to hemorrhagic necrosis and post-wounding neurological deficits. J. Neurosurg. 36, 380–394.

Osterholm, J.L., Mathews, G.J. (1972b). Altered norepinephrine metabolism following experimental spinal cord injury. II. Protection against traumatic spinal cord hemorrhagic necrosis by norepinephrine synthesis blockade with alpha methyl tyrosine. J. Neurosurg. 36, 395–401.

Patel, U., Bernstein, J.J. (1983). Growth, differentiation and viability of fetal rat cortical and spinal cord implants into adult rat spinal cord. J. Neurosci. Res. 9, 303–310.

Perkins, L., Babbini, A., Freeman, L.W. (1964). Distal-proximal nerve implants in spinal cord transection. Neurology 14, 949–954.

Pettegrew, R.K. (1980). Evaluation of the use of enzymes for functional restitution after spinal cord severance in the rat. Exp. Neurol. 68, 284–294.

Puchala, E., Windle, W.F. (1977). The possibility of structural and functional restitution after spinal cord injury. Exp. Neurol. 55, 1–42.

Ramon y Cajal, S. (1928). Degeneration and Regeneration in the Nervous System, Vols. I and II. May, R.M. (trans. and ed.), New York: Hafner (reprinted 1959).

Rawe, S.E., Lee, W.A., Perot, P.L., Jr. (1978). The histopathology of experimental spinal cord trauma. The effect of systemic blood pressure. J. Neurosurg. 48, 1002–1007.

Richardson, H.D., Nakamura, S. (1971). An electron microscopic study of spinal cord edema and the effect of treatment with steroids, mannitol, and hypothermia. Proc. 18th V.A. Spinal Cord Injury Conf. 10–16.

Sandler, A.N., Tator, C.H. (1976). Effect of acute spinal cord compression injury on regional spinal cord blood flow in primates. J. Neurosurg. 45, 660–676.

Schramm, J., Hashizume, K., Fukushima, T., Takahashi, H. (1979). Experimental spinal cord injury by slow, graded compression. J. Neurosurg. 50, 48–57.

Scott, D., Jr., Clemente, C.D. (1955). Regeneration of spinal cord fibers in the cat. J. Comp. Neurol. 102, 633–669.

Seuter, H.J., Venes, J.L. (1979). Loss of autoregulation and post-traumatic ischemia following experimental spinal cord trauma. J. Neurosurg. 50, 198–206.

Shimizu, T. (1983). Transplantation of cultured cerebellar autografts into the spinal cords of chronic paraplegic dogs. In: Spinal Cord Reconstruction. Kao, C.C., Bunge, R.P., Reier, P.J. (eds.). New York: Raven Press, pp. 359–366.

Shirres, D.A. (1905). Regeneration of the axones of the spinal neurones in man. Montreal Med. J. 34, 239–249.

Stelzner, D.J., Ershler, W.B., Weber, E.D. (1975). Effects of spinal transection in neonatal and weanling rats: Survival and function. Exp. Neurol. 46, 156–177.

Stenevi, U., Björklund, A., Svendgaard, N.A. (1976). Transplantation of central and peripheral monoamine neurons to the adult brain: Techniques and conditions for survival. Brain Res. 114, 1–20.

Sugar, O., Gerard, W. (1940). Spinal cord regeneration in the rat. J. Neurophysiol. 3, 1–19.

Tarlov, I.M. (1972). Acute spinal cord compression paralysis. J. Neurosurg. 36, 10–20.

Tarlov, I.M. (1957). Spinal Cord Compression: Mechanisms of Paralysis and Treatment. Springfield, Il: Charles C. Thomas.

Tarlov, I.M., Klinger, H., Vitale, S. (1953). Spinal cord compression studies. I. Experimental techniques to produce acute and gradual compression. Arch. Neurol. Psychiat. 70, 813–819.

Tator, C.H. (1971). Experimental circumferential compression injury of primate spinal cord. Proc. 18th V.A. Spinal Cord Injury Conf. 2–5.

Tator, C.H. (1972). Acute spinal cord injury: A review of recent studies of treatment and pathophysiology. Can. Med. Assoc. J. 107, 143–150.

Tator, C.H. (1973). Acute spinal cord injury in primates produced by an inflatable extradural cuff. Can. J. Surg. 16, 222–230.

Turbes, C.C., Freeman, L.W. (1958). Peripheral nerve-spinal cord anastomosis for experimental cord transection. Neurology 8, 857–861.

Vahlsing, H.L., Feringa, E.R. (1980). A ventral uncrossed cortico-spinal tract in the rat. Exp. Neurol. 70, 282–287.

Veraa, R.P., Grafstein, B. (1981). Cellular mechanisms for recovery from nervous system injury: A conference report. Exp. Neurol. 71, 6–75.

Wagner, F.C., Dohrmann, G.J., Bucy, P.C. (1971). Histopathology of transitory traumatic paraplegia in the monkey. J. Neurosurg. 35, 272–276.

Wakefield, C.L., Eidelberg, E. (1975). Electron microscopic observations of the delayed effects of spinal cord compression. Exp. Neurol. 48, 637–646.

White, R.J., Albin, M.S., Harris, L.S., Yashon, D. (1969). Spinal cord injury: Sequential morphology and hypothermic stabilization. Surg. Forum 20, 432–434.

Windle, W.F. (1956). Regeneration of axons in the vertebrate central nervous system. Physiol. Rev. 36, 427–440.

Windle, W.F. (1980). Concussion, contusion, and severance of the spinal cord. In: The
    Spinal Cord and Its Reaction to Traumatic Injury. Windle, W.F. (ed.). New York/
    Basel: Marcel Dekker, pp. 205–217.
Windle, W.F., Chambers, W.W. (1950). Regeneration in the spinal cord of the cat and
    dog. J. Comp. Neurol. 93, 241–257.
Windle, W.F., Clemente, C.D., Chambers, W.W. (1952a). Inhibition of formation of a
    glial barrier as a means of permitting a peripheral nerve to grow into the brain. J.
    Comp. Neurol. 96, 359–369.
Windle, W.F., Clemente, C.D., Scott, D., Jr., Chambers, W.W. (1952b). Induction of
    neuronal regeneration in the central nervous system of animals. Trans. Am.
    Neurol. Assoc. 77, 164–170.
Windle, W.F., Smart, J.O., Beers, J.J. (1958). Residual function after subtotal cord
    transection in adult cats. Neurology 8, 518–521.
Woodward, J.S., Freeman, L.W. (1956). Ischemia of the spinal cord: An experimental
    study. J. Neurosurg. 13, 63–72.
Yashon, D., Bingham, W.G., Jr., Faddoul, E.M., Hunt, W.E. (1973). Edema of the
    spinal cord following experimental impact trauma. J. Neurosurg. 38, 693–697.

Chapter 2

Unequivocal Regeneration of Rat Optic Nerve Axons into Sciatic Nerve Isografts

MARTIN BERRY,* LOWELL REES,* and JOBST SIEVERS†

Introduction

It is now established that central axons grow for long distances within a peripheral nerve when the latter is implanted into the central nervous system (CNS) (Aguayo et al. 1979, 1982, 1983, 1984, Richardson et al. 1980, 1981, 1984, Benfey and Aguayo 1982). However, peripheral axons poorly penetrate grafts of CNS tissue implanted between the cut ends of a peripheral nerve (Aguayo et al 1978, Weinberg and Spencer 1979, Perkins et al 1980), and few regenerate past the root/cord junction after dorsal root injury (Kimmel and Moyer 1947, Moyer et al. 1953, Stensaas et al. 1979), while CNS axons growing in peripheral nerve bridges extend for only short distances beyond both CNS/PNS interfaces (David and Aguayo 1981, Aguayo et al. 1982, 1984). Moreover, central axons growing in a peripheral nerve graft behave like peripheral nerve axons if they are damaged in this site, that is, they readily regenerate (David and Aguayo 1985). This distinctively different behavior of growing central axons in the two environments suggests that growth fails in the CNS either because factors normally required for elongation are absent from the mature CNS or because other possibilities are operating, e.g., inhibitors act by blocking receptor sites for trophic substances on axonal membrane (Berry 1983, 1985).

One limitation of the peripheral nerve grafting model is the uncertain status of central axons growing in the graft, because it is impossible to ascertain if such fibers are either regenerating within the nerve following severence in the CNS, during the implantation procedure, or growing collaterals of undamaged axons contained in intact central tracts lying in the vicinity of the implanted peripheral nerve stump. Thus, in experiments designed to study unequivocal central regeneration into peripheral nerves, ideally the graft is implanted into a

* Anatomy Department, Guy's Hospital Medical School, London SE1 9RT U.K.
† Anatomy Department, University of Kiel, 2300, Kiel, F.G.R.

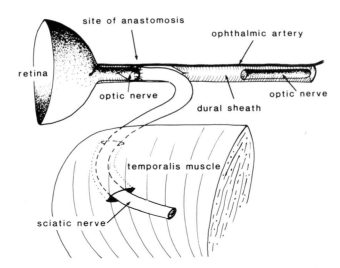

Figure 2-1. Diagram illustrating the operative technique for anastomosing a segment of sciatic nerve to the cut retinal end of the optic nerve. The sciatic nerve leaves the orbit through the temporalis muscle and HRP is subsequently applied to the nerve on the surface of this muscle.

unidirectional central tract that is isolated from other CNS fibers, whose constituent axons are readily transectable *in toto* and whose parent central neurons are tightly grouped within a single circumscribed region of the CNS. Retinal ganglion cells and their axon projections in the retina and optic nerve fulfill these criteria, and this paper describes true regeneration of such axons in the rat, within long segments of sciatic nerve anastomosed either to the cut end of the completely transected optic nerve or implanted into the retina through the sclera.

Materials and Methods

WAG albino rats of either sex, weighing 250 g, were used. Twelve animals, designated the optic nerve section (ONS) group, were killed 30 days post-lesion (dpl). In a further 24 rats, a sciatic nerve segment from a donor animal was anastomosed to the retinal stump of the transected optic nerve. This group was called the optic nerve anastomosis (ONA) group. An additional group of 12 rats all received retinal lesions using a needle introduced through the vitrous (McConnell and Berry 1982) to interrupt the ganglion cell fiber layer. Of these, 6 rats were left for 30 dpl, and in the other 6 a segment of sciatic nerve was implanted immediately into the retinal lesion through a window in the sclera and the rats left for a survival time of 30 dpl.

    All operations were performed under Avertin (tribromoethanol in amylene hydrate) anaesthesia (Figure 2-1). The dural sheath of the optic nerve was exposed through the upper lid after removing the levator palpebrae superioris, superior oblique, superior rectus, and retractor bulbi (superior fibers) muscles. The lateral or superior aspect of dura and arachnoid were incised longitudinally to expose the optic nerve avoiding the subarachnoid branches of the ophthalmic artery and vein. Scissors were used to transect the optic nerve completely 2 mm from the bulb, and a 2-mm proximal segment of optic nerve was removed. The integrity of the blood supply to the retina through the ophthalmic artery (which usually lies on the medial aspect of the sheath and is not damaged by the operative procedure) was verified by applanation ophthalmoscopy (Wise et al. 1971) in every case. The cut optic nerve of ONA animals was anastomosed to a 15-mm length of sciatic nerve by 10/0 atraumatic nylon sutures securing epineurium to pia-arachnoid. One end of the sciatic nerve was introduced into the posterolateral region of the orbit through the temporalis muscle; the other distal end remained in a subcutaneous position on the surface of the muscle (Figure 2-1).

In experiments where 15-mm lengths of sciatic nerve were introduced into retinal lesions, the nerve was positioned as in the ONA rats, inserted into the retinal lesion through a window in the sclera 1.0–1.5 mm dorsal to the optic nerve head, and epineurium affixed to sclera by 10/0 atraumatic nylon sutures.

The site of anastomosis in ONA rats was wax-embedded, and serial sections, 5 μm thick, were examined after silver staining (Nonidez 1939). Whole retinae were fixed for 3–4 hours in 10% neutral formalin, dry mounted on gelatin subbed slides, and ganglion cells stained with cresyl fast violet and ganglion cell axons impregnated with silver by the physical developer technique of Kiernan (1981). A 4% HRP–WGA (Triticium vulgaris-Sigma L2384) conjugate was injected into an area of crush on the sciatic nerve in 6 ONA rats, immediately after forming the anastomosis and in a further 6 ONA rats 30 dpl. Injections were placed 10 mm from the site of anastomosis in that part of the nerve well outside the orbit on the surface of the temporalis muscle. Animals were left for 36 hours before perfusion for 10 minutes with cold (4°C) buffered saline. Both retinae were dissected from the eyes of each rat in cold buffered saline, fixed for 2–3 minutes by immersion in cold 1.0% paraformaldehyde and 1.25% gluteraldehyde in 0.1 M phosphate buffer (pH 7.4), and pairs of retinae from each rat whole mounted onto subbed glass slides. The HRP was developed using the TMB reaction described by Mesulam (1982). Controls for shrinkage and systemic uptake of HRP were provided by mounting normal and treated retinae on the same slide. Controls for diffusion of HRP were rats injected with tracer immediately after sciatic/optic nerve anastomosis. The HRP–WGA solution was also injected into a crush site along the optic nerve, 2 mm from the globe in adult (250 g) intact WAG rats, to assess the normal density of labeled ganglion cells after immediate uptake by the entire axon population of the optic nerve. The untreated eye acted as a control for systemic uptake as described above.

Estimates of the total number of axons surviving 30 dpl in ONA and ONS rats were attempted by counting axons about the optic nerve head in silver-stained whole mounts. The frequencies of different sizes of ganglion cells were quantified using a MOP videoplan (Kontron) image analysis system. A graticule enclosing a total sampling area of 22,500 μm^2 was placed over the projected image of the retina in standard sites, near the optic disc, at the periphery, and midway between these two sites, along standard radii in the temporal, nasal, superior, and inferior quadrants. The means of these 12 counts, in normal and treated retinae from each animal, were used to estimate percentage reductions and accumulations of ganglion cells over all sizes at arbitrary intervals of 6.6 μm^2. The total numbers of HRP-filled ganglion cells were recorded in ONA rats by scanning the entire surface of retinal whole mounts at 100 × magnification.

Results

Examination of silver preparations of the site of anastomosis between the optic nerve and sciatic nerve showed good approximation of the two nerves with little intervention of scar tissue. Large numbers of axons were clearly seen passing between the cut ends of the two nerves (Figure 2-2). Axons survived in the ganglion cell fiber layer of the retina of both ONA and ONS animals although their frequency was greatly reduced when compared with normal.

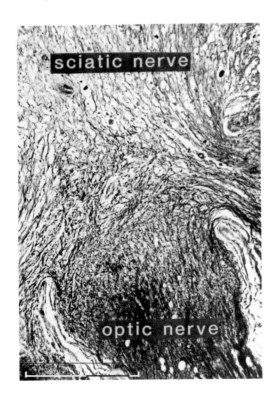

Figure 2-2. Example of the site of anastomosis, 80 dpl. Note the absence of scar tissue and the many axons that bridge the two nerves. (Nonidez silver method; marker = 250 μm.)

Table 2-1. Total Number of
HRP-Labeled Ganglion Cells
Counted in ONA Retinae

Rats	Total no. HRP
1	1,611
2	1,856
3	789
4	1,558
5	513
6	615
Mean	1,207
S.E.	220

Quantitative estimates of the number of axons in the fiber layer were aban-
doned because of inaccuracies imposed by obscuration and an inability to
resolve the individual axons contained in many of the fascicles. Qualitatively, it
was impossible to distinguish ONS retinae from those of ONA rats (Figure 2-3).

HRP-filled ganglion cells, representing all sizes, were found in all ONA
retinae 30 dpl (Figure 2-4 & Table 2-1), but none were detected at 0 dpl. The
spatial distribution of labeled cells appeared normal, with the greatest frequency near the optic disc and a uniform decline in density radially towards the
periphery of the retina (Figure 2-5).

In both ONA and ONS rats, the number of ganglion cells is reduced and their

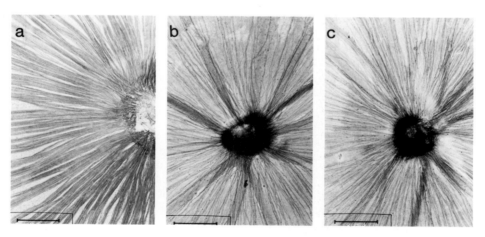

Figure 2-3. Representative examples of axons about the optic nerve head in (a) normal
retina, (b) ONA retina, and (c) ONS retina, 30 dpl. Note that the density of fibers in the
ganglion cell fiber layer in ONS and ONA retinae appears equally reduced. (Silver-
stained retinal whole mounts; marker = 50 μm.)

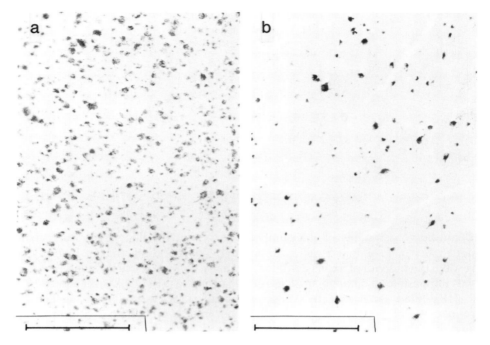

Figure 2-4. (a) Density of HRP-labeled ganglion cells 36-hours after injection of the optic nerve in an unoperated control rat; (b) density of HRP-labeled ganglion cells 36 hours after injection of a sciatic nerve graft 10 mm from the point of anastomosis. (Retinal whole mounts; marker = 250 μm.)

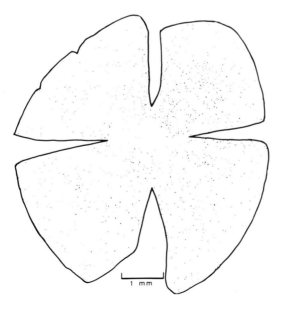

Figure 2-5. Distribution of HRP-labeled ganglion cells in the retina of rat 4 (see Table 2-1) after injection of HRP into a crushed region of the sciatic nerve 10 mm from the site of anastomosis at 30 dpl and killed 36 hours later. Note that cells ranging in size from large to small are all represented and equally distributed throughout the retina. (Camera lucida drawing of the retinal whole mount.)

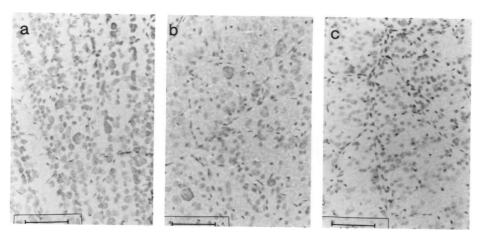

Figure 2-6. Ganglion cells in the retinae of normal (a), ONA (b), and ONS (c) rats. Note the reduced numbers of ganglion cells, the absence of cell columns in (b) and (c), and the differential survival of large cells in (b), relative to (c). (Cresyl violet stained retinal whole mount preparations; marker = 250 μm.)

normal radial alignment is no longer recognizable. Large ganglion cells are rarely seen in ONS retinae, but large numbers do survive in those of ONA rats (Figures 2-6). The percentage reduction in the number of ganglion cells in ONA and ONS retinae is shown in Figure 2-7 where it is clear that 10% (p = 0.01–0.001) more ganglion cells survive in ONA retinae than in those of ONS rats.

The normal frequency distribution of different-sized ganglion cells is unimodal; most cells are smaller than 150 μm^2 in diameter. A smaller number of large cells form a long tail to the distribution with the largest cells attaining

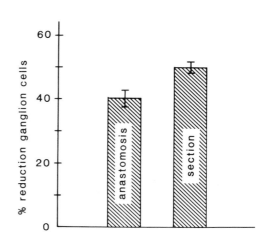

Figure 2-7. Percentage reduction in the number of ganglion cells in ONA and ONS retinae. See text for further details.

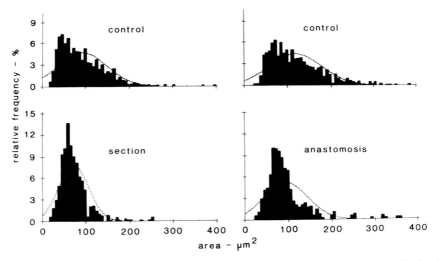

Figure 2-8. Relative percentage distributions of different-sized ganglion cells in the retinae of ONS and ONA treated rats and their controls. Note that ONS rats show a greater shift in the distribution toward smaller sized cells than the ONA group. In each case the Gaussian curve has been fitted to the distribution and confirms this observation.

sizes of 450 μm^2 (Figure 2-8). In both ONA and ONS rats, there is a shift to the left in this distribution because most cells in the experimental eyes are small in size. The shift is least in ONA retinae because some large cells survive (Figure 2-8). Computation of the percentage cumulative frequency of ganglion cells (using serial increments of 6.6 μm^2) confirms the above observation that a complete spectrum of cell sizes survives in ONA retinae but that ONS rats possess only small-sized ganglion cells. (Figure 2-9).

Ganglion cell axons in the fiber layer of the retina regenerate after injury. They grow randomly and by 30 dpl form a mass of entangled axons distal to the lesion within the fiber layer and inner plexiform layer (Figure 2-10a). Some axons grow proximally, skirting the margins of the lesion, approaching the optic disc circuitously by looping between fascicles. However, few axons gain the papilla because they are equally likely to grow away from the optic nerve head as toward it and are not constrained within the confines of fascicles but readily leave to enter another or run randomly within this layer or deeper within the inner plexiform layer (Figure 2-10b). HRP injected into the optic nerve of rats with retinal lesions confirms that few if any regenerating axons grow into the optic nerve (Figure 2-11).

Placing a peripheral nerve in a retinal lesion alters the behavior of regenerating axons. They no longer grow randomly about the lesion but directly traverse

Figure 2-9. Comparison of the percentage cumulative frequency distribution of different-sized ganglion cells between normal, ONS retinae, and ONA retinae, and between ONS and ONA retinae. See text for further details.

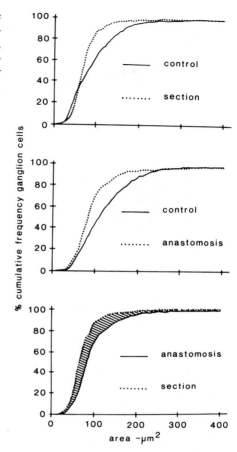

the area of damage to enter the peripheral nerve transplant (Figure 2-12). At present, we have no measure of the number of fibers regenerating into the sciatic nerve segment or of the number of ganglion cells surviving injury compared to those in simple retinal lesions.

Discussion

By 30 days after optic nerve section, retinal ganglion cell axons are still present in both the ganglion cell fiber layer and proximal optic nerve stump. The density of cells in the ganglion cell layer is greatly reduced below normal levels, and large- and medium-sized ganglion cells have largely disappeared. The effects on ganglion cell survival of anastomosing a segment of sciatic nerve to the proximal stump of the completely transected optic nerve are not obviously

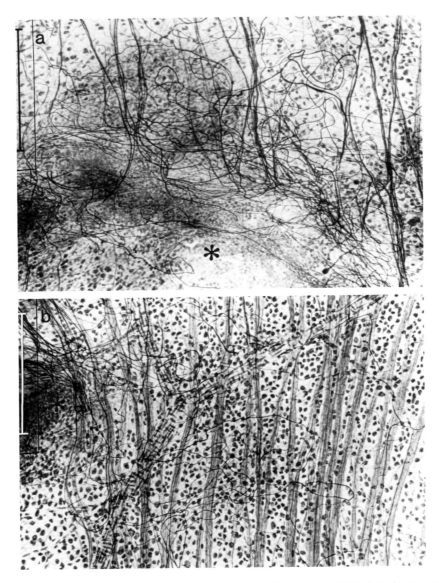

Figure 2-10. (a) Randomly growing axons about a retinal lesion (*) 30 dpl. (b) Axons to the right of the lesion grow for short distances within the radial fascicles of the fiber layer but never remain in them for long distances. Note that regenerating axons in the fascicles either grow toward (bottom edge) or away from the optic disc and after leaving a fascicle continue to course randomly through the retina. (Silver-stained retinal whole mounts; marker = 250 μm.)

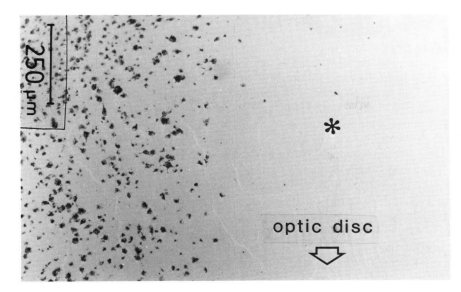

optic disc

Figure 2-11. HRP-filled retinal ganglion cells juxtaposed to an area of retina in which ganglion cell axons have been injured more proximally in the fiber layer. The HRP was applied to the optic nerve and the absence of filled cells in the segment of the retina (*), distal to the retinal fiber layer lesion, demonstrates that few, if any, regenerating ganglion cell axons fail to grow into the optic nerve.

Figure 2-12. Representative example of retinal axons invading a sciatic nerve graft implanted into a retinal lesion. Note that ganglion cell axons do not grow randomly about the retinal lesion, as in Figure 2-10, but directly enter the graft and that qualitatively the number of ganglion cell axons surviving is similar to the number surviving in retinal lesions without a sciatic nerve implant (Figure 2-10).

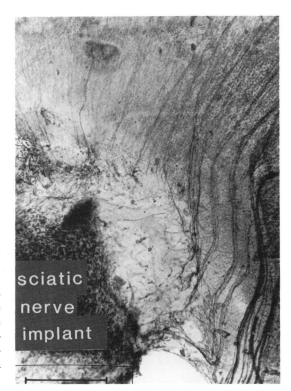

sciatic
nerve
implant

different from those seen in ONS retinae. Neither the numbers of axons in the fiber layer nor the density of ganglion cells in ONA and ONS retinae appear qualitatively different although the presence of a few large ganglion cells is a feature that distinguishes ONA retinae from those of ONS animals. Nonetheless, our HRP study does show that retinal ganglion cell axons do invade the sciatic nerve graft and grow in small numbers for up to 10 mm along the length of the nerve to imbibe the HRP. Negative labeling at 0 dpl and in the unoperated eye excludes passive diffusion and systemic uptake, respectively, as possible causes of ganglion cell labeling. Since all optic nerve fibers have been severed, the presence of retinal ganglion cell axons in the graft is the first unequivocal demonstration of true regeneration of severed central axons into a peripheral nerve. The small numbers of axons regenerating into the graft cannot be explained by malapproximation of sciatic and optic nerve stumps because epineurium and pia-arachnoid were anastomosed and histological evaluation of all anastomotic sites at 30 dpl showed axons bridging the stumps with no intervening glial/collagen cicatrice. Inadequate blood supply to the retina or proximal optic nerve stump is also unlikely to account for the poor regenerative response because the ophthalmic artery was left intact, postoperative bleeding was minimal, and direct observation of blood vessels over the optic nerve and vitreal surface of the retina confirmed the presence of a normal, patent vasculature. The poor regenerative response despite such favorable conditions might indicate that either trophic influences are absent and/or that axon growth is actively inhibited.

It has been proposed that the release of axon growth inhibitory factors by CNS myelin/oligodendrocytes could account for the failure of CNS regeneration (Berry 1982, 1983, 1984) and that such an explanation readily accounts for the paradox of growth failure in the injured, myelinated optic nerve of the rat but the florid regrowth of unmyelinated axons after injury in the retina (McConnell and Berry 1982). Our findings confirm those of McConnell and Berry (1982) and provide evidence for the presence of diffusable factors emanating from the peripheral nerve implant (Williams et al 1984) that might act as a positive stimulus to direct regenerating ganglion cell axons into the implanted sciatic nerve segment. The small number of optic nerve fibers growing in the sciatic nerve graft may thus be explained by postulating that, in the environment of degenerating central myelin, axons may be influenced by factors having diametrically opposing effects on growth. Thus, successful entry into and continued elongation along the sciatic nerve may only be possible for those axons exposed to a net stimulatory effect. Such favored axons may be those closest to the anastomosed sciatic nerve stump which most rapidly escape inhibition by passing into the graft.

The numbers of fibers in the optic nerve are usually estimated to be less than the total number of neurons in the ganglion cell layer of retina (Hughes and Wassle 1976, Vaney and Hughes 1976, Tiao and Blakemore 1976, Hughes 1977). Indeed, retrograde HRP tracing labels about half of the neurons in the ganglion cell layer of normal rats (Cowey and Perry 1979). The discrepancy is probably explained by an inability to distinguish amacrine cells, displaced into the ganglion cell layer (Perry 1979, 1981), from ganglion cells (Stone 1965, 1978, Hughes 1975, 1977). Assuming that the counts by Hughes (1977) of both neurons in the ganglion cell layer (190,000) and of fibers in the optic nerves (120,000) of agoute rats are similar to those of WAG rats, the total number of displaced amacrine cells in the WAG rat retina is 70,000. We have recorded a reduction in the ganglion cell population of 50% and 40% in ONS and ONA rats, respectively. Thus, the total number of neurons in the ganglion cell layer in each group would be 95,000 and 114,000, respectively. [The amacrine cell population is likely to be unaffected by optic nerve section, the axons of these cells do not leave the retina (Allcutt et al. 1984a,b, Graftstein and Ingoglia 1982, Miller and Oberdorfer 1981, Misantone et al. 1984), the actual number of ganglion cells in ONS and ONA retinae is 25,000 and 44,000, respectively.] Thus, 16% (19,000) more cells remain viable in the ONA group compared to the number present in the ONS group. Of the 44,000 ganglion cells surviving in the ONA group, on average only 3% (1,207) of their axons regenerate 10 mm along the sciatic nerve graft to the site of HRP injection by 30 dpl. It is difficult to explain this numerical discrepancy, unless axons of most surviving neurons occupy more proximal parts of the sciatic nerve. Alternatively, both tropic and trophic influences might be required for successful regeneration. The tropic influences offered to CNS axons by a peripheral nerve graft might be mediated by nondiffusable molecules bound to the inner surface of the basal lamina tubes of Schwann cells (Ide et al. 1976, Keynes et al 1984). Diffusable trophic factors might emanate from Schwann cells and, in addition to guiding axons over concentration gradients, would increase cell survival and maintain cell size. The latter two effects might be independent of the first and less sensitive to growth inhibitory molecules.

The shift in cell size in favor of smaller cells seen in both ONA and ONS rats might be brought about by cell death differentially affecting larger cells or by cell shrinkage. Retinal ganglion cell shrinkage has been observed following axonal transection (Graftstein and Ingoglia 1982, Miller and Oberdorfer 1981, Misantone et al. 1984). The maintenance of ganglion cell size in the ONA group might thus be related to an increase in protein synthetic activity initiated by trophic factors retrogradely transported by regenerating axons in the sciatic graft.

The survival and regrowth of axons in the retina after injury (McConnell and Berry 1982) is in marked contrast to regenerative failure and degeneration when damaged in the optic nerve. Thus, in the visual system at least, the most plausible explanation for this differential spatial response is that axon growth inhibition occurs in the optic nerve but not in the retina. The alternative explanation that growth factors supporting ganglion cell axon regrowth are present in the retina but not the optic nerve seems unlikely. The thesis that growth factors are present in both sites but that their efficacy is neutralized in the optic nerve by factors released from the damaged tissue that block the receptors of such growth-promoting factors is implied by the axon growth inhibitory hypothesis (Berry 1982, 1983, 1984). The random growth of regenerating retinal fibers is presumably due to a lack of guidance. Our HRP tracing study shows that, by 30 dpl, few of the randomly growing axons penetrate any distance into the optic nerve. The behavior of the axons is dramatically changed by placing a peripheral nerve into the retinal lesion, when most severed ganglion cell axons regrow directly into the graft. Presumably, the initial growth towards the center of the wound, observed by McConnell and Berry (1982), is sufficient to bring most axons under the trophic influence of the sciatic nerve, before they loop back away from the lesion. Although we have the impression that ganglion cell survival is probably not affected by the presence of the graft, it is difficult to come to definitive conclusions without quantitation or further HRP tracer studies.

Conclusions

Optic nerve fibers regenerate into a segment of sciatic nerve for at least 10 mm by 30 dpl. Since all axons are severed in the optic nerve before anastomosis, the presence of optic nerve fibers in the sciatic graft is an unequivocal demonstration of regeneration of retinal ganglion cell axons. The number of fibers regenerating is a very small proportion of the total number of axons surviving, indicating that presumed trophic influences, emanating from the peripheral nerve as diffusable molecules, are largely overridden by a growth inhibitory factor produced by the damaged optic nerve. The number of ganglion cells surviving is greater than the number of axons that have regenerated at least 10 mm into the sciatic graft, from the point of anastomosis, suggesting either that most regenerating axons have attained lengths of less than 10 mm or that cell survival and cell size are independent of regeneration and influenced by different trophic molecules. Implantation of a peripheral nerve into the retina directs the random growth of regenerating retinal fibers so that regrowing severed fibers enter the peripheral nerve graft. This observation is strong evidence for the production of trophic factors by the peripheral nerve segment.

Acknowledgments. We thank Kevin Fitzpatrick and Sara Smith for the photography, Tony Finch and Mass N'Jie for the histology, and Margaret Collins for preparing the manuscript. The work was supported by the M.R.C., U.K.

References

Aguayo, A.J., Benfey, M., David, D. (1983). A potential for axonal regeneration in neurons of the adult mammalian nervous system. Birth Defect: Original Article Series 19, 327–340.

Aguayo, A.J., Björklund, U., Stenevi, U., Carlsted, T. (1984). Fetal mesencephalic neurons survive and extend long axons across peripheral nervous system grafts inserted into the adult rat striatum. Neurosci. Lett. 45, 53–58.

Aguayo, A.J., Bray, G.M., Perkins, C.S., Duncan, I.D. (1979). Axon-sheath cell interactions in peripheral and central nervous system transplants. Soc. Neurosci. Symp. 4, 361–383.

Aguayo, A.J., David, S., Richardson, P., Bray, G.M. (1982). Axonal elongation in peripheral and central nervous system transplants. In: Advances in Cellular Neurobiology. Federoff, S., Hertz, L. (eds). New York: Academic Press, pp. 215–234.

Aguayo, A.J., Dickson, R., Trecarten, J., Attiwell, M., Bray, G.M., Richardson, P. (1978). Ensheathment and myelination of regenerating PNS fibres by transplanted optic nerve glia. Neurosci. Lett. 9, 97–104.

Allcutt, D., Berry, M., Sievers, J. (1984a). A quantitative comparison of the reaction of retinal ganglion cells to optic nerve crush in neonatal and adult mice. Brain Res. 16, pp. 219–230.

Allcutt, D., Berry, M., Sievers, J. (1984b). A quantitative comparison of the reaction of retinal ganglion cells to optic nerve crush in neonatal and adult mice. Brain Res. 16, pp. 231–240.

Benes, V. (1968). Spinal Cord Injury. London: Bailliere, Tindall and Cassell.

Benfey, M., Aguayo, A.J. (1982). Extensive elongation of axons from rat brain into peripheral nerve grafts. Nature 296, 150–152.

Berry, M. (1982). Post-injury myelin-breakdown products inhibit axonal growth: An hypothesis to explain the failure of axonal regeneration in the mammalian central nervous system. Biblthca Anat. 23, 1–11.

Berry, M. (1983). Regeneration of axons in the central nervous system. Prog. Anat. 3, 213–233.

Berry, M. (1985). Regeneration and plasticity in the CNS. In: Scientific Basis of Clinical Neurology. Kennard, C., Swash, M. (eds.). Edinburgh: Churchill Livingston. pp. 658–679.

Brown, J.O., McCouch, G.P. (1949). Abortive regeneration of the transected spinal cord. J. Comp. Neurol. 87, 131–137.

Chi, N.N., Bignami, A., Bich, N.T., Dahl, D. (1980). Autologous sciatic nerve grafts to the rat spinal cord: Immunofluorescence studies with neurofilament and gliofilament (GFA) antisera. Exp. Neurol. 69, 568–580.

Cowey, A., Perry, V.H. (1979). The projection of the temporal retina in rats, studied by retrograde transport of horseradish peroxidase. Exp. Brain Res. 35, 457–464.

David, S., Aguayo, A.J. (1981). Axonal elongation into peripheral nervous system bridges after central nervous system injury in adult rats. Science 214, 931–933.

David, S., Aguayo, A.J. (1985). Axonal regeneration after crush injury of rat central nervous system fibres innervating nerve grafts. J. Neurocytol. 14, 1–12.

Feigin, I., Geller, E.H., Wolf, A. (1951). Absence of regeneration in the spinal cord of the young rat. J. Neuropath. Exp. Neurol. 10, 420–425.

Gamble, H.J. (1976). Spinal and cranial nerve roots. In: The Peripheral Nerve. Landon, D. (ed.). London: Chapman and Hall, p. 330.

Goldberg, S., Frank, F. (1979). The guidance of optic axons in the developing and adult mouse retina. Anat. Rec. 193, 763–774.

Graftstein, B., Ingoglia, N.A. (1982). Intracranial transection of optic nerve in adult mice: Preliminary observations. Exp. Neurol. 76, 318–330.

Hughes, A. (1975). A quantitative analysis of the cat retinal ganglion cell topography. J. Comp. Neurol. 163, 107–128.

Hughes, A. (1977). The pigmented rat optic nerve: Fibre count and fibre diameter spectrum. J. Comp. Neurol. 176, 263–268.

Hughes, A., Wassle, H. (1976). The cat optic nerve: Fibre total count and diameter spectrum. J. Comp. Neurol. 169, 171–184.

Ide, C., Tohyama, K., Yokota, R., Nitatori, T., Onodera, S. (1976). Schwann cell basal lamina and nerve regeneration. Brain Res. 288, 61–75.

Kao, C.C. (1974). Comparison of healing process in transected spinal cords grafted with autogenous brain tissue, sciatic nerve and nodose ganglion. Exp. Neurol. 44, 424–439.

Kao, C.C., Chang, L.W., Bloodworth, J.M.B. (1977a). Electron microscopic observations of the mechanisms of terminal club formation in transected spinal cord axons. J. Neuropath. Exp. Neurol. 36, 140–156.

Kao, C.C., Chang, L.W., Bloodworth, J.M.B. (1977b). Axonal regeneration across transected mammalian spinal cord. An electron microscopic study of delayed microsurgical nerve grafting. Exp. Neurol. 54, 591–615.

Kao, C.C., Shimizer, Y., Perkins, L.C., Freeman, L.W. (1970). Experimental use of cultured cerebellar cortical tissue to inhibit the collagenous scar following spinal cord transection. J. Neurosurg. 33, 127–139.

Keynes, R.J., Hopkins, W.G., Huang, C.L.H. (1984). Regeneration of mouse peripheral nerves in degenerating skeletal muscle: Guidance by residual muscle fibre basement membrane. Brain Res. 295, 275–281.

Kiernan, J.A. (1971). Pituicytes and the regenerative properties of neurosecretory and other axons in the rat. J. Anat. 109, 97–114.

Kiernan, J.A. (1981). Histological and Histochemical Methods: Theory and Practice. Oxford: Pergamon Press, pp. 272–273.

Kimmel, D.L., Moyer, E.K. (1947). Dorsal roots following anastomosis of the central stump. J. Comp. Neurol. 87, 289–319.

Le Gros Clark, W.E. (1943). The problem of neuronal degeneration in central nervous system. II. The insertion of peripheral nerve stumps into the brain. J. Anat. 77, 251–259.

Lugaro, E. (1906). Sulla presentarigenerazione autogena delle radici posteriori. Rev. Pat. Nerv. Men. 11, 337–340.

McConnell, P., Berry, M. (1982). Regeneration of ganglion cell axons in the adult mouse retina. Brain Res. 241, 362–365.

McCouch, G.P. (1955). Comments on regeneration of functional connections. In: Regeneration in the Central Nervous System. Windle W.F. (ed.). Springfield, Ill.: Charles C. Thomas, pp. 171–175.

Mesulam, M.M. (1982). Principles of horseradish peroxidase neurohistochemistry and their application for tracing neural pathways—axonal trasport, enzyme histochemistry and light microscopical analysis. In: Tracing Neural Connections with Horseradish Peroxidase. Mesulam, M.M. (ed). Chichester: John Wiley and Sons, pp. 1–152.

Miller, N.M., Oberdorfer, M. (1981). Neuronal and neuroglial responses following retinal lesions in the neonatal rats. J. Comp. Neurol. 202, 493–504.

Misantone, L.J., Gershenbaum, M., Murray, M. (1984). Viability of ganglion cells after optic nerve crush in rats. J. Neurocytol. 13, 449–465.

Moyer, E.K., Kimmel, D.L., Winborn, L.W. (1953). Regeneration of sensory nerve roots in young and in senile rats. J. Comp. Neurol. 198, 283–308.

Nonidez, J.F. (1939) Studies on the innervation of the heart. I. Distribution of the cardiac nerves, with special reference to the identification of the sympathetic and parasympathetic postganglionics. Am. J. Anat. 65, 361–413.

Paskind, H.A. (1936) Regeneration of posterior root fibres in cat. Arch. Neurol. Psychiat. 36, 1077–1084.

Perkins, C.S., Carlstedt, T., Muzimo, K., Aguayo, A.J. (1980). Failure of regenerating dorsal root axons to regrow into the spinal cord. Can. J. Neurol. Sci. 7, 323.

Perry, V.H. (1979) The ganglion cell layer of the retina of the rat: Golgi study. Proc. R. Soc. Lond. B. 204, 363–375.

Perry, V.H. (1981). Evidence for an amacrine cell system in the ganglion cell layer of the rat retina. Neuroscience 6(5), 931–944.

Richardson, P.M., Aguayo, A.J., McGuinness, V.M. (1981). Role of sheath cells in axonal regeneration. In: Proceedings of the 10th Annual Symposium on Special Cord Reconstruction. Kao, C., Bunge, R.P., Reier, P. (eds.). New York: Raven Press, pp. 293–304.

Richardson, P.M., Issa, V.M.K., Aguayo, A.J. (1984). Regeneration of long axons in the rat. J. Neurocytol. 13, 165–182.

Richardson, P.M., McGuinness, V.M., Aguayo, A.J. (1980). Axons from CNS neurones regenerate into PNS grafts. Nature 284, 264–265.

Sager, O., Marcovic, G. (1972). Regeneration in the central nervous system. Rev. Roumanian Neurol. 9, 23–29.

Stensaas, L.J., Burgess, P.R., Horch, K.W. (1979). Regenerating dorsal root axons are blocked by spinal astrocytes. Soc. Neurosci. Abst. 5, 684.

Stone, J. (1965). A quantitative analysis of the distribution of ganglion cells in the cat's retina. J. Comp. Neurol. 180, 753–772.

Stone, J. (1978). The number and distribution of ganglion cells in the cat's retina. J. Comp. Neurol. 180, 753–769.

Sugar, O., Gerard, R.W. (1940). Spinal cord regeneration in the rat. J. Neurophysiol. 3, 1–19.

Ten Cate, J. (1932) Refunde nach der experimentellen Isoherung eines Ruckenmarksabschmittes. Arch. Neere Physiol de l'Homme et des Animaux 17, 149–238.

Tiao, Y.C., Blakemore, C. (1976). Regional specialisation in the golden hamster's retina. J. Comp. Neurol. 168, 439–458.

Tower, S.S. (1931). A search for trophic influences of posterior spinal roots on skeletal muscle, with a note on the nerve fibres found in the proximal stumps of the roots after excision of the root ganglion. Brain 54, 99–110.

Vaney, D.I., Hughes, A. (1976). The rabbit optic nerve: Fibre spectrum, fibre count and comparison with a retinal ganglion cell count. J. Comp. Neurol. 170, 241–252.

Weinberg, E.L., Spencer, P.S. (1979). Studies on the control of myelinogenesis. 3. Signalling of oligodendrocyte myelination by regenerating peripheral axons. Brain Res. 162, 273–279.

Westbrook, W.H.L., Tower, S.S. (1940). An analysis of the problem of emergent fibers in the posterior spinal root, dealing with the rate of growth of extraneous fibers into the roots after ganglionectomy. J. Comp. Neurol. 72, 383–397.

Williams, L.R., Powell, H.C., Lundborg, G., Varon, S. (1984). Competence of nerve tissue as distal insert promoting nerve regeneration in a silicone chamber. Brain Res. 293, 201–211.

Wise, G., Dollery, C., Henkinb P. (1971). The Retinal Circulation. New York: Harper and Row.

Chapter 3

The Differentiation of Non-Neuronal Elements in Neocortical Transplants

LESLIE M. SMITH and FORD F. EBNER*

Introduction

Background

Brain tissue transplantation is a versatile technique with the potential to identify cellular mechanisms that control developing as well as mature functions of
neurons and glia. We are currently interested in how the continued differentiation of embryonic donor tissue affects the ingrowth of adult host axons into
these transplants. Two important variables are the type of host fiber and the age
of the donor tissue at the time of transplantation. For example, axons labeled
by acetylcholinesterase (AChE) histochemistry always start to grow into the
transplants within a few days and ultimately achieve numerical densities comparable to the normal cortex (Hohmann and Ebner 1982, Park, et al. 1984).
Monoamine fibers visualized by histofluorescence, in contrast, are not detectable for 3–4 weeks and never reach normal densities in these neocortical transplants (Park et al. 1984). Only rare thalamic and commissural fibers elongate
across the interface zone into the transplants without special pretreatment
(Smith et al. 1984). Host axons arising from peptidergic neurons have never
been observed entering the transplants at any donor age (Ebner et al. 1984).
Host GABAergic neurons grow into transplants taken from very young donors,
embryonic day 14 or younger, but not at all into older donor tissue (Smith et al.
1984). All types of host fiber systems are damaged to some extent at the time of
transplantation, but these results indicate that each responds to the damage in
very different ways. The precise molecular composition of the donor tissue
may be crucial to successful transplant innervation. For example, cholinergic
axons that initiate an immediate response to damage encounter a set of cell

* Center for Neural Science and Division of Biology and Medicine, Brown University, Providence,
Rhode Island 02912 U.S.A.

surface and matrix molecules that are different from those encountered by slower growing fibers because the embryonic donor tissue is differentiating rapidly after implantation. The type of connections that develop between donor and host tissue therefore may depend upon synchrony of host axon growth with the degree of maturity of transplant cells.

Neurons in neocortical transplants remain immature by several criteria. They do not migrate within the transplant to form six well-defined layers. The transplants from older donors show some lamination because the immature neurons had migrated into the cortical plate before transplantation, but the cell layers are still not normal. Long apical dendrites typical of pyramidal cells in the infragranular layers are rare in the transplants; instead they tend to branch repeatedly near the cell body. Not all transplants develop the same cell types; GABAergic neurons develop in transplants from older donors (embryonic day 17 and older), but not in transplants from younger donors (day 14 or younger) (Smith et al. 1984). All transplant neurons develop incomplete patterns of innervation by extrinsic host fiber systems.

In this chapter we address the question: To what stage of maturity do the transplanted glia and blood vessels progress in the absence of normal differentiation and innervation of the transplant neurons? These "supporting elements," as well as the neurons, may require specific conditions to achieve their mature characteristics. The relative maturity of the non-neuronal elements cannot be determined at the precise time when each type of axon is mounting its maximum growth response following injury, but it is possible to define the time course of maturation of non-neuronal elements in the transplants up to the point where they achieve a relatively stable state. We will first discuss the timing of events during the normal development of mouse neocortex to provide background for a description of the maturational changes in the non-neuronal elements in the transplants. We will then discuss several cases that support our general conclusion that non-neuronal elements remain in a state of incomplete differentiation that is equal to, if not greater than, the degree of immaturity of neuronal differentiation in these transplants.

The Normal Development of Mouse Cortex

The Origin and Migration of Neurons

The normal gestation period of BALB/c mice is 20 days. Neurons in mouse neocortex undergo their final mitotic division in the second half of the gestation period, between embryonic day 11 (E11) and E18 (Figure 3-1) (Angevine and Sidman 1962). The majority of cortical neurons are born between E13 and E16, and the number of new cells decreases sharply on days 17 and 18 (Smart and Smart 1982). In the medial part of neocortex, the immature neurons begin to migrate and define a cortical plate region around E14 to E15 (Smart and Mc-Sherry 1982), even though the migration and cortical plate formation occurs approximately one day earlier in more lateral parts of developing cortex. The medial region of the cortical plate increases in depth and cellular density

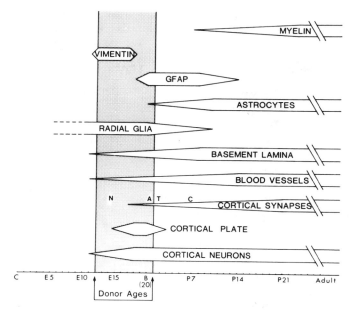

Figure 3-1. Schematic representation of the approximate times of onset (pointed end), and acquisition of adult status (parallel lines) of some events that occur during the normal development of mouse neocortex. The data are taken from studies referenced in the text. Age from conception (C) to birth (B) to maturity is indicated below along the horizontal axis. The stippled zone spanning the range of donor animal ages intersects with the status of each event. The degree of differentiation of the tissue is very different from the youngest (E12) to the oldest (newborn) donor ages. Cortical synapses refer to total numbers (frequency), with the approximate time of initial detection of catecholamine (N), AChE-positive (A), thalamic (T), and corticocortical systems indicated above.

through E18, so that virtually all of the immature neurons are in their final laminar position by the time of birth. The time that neurons require between their last mitotic division and their appearance in the cortical plate increases later in development. In the rat, neurons labeled between E14 and E18 migrate to the cortical plate in about 2 days, while cells labeled near birth (E19–E21 in the rat) take 3 to as long as 10 days to migrate (Hicks and d'Amato 1968). Once in place, many of the immature cortical neurons die during the first 3 postnatal weeks, in concert with a dramatic increase in cortical volume during the same period (Heumann and Leuba 1983).

The Origin of Glial Cells

The origin of glial cells is more difficult to establish than that of neurons because they retain the ability to divide for a much longer period. Germinal cells form and retract processes that contact both the pial and ventricular surfaces during approximately the first half of gestation as they undergo repeated mitotic

division (Sauer 1935). One set of cells, the radial glia, stops dividing and main-
tains processes that span the wall of the telencephalic vesicle. Once present,
the radial glia exhibit closely timed changes in metabolic activity that also may
reflect stages in their cell surface differentiation (Bignami and Dahl 1973). All of
these stages occur before radial glia disappear from the neocortex during the
first 2–3 weeks after birth. Recognizable protoplasmic and fibrous astrocytes
appear in cortex later than neurons, becoming distinguishable just before birth
and increasing rapidly in number duing the first 1–3 postnatal weeks. Current
evidence suggests that astrocytes arise both from cells in the subependymal
layer (Privat and LeBlond 1972) and from the transformation of radial glia into
astrocytes (Levitt and Rakic 1980, Schmechel and Rakic 1979).

Glial cells, in contrast to neurons, show a progressive increase in number
throughout life (Heumann and Leuba 1983). Part of this increase is due to the
continued cell division needed for myelinization. In rat cortex myelin formation
starts around postnatal day 9 (P9) (Caley and Maxwell 1968) and is not complete until P60 (Jacobson 1963).

Radial glia, astrocytes, and perhaps other cells in the CNS synthesize structural proteins, such as intermediate filaments, at different times during cortical
development. Cytoskeletal proteins may provide clues to the state of cell surface molecules that in turn may be important for axon guidance. Intermediate
filaments composed of vimentin are expressed in radial glia and immature glia
(Dahl et al. 1981) and are detectable by immunocytochemical localization as
early as E11 (Schnitzer et al 1981). Other intermediate filaments, such as those
composed of glial fibrillary acidic protein (GFAP)(Bignami et al. 1972, Eng and
DeArmond 1981), become detectable at E18 in mouse cortex, and the radial glia
and astrocytes remain strongly GFAP-positive until P7 to P14 (Woodhams et al
1981). Mature cortical astrocytes decrease their GFAP content below detectable levels, except for a few GFAP-positive astrocytes in layer 1, around blood
vessels, and in the subcortical white matter (Figure 3-2). The transition from
glial cell production of vimentin to synthesis of GFAP occurs around the time
of birth (Dahl 1981). Extracellular influences may control these fluctuations in
the rate of cortical GFAP synthesis, such as hormones and other blood-borne
molecules (Fischer et al. 1982, Morrison et al. 1984). The mature astrocytes in
the hippocampus only a few hundred microns distant are dramatically more
GFAP-positive than in the neocortex (Figure 3-2). An odd corollary of normal
GFAP expression is that prior to P8 astrocytes are incapable of synthesizing
increased amounts of GFAP in response to mechanical damage to cortex, but
after P8 they become intensely GFAP-positive in response to injury and stay
that way for months to years around the residual scar (Berry et al. 1983 and
Figure 3-6).

The Formation of Connections in Neocortex

The first morphologically discernible synapses in neocortex appear around
E16–E18 in the marginal zone and subplate region in the rat (Blue and Parnave-

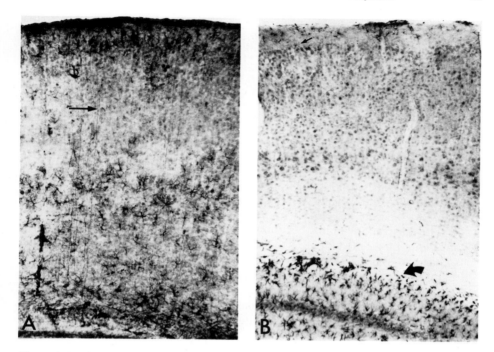

Figure 3-2. The appearance of GFAP-containing cells in normal mouse neocortex at P8 (A) and in the adult (B). At P8 both radial glia (arrow) and astrocytes (mostly in layers I, V, VI, and white matter) are labeled. In the adult brain only a few astrocytes show immunocytochemically detectable GFAP in neocortex (arrow in layer I), in contrast to the hippocampus, part of which is shown at the bottom of B.

las 1983a, Wolff 1976), and it is reasonable to assume that the synapses in mouse cortex first occur around the same time. Synaptogenesis is mainly a postnatal event in the rat cortex. Synaptic frequency increased from around 2% of adult levels at the time of birth to adult levels by 3 weeks after birth (Blue and Parnavelas 1983b, Kristt and Molliver 1976). Both morphological categories of synapses (i.e., terminals with round vesicles forming asymmetrical contacts and terminals with "flattened" vesicles forming symmetrical contacts) develop during the first 3 postnatal weeks. The earliest extrinsic fibers to arrive in mouse cortex have been identified by catecholamine fluorescence on E14 (Caviness and Korde 1981), slightly earlier than in the rat (Levitt and Moore 1979). AChE-labeled fibers are not detectable until near the time of birth (E18) in mice (Hohmann and Ebner 1985). Thalamic fibers from the ventral nucleus have been shown recently by Crandall and Caviness (1984) to be present in the white matter of mouse cortex by E15–16, but the exact time when the thalamic fibers of each type make their first synapses in mouse cortex is unknown. As in other mammals, corticocortical connections in the mouse are the last fiber systems to mature.

Vascularization of Neocortex

The maturation of the cortical blood supply takes place over a long period of development beginning as early as E11 (Strong 1964). Initially a sinus-like plexus of vessels forms over the surface of cortex. From these cisternae, stem vessels sprout perpendicular to the cortical surface down to the subependymal zone where they form what Strong (1964) called the "subependymal plexus" in the developing rabbit brain. The subependymal plexus is developed as early as E13 in the rat (Wolff et al. 1975).

Cortical blood vessels characteristically develop as solid cords of mesodermal cells surrounded by an incomplete basement lamina. The cellular cords later develop a narrow lumen and then increase in size over a period of several days (Caley and Maxwell 1970, Kramer and Lierse 1967). The strands of mesodermal cells become enveloped by astroglial processes only near the time of birth. The basement lamina becomes more complicated at that time, some constitutents being provided by the astrocytes and some by the mesodermal cells (Bar and Wolff 1972). A surge of capillary sprouting occurs in the early postnatal period. Sprouting increases most rapidly in the marginal layer a few days after birth, and again in the middle layers at P8 (Rowan and Maxwell 1981). The transient decrease in vascular length density that we find between P2 and P10 (Figure 3-6) may be associated with the rapid decrease in neuronal density observed between P5 and P10, a period when the cortical volume is doubling (Heumann and Leuba 1983). The postnatal formation of capillaries occurs in conjunction with the increased metabolic demands prompted by the switch to aerobic glycolysis at birth, the development of cortical circuitry (Wise and Jones 1978), and the onset of cortical cell responses to cutaneous stimulation during the early postnatal period (P7) (Armstrong-James 1975). Cortical transplants from prenatal donors thus will contain a germinal matrix of blood vessel-related mesodermal cells even when we take special care to remove meningeal membranes and surface blood vessels.

The Response of Normal Adult Neocortex to Mechanical Damage: The Surgical Procedure without a Transplant

In our transplant procedure described below, the passage of a capillary tube through the adult mouse brain for 4–5 mm breaks numerous small- to medium-sized blood vessels, cuts all types of axons of extrinsic and intrinsic neurons, and damages glial cells. The damage is confined almost entirely to the cortical gray matter; the tunnel formed by the capillary rarely encroaches on the white matter and never damages the ependyma or enters the ventricle. Host cortex is forced into the invading tube and a core of host brain tissue is extruded. Small-caliber arteries and veins seal off rapidly, aided in the mouse by a remarkably short (15 seconds) clotting time. Astrocytes lining the tunnel swell rapidly and increase their production of structural and enzymatic proteins in a relatively stereotyped sequence. After injury, cortical astrocytes show a marked increase in their content of GFAP. Initially, only those cells near the injury become

GFAP-positive, but over the first 7 days following cortical lesions, the GFAP synthesis increases in astrocytes throughout the hemisphere. Within 3 weeks the reaction is reduced in extent to the area around the lesion. A scarlike rim of GFAP-labeled astrocytes remains around the cavity for months (Figure 3-7A). The astrocytes recreate a new cortical "surface" by lining the lesion cavity with basement lamina that in some instances becomes contiguous with the preexisting basement lamina of the hemisphere (see Barry et al. 1983 for a description of the reaction of cortex to injury).

Immediately after mechanical disruption of the cortex the area is hemorrhagic, and several cellular responses are initiated that reach maximum levels at different times. Blood-borne macrophages are present in peak numbers at 4 days post-lesion, fibroblasts peak at 8–10 days, while basement lamina, type I and III collagen, and new blood vessels achieve highest densities sometime after the first week. The basement membrane formed by type IV and V collagen is clearly present by 8 days after lesions (Berry et al. 1983). It may form part of or fuse with the astrocytic basement lamina that is composed, at least in part, of the protein laminin (Liese 1984, Liese et al. 1983). Thus, mesodermal cells and astrocytes both contribute to the scar formation around lesions in cortex.

Methods: Transplantation Surgery

The procedure of transplantation begins with the surgical removal of an embryo from the uterus of a pregnant BALB/c mouse after a timed gestation period. Tissue is removed for transplantation from embryos as young as E12, when the cortical tissue first can be readily separated from the overlying meninges and skin, through P3, after which the donor tissue will not survive in an adult host. A dorsomedial region of the telencephalic vesicle (lateral to the estimated border of cingulate cortex and medial to the developing striatum where it can be seen bulging into the ventricle) is dissected free into a drop of Eagles minimal essential medium tissue culture fluid containing 0.04% DNAase (Figure 3-3a). The ventricle remains open under this region of the immature cortex until the time of birth. Therefore, the thickness of the cortex can be easily measured from ependyma to pia, and the radial glial cells can be kept intact, if the approximately $0.5 \times 0.5 \times 3$ mm piece of tissue is handled carefully.

The donor tissue is gently sucked into a square capillary tube for 2–3 cm by hydraulic pressure for later delivery into the adult host brain. The capillary is held in a micromanipulator for control over positioning and insertion into the host brain.

The adult host is prepared to receive the donor tissue by placing the deeply anesthetized animal into a simple headholder and exposing the dorsolateral surface of the cerebral hemisphere. The head is positioned so that the surface of the cortex is nearly parallel to the capillary tube in the micromanipulator. A hole is made in the meninges near the lateral border of the bone opening, and the capillary is advanced through the host cortex to the medial border of the bone opening (Figure 3-3b). A second small opening is made in the host brain

PROCEDURE FOR TRANSPLANTATION

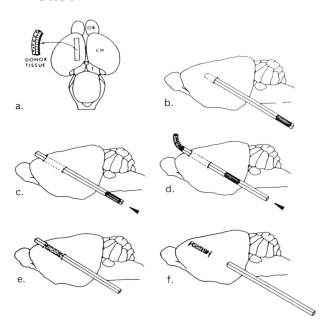

Figure 3-3. Shows the area of the embryonic neocortex removed for transplantation (a) and how the donor tissue is inserted into the adult host brain (b–f). Two tissues are illustrated in the capillary tube in d; the host cortex is shown being extruded from the capillary and the donor tissue is still within the tube. The donor tissue is still in the capillary in e, just prior to its extrusion as the capillary is retracted in f. OB = olfactory bulb; CH =cerebral hemisphere (telencephalic vesicle); T = thalamus.

meninges over the buried end of the tube (Figure 3-3c), and the core of host cortex that was forced into the capillary during its advance through the brain is expelled out of the tip of the tube by positive hydraulic pressure (Figure 3-3d). Without the host tissue to block the flow of fluid out of the capillary, the transplant tissue can be floated to the buried end of the capillary (Figure 3-3e). The donor tissue is then prevented from slipping backward by positive fluid pressure while the capillary tube is retracted simultaneously by the microma-nipulator (Figure 3-3f). The swelling of the damaged host cortex appears to close the space around the transplant left behind by the wall of the receding capillary tube so that the donor tissue remains in place but is not deformed by compression forces. Removal of the host tissue also eliminates the normal targets of the damaged thalamic, commissural and other fibers to that region, and the embryonic tissue provides new postsynaptic surfaces as alternative synaptic sites. The skin is sutured together without attempting to replace the bond flap, and the animals almost always recover uneventfully. No drugs of any kind are given postoperatively.

This surgical procedure leaves a minimally damaged embryonic tissue to differentiate in the environment of a lesioned adult brain. Instead of growing in parallel with the contiguous embryonic donor tissue and being nourished by fetal CSF and blood flow, the donor tissue is initially surrounded by hemorrhage, broken blood vessels, and the debris of disintegrating neurons and glia. Up to the time of transplantation the host cortex constituted a stable environment for the normal functioning of mature neurons and glia, and after transplantation the host mounts an attempt to restore that condition.

Results: Events that Follow Transplantation

Differentiation of the Donor Tissue

Following implantation of embryonic tissue into the tunnel formed by the capillary tube many of the implanted cells survive and continue to differentiate. We can follow the differentiation of neurons and glia using a variety of labels, and it is clear that some events occur considerably earlier and some later than during normal development; some important events never take place at all in the transplanted tissue.

Development of Vasculature in the Transplant

Vascularization is crucial to the viability of the implanted cells, and it is initiated immediately in transplants that survive. At the time of transplantation, the donor tissue is immersed in an abnormal fluid environment. It is saturated during the transfer from donor to host with a fluid containing only salts, amino acids, glucose, and vitamins (Eagles MEM), and then it is immersed in the cellular debris of damaged adult neurons and glia, blood cells, and serum proteins. The fluid dynamics of the first few days after implantation can be reconstructed only roughly, but evidence of blood vessel growth has been reported in hippocampal transplants by Indian ink labeling of the host blood vessels within the first 24 hours after transplantation (Lawrence et al 1984). In addition, these studies demonstrate by immunocytochemical labeling of type IV collagen that the basement lamina around the host blood vessels is expanding and forming new fingerlike evaginations within 24 hours after surgery.

In neocortical transplants, tissue from all donor ages contain a subependymnal plexus of vessels, the remnants of which are inserted into the host brain with the more obvious neurons and glia. The normal progression of anastomosis and selective necrosis described in normal prenatal development (Strong 1964) presumably continues, at least in some modified form, in the transplant. Whether some or all of these donor vessels link up with ingrowing host vessels remains unknown.

By 3–5 days post-transplantation (DPT), the vessels around the perimeter of the transplant develop bulbous swellings and appear to be growing some distance into the donor tissue (Figure 3-4A). By 8–9 DPT the vessels appear

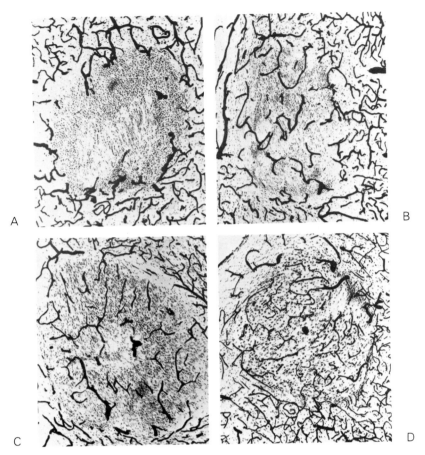

Figure 3-4. Vascularization of transplanted neocortex (E17 donor) is shown at 5 days (A), 8 days (B), 9 days (C), and 11 days (D) after transplantation. Preparations were made by Indian ink perfusion of the host circulation followed by Nissl stain of the section. See text for details.

throughout the transplant (Figures 3-4B and C). Solid cores of mesodermal cells that continue to develop in the transplant during these few days may fuse with the sprouting host vessels to produce the sudden onset of patent vasculature. By 11 DPT the density of blood vessels has increased to near maximum levels, with a slight increase over the next several months (Figure 3-4D). The final density of blood vessels is presumably determined by many factors, but in our transplants the vasculature never achieves the length density of blood vessels in the surrounding host or normal cortex regardless of the donor age. The type of vessels that are formed in the transplant appear quite normal in some areas (Figure 3-5). Blood vessels arborize and anastomose in the donor tissue during the first 2 weeks after transplantation, but capillary networks

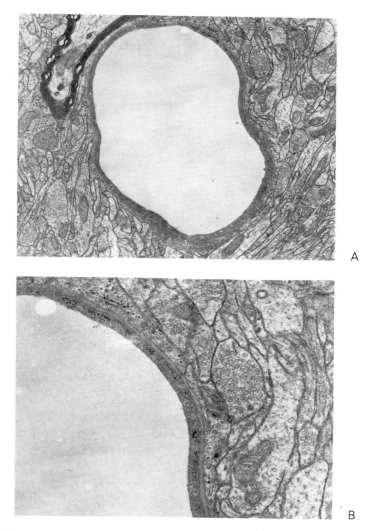

Figure 3-5. (A) The fine structure of a small blood vessel in a mature (>60 days postoperative) transplant. The thin endothelial cells show a junctional "seam" and are surrounded by a basement lamina. (B) Enlargement of one sector shows the endothelial, basement lamina, and astrocytic layers separating the vessel lumen from the surrounding neuropil.

comparable to the surrounding host brain rarely develop. The transplants do not show the expected surge of capillary formation at 1–2 weeks after transplantation (Figure 3-6).

Less than normal vascular density in the transplant may be correlated with low metabolic activity, such as has been observed in similar transplants by showing very low levels of 2-deoxyglucose uptake (Sharp and Gonzalez 1984).

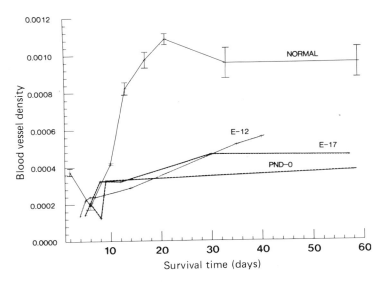

Figure 3-6. Graph of the length density of blood vessels during normal development (NORMAL) and in transplants from three different donor ages (E-12, E-17, and within the first 24 hours after birth [PND-0]. There is a marked divergence in the development of vascular density at 1 week after birth such that the transplants never achieve "normal" length densities of vascularization. Units on the ordinate are $\mu m/\mu m^3$. Variance is SEM. Each data point is the mean value for counts from 3 normal cortices or 3 transplants.

Some endothelial cells appear abnormal, the basement lamina appears incomplete in some areas around the endothelial cells, and smooth muscle cells are rarely present around transplant vessels. Axon fascicles or synaptic vesicle-filled axon segments are rarely present beneath the vascular basement lamina. The absence of axons around vessels is not unexpected since the ingrowth of catecholamine containing fluorescent axons from any source is minimal in these transplants even after survival periods of several months (Park et al. 1984). Immunocytochemical localization of tyrosine hydroxylase (TH) confirms the spareness of catecholaminergic fibers in the transplants and provides a clear indication that even the sparse TH-positive fibers seen in the transplants are not intimately associated with blood vessels in the transplants as they are in the surrounding host brain (unpublished observations).

These results taken together suggest that the transplants are perfused by the host brain circulation but that they never achieve adult length densities or mature morphology. The status of the blood–brain barrier has not been studied yet in the mature transplants, but the apparent discontinuity of the basement lamina and the astrocytic foot processes around some blood vessels supports the interpretation that the blood–brain barrier is incompletely formed in some areas of the transplants similar to the condition found a few days after birth during normal development. We have not examined the transplant capillaries after L-dopa injections (Svendgaard et al. 1975), but our preliminary results from immunohistochemical labeling of serum proteins suggest that the blood–brain barrier is deficient in some vessels, especially near the transplant-host interface.

The Fate of Radial Glia and the Appearance of Astrocytes.

The fate of radial glia and astrocytes in transplanted embryonic neocortex may provide important clues to the nature of the environment encountered by axons as they attempt to grow into the transplants. GFAP synthesis is already induced in the radial glial cells of older E17–E19 donor tissue but is not expressed yet in the E12–E14 donor tissue at the time of transplantation. During normal development, GFAP synthesis would be expected to continue at a high level after E13 for approximately another 2 weeks before it is sharply decreased.

By 7 days after transplantation, donor tissues of all ages still contain almost exclusively GFAP immunoreactive radial glial cells. This indicates that the radial glia are not destroyed by the transplant procedure and that they are not converted immediately to astrocytes or other cell types. Most of the labeled processes continue to span the depth of cortex (in reality the width of the transplant) and because the embryonic tissue is frequently folded in a fan shape, the radial glia often appear the emanate from one locus and to distribute in a radial pattern. Since GFAP would not normally be detectable in the E13 donor tissue for another 5 days, the appearance of GFAP-positive cells in these transplants by 7 days after surgery indicates that the experimental conditions induce the synthesis of GFAP at approximately the expected time.

By 14 days after transplantation, both radial glia and typical astrocytes are present in the transplants (Figure 3-7). Cells with both protoplasmic and fibrous astrocytic morphology can be easily recognized, the fibrous type typically being associated with fascicles of axons in the transplants. Between 2 and 4 weeks the radial glia disappear completely and astrocytes alone remain as the only GFAP-positive cells. The most unusual feature of the cortical astrocytes in the transplants is that most of them remain GFAP-positive for up to 1 year after transplantation. Our interpretation of this observation is that mechanisms which normally suppress cortical GFAP synthesis during the first 1–2 weeks after birth do not operate on the transplant cells when they are in the adult brain environment. We cannot distinguish between arrested development and continued post-traumatic reactiveness of the astrocytes as the basis for prolonged GFAP production. However, the astrocytes stay in this state in newborn hosts (Björklund et al. 1983) as well as in adult hosts, and this state of prolonged GFAP synthesis may be an important element in promoting or inhibiting the ingrowth of some types of axons. In the early post-tranplant period, successful axons begin to invade the transplants within 7 days when the astrocytes are not yet present and the only GFAP-positive cells are radial glia. Stabilization of

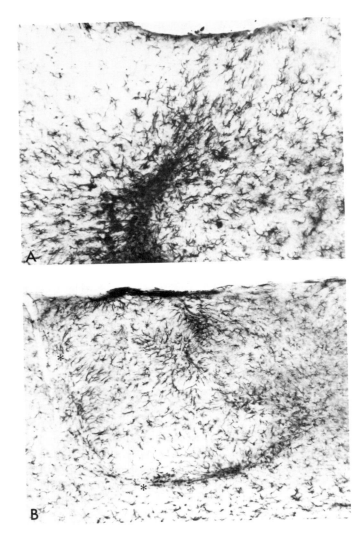

Figure 3-7. GFAP immunoreactivity in a cortical scar (A) and in a cortical transplant (B) at 60 and 45 days after transplantation, respectively. The asterisks mark two locations along the interface between the donor and host tissue.

astrocytes in a perpetual state of GFAP production is at least consistent with the interpretation that this is a state of prolonged immaturity of the astrocytes. We would predict that vimentin would show a similar pattern, because vimentin is expressed for long periods when embryonic cortex is transplanted to the anterior chamber of the eye; that is, astrocytes remain vimentin-positive as well as GFAP-positive for long periods after transplantation (Björklund et al. 1984).

The Maturation of Oligodendroglia

Myelination of axons in neocortical transplants never achieves host levels. This fact is visualized most clearly when the white matter of the transplant faces the white matter of the host cortex (Figure 3-8).

The majority of the axons in the host cortex are myelinated and run in parallel fascicles beneath the cortical cells. In contrast, the white matter of the transplant contains only a few myelinated axons, mostly of a smaller diameter than in the host, embedded in a profuse tangle of completely bare axons. The appearance of the "mature" transplant (older than 30 days) is typical of the

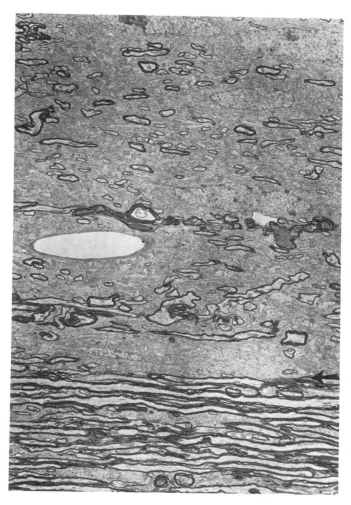

Figure 3-8. The fine structure of white matter in the host (below the arrow) and donor (above the arrow) tissue. Note the large number of unmyelinated axons in the transplant.

host white matter during the first few weeks of postnatal development. The difference is that in normal development the degree of myelination progresses rapidly to the adult condition during the first two postnatal months (Jacobson 1963). We have never identified oligodendroglia that are GFAP-positive for short or prolonged periods (Choi and Kim 1984), but this possibility requires more careful study.

The Occurence of Ependymal Epithelial Cells

After the radial glia can no longer be visualized during normal cortical development, the cells closest to the ventricle remain as a row of ependymal epithelium lining the ventricle. The ependymal epithelium becomes GFAP-positive for a short period late in gestation, at least in the human brain (Roessmann et al. 1980). Ependymal epithelium does not develop in neocortical transplants, but a small cluster of more or less cuboidal-shaped cells is present in one location near the white matter of the transplant in every case. When viewed in the electron microscope, these cells show a characteristically dense granular cytoplasm and contain or are bounded by unusual spaces (Figure 3-9). These cell clusters have never been identified in GFAP-stained preparations, and if they are transiently GFAP-positive in the transplants, we have not observed them at the proper time.

The Fate of Embryonic Connective Tissue

Most parts of the neocortical transplants are not in contact with the surface of the host brain, and they do not accumulate connective tissue elements at the interface between the donor and host tissue. Occasionally, focal zones remain along the interface that contain macrophages, dense aggregates of GFAP-positive astrocytic processes, and other unidentified fibrous material. After examining many regions of the interface between host and donor cells in the electron microscope, however, we have never encountered collagen fibrils within the substance of the host brain. One unanswered question is whether the connective tissue attached to the embryonic donor tissue survives in any form in the adult host and if so, where it is located.

The Response of the Adult Host Brain to the Transplant

The response of the adult brain to injury is modified by the presence of the transplant tissue in several ways that we can specify and most likely in many ways that remain to be discovered.

One of the modifications is manifested by the host astrocytes. Following transplantation, the usual reaction is for GFAP-positive astrocytes to appear throughout the hemisphere. After 21 days the reactive cells are restricted to the region surrounding the transplant. Instead of forming a permanent ring of scarlike glial processes around the border zone (Figure 3-7A), the GFAP-labeled astrocytes decrease in many regions to undetectable levels on the host

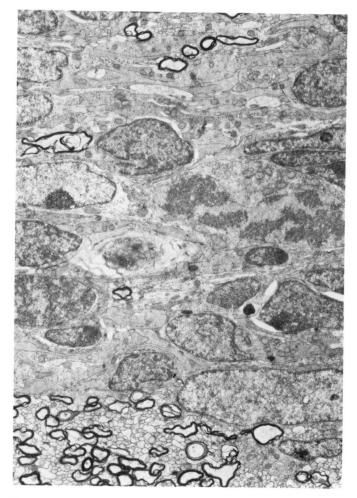

Figure 3-9. Electron micrograph of a cluster of cells that appear in every transplant near the white matter. They are usually detected at low magnifications as a cluster of electron dense cells surrounded by focal zones of widened extracellular spaces.

side of the interface (Figure 3-7B). This absence of scarring along the border zone suggests that the transplant inhibits the post-traumatic response of the host which is to maintain a thick interface barrier. Host astrocytes return to low levels of GFAP production as seen in normal cortex. The volume density of astrocytes in the transplants does not appear greater than in the host cortex at the height of the GFAP response, except in occasional small foci of scarring along the border between transplant and host tissue. The continued production of GFAP by transplant astrocytes makes a striking contrast to the minimal continued GFAP response in the host brain.

Summary and Conclusion

The non-neural elements of donor and host neocortical tissue respond to transplantation in very different ways. The host circulation perfuses the donor tissue within a few days after transplantation. The host astrocytes respond as usual to the surgery, but the presence of the transplant greatly diminishes the permanent astrocytic scarring around the lesioned area. Remnants of connective tissue cells, collagen, and basement lamina have not been found in the interface region between donor and host tissue. Thus, usual physical barriers to axon growth from the adult host into the transplant are minimal, and the absence of axonal ingrowth by specific fiber systems such as those from the thalamus must be explained by the failure of other unknown mechanisms. Hypotheses to explain the paucity of ingrowth by host fiber systems include retrograde degeneration leading to death of the damaged neurons, the absence of appropriate molecules on the transplant cell surfaces for axonal guidance, or competition between axonal systems that grow into the transplants.

The cell surfaces of the immature neurons and glia are the best candidates for creating a substrate pathway that supports axonal ingrowth from the host into the transplant. The radial glia persist for several days in the transplant before astrocytes can be detected. Once GFAP-positive astrocytes appear they replace the radial glia and then remain clearly labeled in the transplants for long periods. The cortical neurons in the transplants do not receive their normal thalamocortical and corticocortical connections, but this impoverishment does not prevent them from forming synapses with each other in numerical densities that approach that of normal adult cortex (Smith and Ebner 1982). Neuronal cell surfaces, therefore, achieve some features of mature cortical neurons within 1–2 months after transplantation and do not appear to change (or degenerate) in any way that we can detect over the next 6–12 months.

In contrast, non-neuronal elements in the transplants remain surprisingly immature. The length density of transplant blood vessels is always less than normal adult controls. Blood vessels remain uninnervated by sympathetic axons. In some instances the basement lamina surrounding blood vessels is missing. Axons remain either unmyelinated or are ensheathed by abnormally thin myelin coverings. Astrocytes fail to diminish their GFAP production as they would in normal adult neocortex. The conclusion that the supporting cells remain in a permanent state of incomplete differentiation suggests that glial surface molecules important to the growth and guidance of specific fiber systems are not expressed, and as a result these axons do not grow into the transplants. This interpretation raises the question of whether the state of differentiation of any of these non-neuronal elements could be manipulated through experimental procedures aimed at changing the final degree of cell surface maturation. It is possible that the state of differentiation of supporting elements is linked together and that the missing factor might be the absence of a small number of inductive events. The transplantation paradigm is particularly well suited to study factors that influence development because "normal" developmental events, such as enzyme induction, are interrupted at an identified point in time when the cortical cells can be removed. The embryonic tissue can be exposed to various treatments before development is allowed to continue again in a normal or experimentally altered adult host brain environment. An important application of this paradigm would be to determine the degree of transplant cell differentiation that is optimal for the ingrowth of specific sensory and other axonal systems.

Acknowledgments. Special thanks are due Mr. Perry Busalacchi who, as an undergraduate, made a major contribution to the study of the vascularization of neocortical transplants. We thank Dr. L. Eng for generously supplying the antiserum to GFAP for these studies, Mary Ellen Flinn for her patience and help in preparing the manuscript, and Ms. Maura DiPrete for her technical assistance. These studies have been supported by grant #NS13031.

References

Angevine, J.B., Sidman, R.L. (1962). Autoradiographic study of histogenesis in the cerebral cortex of the mouse. Anat. Rec. 142, 210.

Armstrong-James, M.A. (1975). The functional status and columnar organisation of single cells responding to cutaneous stimulation in neonatal rat somatosensory cortex (SI). J. Physiol. 246, 501–538.

Bar, T., Wolff, J.R. (1972). The formation of capillary basement membranes during internal vascularisation of the rat's cerebral cortex. Z. Zellforsch. 133, 231–248.

Berry, M., Maxwell, W.L., Logan, A., Mathewson, A., McConnell, P., Ashhurst, D.E., Thomas, G.H. (1983). Deposition of scar tissue in the central nervous system. Trauma 3, 31–53.

Bignami, A., Dahl, D. (1973). Differentiation of astrocytes in the cerebellar cortex and the pyramidal tracts of the newborn rat: An immunofluorescence study with antibodies to a protein specific to astrocytes. Brain Res. 49, 393–402.

Bignami, A., Eng, L.F., Dahl, D., Uyeda, C.T. (1972). Localization of the glial fibrillary acidic protein in astrocytes by immunofluorescence. Brain Res. 43, 429–435.

Björklund, H., Dahl, D., Haglid, K., Rosengren, L., Olson, L. (1983). Astrocytic development in fetal parietal cortex grafted to cerebral and cerebellar cortex of immature rats. Dev. Br. Res. 9, 171–180.

Björklund, H., Dahl, D., Olson, L. (1984). Morphometry of GFA- and vimentin-positive astrocytes in grafted and lesioned cortex cerebri. Int. J. Dev. Neurosci. 2, 181–192.

Blue, M.E., Parnavelas, J.G. (1983a). The formation and maturation of synapses in the visual cortex of the rat. I. Qualitative analysis. J. Neurocytol. 12, 599–616.

Blue, M.E., Parnavelas, J.G. (1983b). The formation and maturation of synapses in the visual cortex of the rat. II. Quantitative analysis. J. Neurocytol. 12, 697–712.

Caley, D.W., Maxwell, D.S. (1968). An electron microscopic study of the neuroglia during postnatal development of the rat cerebrum. J. Comp. Neurol 133, 45–70.

Caley, D.W., Maxwell, D.S. (1970). Development of the blood vessels and extracellular spaces during postnatal maturation of rat cerebral cortex. J. Comp. Neurol. 138, 31–48.

Caviness, V.S., Korde, M.G. (1981). Monoaminergic afferents to the neocortex: A developmental histofluorescence study in normal and reeler mouse embryos. Brain Res 209, 1–9.

Choi, B.H., Kim, R.C. (1984). Expression of glial fibrillary acidic protein in immature oligodendroglia. Science 223, 407–409.

Crandall, J.E., Caviness, V.S. (1984). Thalamocortical connections in newborn mice. J. Comp. Neurol. 228, 542–556.

Dahl, D. (1981). The vimentin-GFA protein transition in rat neuroglial cytoskeleton occurs at the time of myelination. J. Neurosci. Res. 6, 741–748.

Dahl, D., Rueger, D.C., Bignami, A., Weber, K., Osborn, M. (1981). Vimentin, the 57,000 dalton protein of fibroblast filaments, is a major cytoskeletal component in immature glia. Eur. J. Cell. Biol. 24, 191–196.

Ebner, F.F., Olschowka, J.A., Jacobowitz, D.M. (1984). The development of peptide-containing neurons within neocortical transplants in adult mice. Peptides 5, 103–113.

Eng, L.F., DeArmond, S.J. (1981). Glial fibrillary acidic (GFA) protein immunocyto-chemistry in development and neuropathology. Prog. Clin. Biol. Res. 59A, 65–79.

Fischer, G., Leutz, A., Schachner, M. (1982). Cultivation of immature astrocytes of mouse cerebellum in a serum-free, hormonally defined medium. Appearance of the mature astrocyte phenotype after addition of serum. Neurosci. Lett. 29, 297–302.

Heumann, D., Leuba, G. (1983). Neuronal death in the development and aging of the cerebral cortex of the mouse. Neuropath. Appl. Neurobiol. 9, 297–311.

Hicks, S.P., D'Amato, C.J. (1968). Cell migrations to the isocortex in the rat. Anat. Rec. 160, 619–634.

Hohmann, C.F., Ebner, F.F. (1982). The development of cholinergic markers in normal and transplanted mouse neocortex. Neurosci. Abs. 8, 865.

Hohmann, C.F., Ebner, F.F. (1985). Development of cholinergic markers in mouse forebrain. I. Acetylcholinesterase histochemistry and cholineacetyltransferase en-zyme activity. Dev. Br. Res. In press.

Jacobson, S. (1963). Sequence of myelinization in the brain of the albino rat: Cerebral cortex, thalamus, and related structures. J. Comp. Neurol. 121, 5–29.

Kramer, J., Lierse, W. (1967). Die postnatale entwicklung der kapillarisation im gehirn der maus (Mus musculus L.) Acta Anat. (Basel) 66, 446–459.

Kristt, D.A., Molliver, M.E. (1976). Synapses in newborn rat cerebral cortex: A quanti-tative ultrastructural study. Brain Res. 108, 180–186.

Lawrence, J.M., Huang, S.K., Raisman, G. (1984). Vascular and astrocytic reactions during establishment of hippocampal transplants in the adult host brain. Neurosci. 12, 745–760.

Levitt, P., Moore, R.V. (1979). Development of the noradrenergic innervation of neo-cortex. Brain Res. 162, 243–259.

Levitt, P., Rakic, P. (1980). Immunoperoxidase localization of glial fibrillary acidic protein in radial glial cells and astrocytes of developing rhesus monkey brain. J. Comp. Neurol. 193, 815–840.

Liesi, P. (1984). The major matrix glycoproteins, laminin and fibronectin, in cultured cells from mammalian brain. In: Transplantation in the Mammalian CNS. Björklund, A., Stenevi, U. (eds.). p. 27.

Liesi, P., Dahl, D., Vaheri, A. (1983). Laminin is produced by early rat astrocytes in primary cultures. J. Cell Biol. 96, 920–924.

Morrison, R.S., de Vellis, J., Lee, Y. L., Bradshaw, R.A., Eng, L.F. (1984). Hormones and growth factors regulate the biosynthesis of glial fibrillary acidic protein in rat brain astrocytes. J. Cell Biol. In press.

Park, J., Clinton, R.J., Ebner, F.F. (1984). The growth of catecholamine- and AChE-containing fibers into neocortical transplants. Neurosci. Abs. 10, 1083.

Privat, A., LeBlond, C.P. (1972). The subependymal layer and neighboring region in the brain of the young rat. J. Comp. Neurol. 146, 277–302.

Raju, T., Bignami, A., Dahl, D. (1981). *In vivo* and *in vitro* differentiation of neurons and astrocytes in the rat embryo: Immunofluorescence study with neurofilament and glial filament antisera. Dev. Biol. 85, 344–357.

Roessmann, U., Velasco, M.E., Sindely, S.D., Gambetti, P. (1980). Glial fibrillary acidic protein (GFAP) in ependymal cells during development, and immunocyto-chemical study. Brain Res. 200, 13–21.

Rowan, R.A., Maxwell, D.S. (1981). Patterns of vascular sprouting in the postnatal development of the cerebral cortex of the rat. Am. J. Anat. 160, 247–265.

Sauer, F.C. (1935). Mitosis in the neural tube. J. Comp. Neurol. 62, 377–405.

Schmechel, D., Rakic, P. (1979). A Golgi study of glial cells in developing monkey telencephalon: Morphogenesis and transformation into astrocytes. Anat. Embryol. 156, 115–152.

Schnitzer, J., Franke, W.W., Schachner, M. (1981). Immunocytochemical demonstra-tion of vimentin in astrocytes and ependymal cells of developing and adult mouse nervous system. J. Cell Biol. 90, 435–447.

Sharp, F.R., Gonzalez, M.F. (1984). Fetal frontal cortex transplant (^{14}C) 2-deoxyglu-cose uptake and histology: Survival in cavities of host rat brain motor cortex. Neurol. 34, 1305–1311.

Smart, I.H.M., McSherry, G.M. (1982). Growth patterns in the lateral wall of the mouse telencephalon. II. Histological changes during and subsequent to the period of isocortical neuron production. J. Anat. 134, 415–442.

Smart, I.H.M., Smart, M. (1982). Growth patterns in the lateral wall of the mouse telencephalon: I. Autoradiographic studies of the histogenesis of the isocortex and adjacent areas. J. Anat. 134, 273–298.

Smith, L.M., Ebner, F.F. (1982). The fine structure of embryonic neocortex trans-planted into adult mouse neocortex. Neurosci. Abs. 8, 865.

Smith, L.M., Ebner, F.F. (1984). The expression of GFA protein synthesis in donor and host astrocytes following transplantation. Neurosci. Abs. 10, 983.

Smith, L.M., Hohmann, C.F., Ebner, F.F. (1984). The development of specific cell types and connectivity in neocortical transplants. In: Transplantation in the Mam-malian CNS. Björklund, A., Stenevi, U. (ed.). Amsterdam: Elsevier. In press.

Strong, L.H. (1964). The early embryonic pattern of internal vascularization of the mammalian cerebral cortex. J. Comp. Neurol. 123, 121–138.

Svendgaard, N., Björklund, A., Hardebo, J., Stenevi, U. (1975). Axonal degeneration associated with a defective blood–brain barrier in cerebral implants. Nature 255, 334–337.

Wise, S.P., Jones, E.G. (1978). Developmental studies of the thalamocortical and com-missural connections in the rat somatic sensory cortex. J. Comp. Neurol. 178, 187–208.

Woff, J.R. (1976). Quantitative analysis of topography and development of synapses in the visual cortex. Exp. Br. Res. Suppl. 1, 259–263.

Wolff, J.R., Goerz, C., Bar, T., Guldner, F.H., (1975). Common morphogenetic aspects of various organotypic microvascular patterns. Microvasc. Res. 10, 373–395.

Woodhams, P.L., Basco, E., Hajos, F., Csillag, A., Balazs, R. (1981). Radial glia in the developing mouse cerebral cortex and hippocampus. Anat. Embryol. 163, 331–343.

Chapter 4

Uses of Neuronal Transplantation in Models of Neurodegenerative Diseases

FRED H. GAGE,*† ANDERS BJÖRKLUND,* OLE ISACSON,* and PATRIK BRUNDIN*

Introduction

The experimental use of intracerebral neuronal grafting has expanded greatly in the last 10 years, as compared to any other time in history, though the basic methodology has been available for centuries. Early experiments focused on determining whether intracerebral grafting was possible (see, e.g., Saltykow 1905, Thompson 1890, Del Conte 1907, Dunn 1917). Subsequently, the parameters for optimal grafting were sought for a variety of approaches, focusing on issues such as age of donor (Olson et al. 1982, Kromer et al. 1983, Das et al. 1980), age of host (Hallas et al. 1980, Azmitia et al. 1981), cross-species compatibility (Björklund et al. 1982, Freed 1983, Low et al. 1983), host-graft interconnections (Björklund et al. 1976, 1979a, McLoon and Lund 1980a,b), target specificity (Lund et al. 1982), and vascularization (Stenevi et al. 1976). These critical experiments continue, revealing more information about the limits and potentials for graft survival and integration with the host brain.

Presently the reliability and versatility of the general methodology is such that it can be applied to many different experimental situations. As interest and information about the intracerebral grafting technique have increased, investigators in a variety of subareas in the neurosciences, such as developmental neurosciences (Jaeger and Lund 1980, 1981, Das et al. 1980, Wells and McAllister 1982), neuropsychology (Labbe et al. 1983, Björklund et al. 1981, Fray et al. 1983), and neuroendocrinology (Gash et al. 1980, Krieger et al. 1982), have begun to use the technique to solve experimental problems for which the technique may be well suited. In the present paper we will describe the rationale and initial results we have obtained from the use of the transplantation method

* Department of Histology, University of Lund, S-223 62 Lund, Sweden.
† Present address: Department of Neurosciences, University of California, San Diego, La Jolla, California 92093 U.S.A.

to investigate three different animal models of neurodegenerative disease. Each model represents a different application of the grafting technique.

Animal Models of Neurodegenerative Diseases

Animal models of neurodegenerative disease are developed and used because research directly on humans is unethical, illegal, dangerous, or expensive. Three different types of animal models are frequently used. The first type is a homologous model and implies that the same diseases or impairments are present in animals as are present in humans; implicit in such models is the assumption that the cause of the impairments is the same in humans and in animals. This type of model is rare in neurosciences, but it is required in order to investigate the causes of disease because it is the only one that assumes the same etiology.

The second type of model is an analogous model, which is generally based on knowledge concerning the selective damage to the brain that occurs as a result of the disease in the human case and a detailed knowledge of the symptoms. The development of the experimental model is based on experimentally damaging analogous brain structures in the animal and matching the neuropathological, physiological, and behavioral manifestations as closely as possible to the human disease. This model requires that the investigator take into consideration the biological limitations of the analogy, and therefore the behavioral symptoms elicited by the experimental damage are analogous within biological constraints of the experimental animal used. This type of model is often used to investigate the cellular mechanism underlying the experimentally induced physiological and behavioral symptoms.

The third type of model is a correlative model and requires only that one symptom of the animal model be related to the clinical disease. This type of model is most often used as a screening tool to test the effect of some therapy (surgical, pharmacological, or behavioral) in ameliorating experimentally induced symptoms, and in this model the symptoms are not required to be analogous to those observed in the human disease. The three models to be discussed in this paper represent examples from each of the three types of models described above.

Rationale for Intracerebral Grafting Experiments in Models of Neurodegenerative Disease

A standard paradigm for the study of neurological diseases with animal models is to investigate the behavioral, physiological, or biochemical consequences of brain damage, whether induced by the experimenter (analogous or correlative models) or naturally occurring (homologous), as in the degenerative changes that occur with aging. This approach is based on the observations of deficits associated with specific lesions and seeks to identify underlying mechansims necessary for the normal as well as abnormal functional activity. However, such an approach is unsuitable for identifying the sufficiency of individual neuronal mechanisms to sustain specific components of normal function. Additional difficulties associated with interpreting neurodegenerative processes are that the relationships are generally correlative rather than under experimental control and that degeneration of several systems may develop simultaneously.

The intracerebral grafting technique provides a potential resolution of these interpretive problems. First, by using specific neuronal suspension grafts of selected nuclei transplanted to identified brain regions, the neuronal substrate sufficient for normal function can be potentially identified and can be compared with the necessary lesion-induced requirements to produce a given dysfunction. Second, neuronal grafts permit experimental manipulation of individual neuronal populations to overcome the essential interpretive problems associated with correlational analysis. Functional recovery of particular aspects of the many dysfunctions occurring simultaneously in some models, following grafts of certain populations of neurons reinnervating discrete areas of the host brain, would facilitate identification of both the neurochemical systems and the neuroanatomical organization associated with the various components or functional deficits in the animal model. With this strategy in mind, we have embarked upon a series of studies into the anatomy and function of neuronal grafting to three different animals models: (1) aged animals as a homologous model of deficits that can occur in the aging human, (2) bilateral neurotoxic damage of the striatum in the rat as an analogous model of Huntington's chorea, and (3) unilateral neurotoxic damage of the ascending dopaminergic system in the rat as a correlative model of Parkinson's disease. In the remainder of this paper we will summarize our results from these three models.

Aging-Related Impairments

Aging can result in naturally occurring brain damage, with anatomical, biochemical, and functional changes that appear to be substantial yet selective (Bartus et al. 1982, Terry and Katzman 1983, Coyle et al. 1983). Recent advances in the localization and characterization of age-related neurodegenerative changes in both animals and humans have made possible the use of the aged rat as a homologous model for age-related impairments in humans (Gage . et al. 1983a, 1983b, 1984a, Campbell et al. 1980, Wallace et al. 1980). Though cell loss and morphological changes in the aged brain have been reported in numerous cortical (Mountjoy et al. 1983) and subcortical areas (Sabel and Stein 1981), we have focused our attention on cholinergic innervation of the hippocampus and on the dopaminergic innervation of the striatum for the following reasons: (1) Age-related anatomical, biochemical, and functional changes have been repeatedly documented for both of these neurochemical systems (Sims et al. 1982, Cubells and Joseph 1981, Geinisman et al. 1977, Barnes et al. 1983, Marshall and Berrios 1979, Joseph et al. 1983); (2) intracerebral grafts of suspensions of embryonic dopaminergic and cholinergic neurons into young adult rats are known to grow and survive successfully for long periods (Björklund et al. 1980b, Björklund and Stenevi 1977, 1979a); and (3) these same grafts have been demonstrated to restore functional deficits associated with damage to either the cholinergic septohippocampal system or the dopaminergic nigro-striatal system (Björklund et al. 1980a, 1981, Freed et al. 1980, Low et al. 1982, Dunnett et al. 1982).

The first stage in studying transplantation to the aged brain has been to demonstrate the survival of transplants in the aged brain and their ability to provide appropriate reinnervation of the host (Gage et al. 1983a). To this end, neuronal cell suspensions prepared from the ventral mesencephalon and septal-diagonal band of rat embryos were implanted into the depth of the intact neo-striatum or hippocampus of 21- to 23-month-old female rats of the same strain. Graft survival, assessed 3–4 months after grafting, was comparable to that seen in our previous studies of young adult recipients. Fiber outgrowth into the host brain was evaluated in animals that were subjected to lesions of the intrinsic nigrostriatal or septohippocampal system 6–10 days before killing. Dense do-paminergic fiber outgrowth was seen within a zone of up to about 1-mm radius around the nigral implants, and dense outgrowth of acetylcholinesterase (AChE)-positive fibers occurred up to about 2 mm away from the septal im-plants. The overall magnitude of fiber outgrowth was less than that generally seen in previously denervated targets in young adult recipients, but it appeared to be as extensive as in young recipients when the grafts are placed in non-denervated targets. The distribution of the AChE-positive fibers from the septal implants in the host hippocampus suggested that the pattern found in the non-denervated target of the aged recipients was more diffuse, and partly different, from normal, and the age-dependent synapse loss in intrinsic connections may influence the patterning of the graft-derived innervation.

The next stage in studying the effects of transplantation in the aged rat was to determine whether and to what extent the grafts could ameliorate the behav-ioral deficits that we observed in the aged rats prior to transplantation. Two principal deficits were studied in the aged animals: (1) motor coordination skills and (2) spatial learning. Motor coordination skills were assessed on four measures adapted from the battery described by Campbell et al. (1980): (1) the ability to maintain balance on and successfully reach a safety platform at either end of a narrow bridge of square cross-section; (2) the ability to maintain balance on a similar bridge of round cross-section; (3) the period of time that the animal could sustain its own weight clinging suspended from a taut wire; and (4) the ability to descend in a coordinated manner on a vertical pole cov-ered with wire mesh. Prior to transplantation, the aged rats were significantly impaired with respect to the young controls on the four measures. On the square and round bridges, young rats had no difficulty walking and exploring along the rod, and they generally reached the platform within 30–60 seconds. The aged rats before transplantation, by contrast, had greater difficulties main-taining balance. Most animals fell off the bridges or alternatively lay on the bridges without attempting to walk and clung tightly with all four paws or with the forepaws while the hind paws hung freely. Twelve weeks following transplantation the aged rats with nigral grafts, but not the aged control or the septal grafted rats, showed marked and significant improvement in their balance and limb coordination on both the square and round bridges. Typically they could walk along the bridge without falling, displayed gait and posture similar to the young rats, and fell less frequently than the other aged rats. On the wire mesh-covered pole the aged rats descended more rapidly before transplantation than did the young controls, frequently falling, slipping, or sliding down backwards. Although the aged rats with nigral transplants had a tendency to descend in a more controlled and coordinated manner, with head-down orientation as seen in the young controls, the differences from the other aged rats did not reach significance on this measure. The aged rats showed no difference between groups in either body weight or in latency to fall from the taut wire; this suggests that enhanced motor coordination in the aged rats with nigral grafts was not attributable to nonspecific differences in weight or strength of these animals (Gage et al. 1983c).

Spatial learning was assessed in the Morris' water maze task (Morris 1981) 1 week prior to transplantation and 2½–3 months after transplantation. This test requires that a rat use spatial cues in the environment to find a platform hidden below the surface of a pool of opaque water. Normal young rats have no trouble learning this task with speed and accuracy. Because our previous studies using this task (Gage et al. 1984b,c) showed that only a portion (one-quarter to one-third) of our rats were markedly impaired, a pretransplant test served to identify those impaired individuals in the aged rat group. Based on the performance of the young controls, we set the criterion for impaired performance in the aged rats such that the mean escape latency (i.e., swim time to find the submerged platform) should be above an upper 99% confidence limit (Gage et al. 1984a). A subgroup of old rats showed mean swim times greater than the criterion and were thus allocated to the "old impaired" group for transplantation. The remaining subgroup of aged rats constituted the "old nonimpaired" group. This latter group, together with a young control group, served as reference groups. A portion of the "old impaired" group received bilateral suspension grafts prepared from the septal-diagonal band area obtained from 14- to 16-day-old embryos of the same rat strain. Three implant deposits were made stereotaxically into the hippocampal formation on each side. The remaining "old impaired" rats were left unoperated and served as the "old impaired" control group. Both groups of "old impaired" rats had longer escape latencies as compared to the young controls and to the "old nonimpaired" rats. On the second test, 2½–3 months after grafting, the nongrafted groups remained impaired, while the grafted animals, as a group, showed a significant improvement in performance as indicated by escape latency. This improvement of the grafted group was demonstrated by comparisons to its pretransplantation performance as well as to the performance of the nongrafted old controls in the second test.

The ability of the rats to use spatial cues for the location of the platform in the pool was assessed by analyzing their search behavior after removal of the platform on the fifth day of testing. While the young rats and rats in the "old

nonimpaired'' groups focused their search on the fourth quadrant, where the
platform had previously been placed, the ''old impaired'' rats failed to do so in
the pretransplant test. In the posttransplantation test the grafted rats but not
the nongrafted ''old impaired'' group showed significantly improved performance; swim distance in the fourth quadrant was increased 83%, and they
swam significantly more in the fourth quadrant than in the other quadrants of
the pool. By contrast the nongrafted controls showed no significant change
over their pretransplant performance.

These results demonstrate, for the first time, the ability of intracerebral
grafts to ameliorate age-related impairments in complex, cognitive behavior.
The mechanism of action of the septal grafts is not at present clear, but it is
important to note that the intrahippocampal septal grafts identical to the ones
used here had no effect on the motor coordination disabilities described earlier
(see above), while the fetal substantia nigra implanted into the striatum was
effective in reducing these motor-related disabilities. This suggests that the
behavioral effects of the grafts are regionally specific and may be mediated
through a direct action on elements in the surrounding region of the host brain.

In summary, the homologous model provides a unique problem for the investigator, i.e., to identify what neurochemical system or systems are responsible for the observed functional deficits and where they are located in the brain.
This differs from the analogous or correlational model where the experimenter
induces the brain damage based on data and a theory of the etiology of the
neurodegenerative disease. The grafting paradigm has been shown in this case
to be useful in demonstrating a transmitter-related regional specificity in the
amelioration of age-related deficits that coincides with the suggestion of a dopaminergic involvement with motor-related deficits and a cholinergic involvement with cognitively related deficits in the aged rat. Further experiments with
this model of age-related deficits and the ameliorative effects of specific transplants are required to determine more concretely the transmitter specificity of
these transplants on specific behaviors, but clearly the utility of the transplant
paradigm to localize regionally important cell populations for the age-related
deficits has now been demonstrated in this model.

Animal Models of Huntington's Disease

Huntington's disease (HD) or chorea is an inherited autosomal dominant
neurodegenerative disease, where human chromosome nr 4 has recently been
implicated in an as-yet unknown pathogenesis (Gusella et al. 1983). Patients
often display a variety of symptoms ranging from involuntary movements to
complex cognitive and emotional disturbances (Bruyn 1968, 1982, Bird 1980,
Spokes 1980, Garron 1973). The therapy of choice is mainly neuroleptics,
which give some symptomatic relief, but the disease usually develops with
progressively more severe symptoms over a 10 to 20 year period leading to
death. Involvement of the caudate-putamen in the pathology of HD and chorea

became evident in early investigations and is the most frequent neuropathological finding (Alzheimer 1911, Earle 1973). Atrophy of the caudate-putamen has been correlated with the progress of the disease. A related anatomical structure, the globus pallidus, shows atrophy and some slight cell loss (Gebbink 1968, Lange et al. 1976). The substantia nigra pars compacta appears undamaged while, probably as a consequence of the loss of striatal afferents, the pars reticulata does show atrophy (Bird 1980). The nucleus accumbens, nucleus basalis, and other limbic structures are spared, whereas patchy cell loss in the cortex has been reported. A marked decrease of transmitter levels of GABA, acetylcholine, and the neuropeptides intrinsic to striatum has been noted in the striatum and its projection areas as a result of the neuronal degeneration in the striatum.

No homologous animal model of inherited HD exists. Some descriptions of a dyskinetic syndrome with a recessive genetic background have been reported for white rabbits (Nachtsheim 1934, Koestner 1973), but the pathology had only a slight resemblance to HD. Surgical or electrolytic lesions to the striatum can reproduce some hyperkinetic and cognitive symptoms of HD (Whittier and Orr 1962, Divac et al. 1967). Excitotoxic lesions by kainic acid (KA) and ibotenic acid (IA) of the caudate-putamen in experimental animals resemble the neuropathology of Huntington's disease (Coyle and Schwarcz 1976, McGeer and McGeer 1976). Some investigators have speculated on the possibility of endogenous so-called excitotoxins in the pathogenesis of neurodegenerative diseases (Plaitakis et al. 1982). The changes found in transmitter levels in the experimental model are analogous to the findings in post-mortem Huntingtonian brains, especially in the neostriatum and related projections areas (Coyle and Schwarz 1976, McGeer and McGeer 1976). Metabolic studies of regional brain activity in the animal model and in patients with HD indicate that the neostriatum has a decreased metabolic activity both in the model (Metter et al. 1982, Kimura et al. 1980, Kelly et al. 1982) and in patients with the disease.

The behavioral changes found after the excitotoxic neostriatal lesion are, of course, of a more correlative than analogous kind. Overt involuntary movements are not observed in the lesioned rat, whereas this is one of the main symptoms in patients with HD. Neither is it possible to detect in the rat self-neglect, social inappropriateness, or psychotic syndrome, which can be features in the initial diagnosis or misdiagnosis of HD patients (Garron 1973, Bird 1980). However, several behaviors in lesioned rats can be related to the symptoms of HD (Sanberg and Fibiger 1979, Mason and Fibiger 1978, 1979, Pisa et al. 1981); for example, a spontaneous and amphetamine-induced motor hyperactivity (Mason and Fibiger 1979). Spontaneous motor hyperactivity is more pronounced during the rat's naturally active diurnal period, i.e., at night; HD patients' involuntary movements are exaggerated during the day (Mason and Fibiger 1979).

The cognitive functions of the neostriatum have also been demonstrated in lesion studies, where deficits in learning and memory tests occur after excitotoxic lesions to the caudate-putamen (Dunnett and Iversen 1981, Pisa et al.

1981). The functional deterioration evident in HD could well be related to the caudate-putamen damage, but the anatomically and functionally related cortex and mesolimbic systems may also contribute to the cognitive dysfunctions.

Previous work in this laboratory has shown that it is possible to graft striatal primordium to the KA-lesioned neostriatum and that the grafts restore the Glutamic-amino acid decarboxylase (GAD) and choline acetyltransferase (ChAT) enzyme transmitter levels previously decreased by the excitotoxic lesion (Schmidt et al. 1981). Reports of nonspecific damage by KA (Nadler et al. 1978, Ben-Ari et al. 1979, Zaczek et al. 1980) prompted us to develop a large and reproducible lesion of the neostriatum using IA, which is superior to KA in that it does not cause lesions distant to the site of injection (Guldin et al. 1981). The optimal lesion was found to be that of 20 μg IA injected stereotaxically at 4 sites in the caudate-putamen. Four to 7 days after the lesion, during the reactive gliosis of the striatum, we subsequently transplanted fetal rat striatum of 13–15 days gestational age to the previously lesioned sites of the neostriatum. Four to 6 μl of dissociated cell suspension, with cell concentrations of between 75,000–125,000 cells/μl, were transplanted to the lesioned neostriatum to replace the lost intrinsic neurons.

Our results showed that the lesion caused extensive cell loss in the caudate-putamen, sparing only some 5–10% of the normal neuronal tissue (Isacson et al. 1984c). The remaining neostriatum was gliotic with few surviving intrinsic neurons separated by densely packed fiber bundles mainly derived from the internal capsule. In addition, GAD and ChAT enzyme activity levels (expressed per gram protein) were reduced to 30–40% and 40–50%, respectively, compared to the nonlesioned contralateral neostriatum (Schwarcz et al. 1979, Isacson et al. 1985a). There was also a depletion of neuropeptides, substance P, met-enkephalin, somatostatin, and NPY (Dawbarn et al. 1985) in the striatum and consequently met-enkephalin in the deafferentated globus pallidus and substance P in substantia nigra pars reticulata. Both of these latter structures appeared atrophic. Following an initial reactive gliosis soon after the striatum was lesioned with IA, atrophy progressed with a concomitant increase in the size of the lateral ventricle, a pattern that is also seen in HD.

In studies of regional cerebral metabolism using the technique developed by Sokoloff (Sokoloff 1977), we found a decreased (^{14}C) deoxyglucose utilization in the unilaterally lesioned striatum, while the contralateral intact striatum showed an increased glucose use compared to the control striatum (Kelly et al. 1982, Isacson et al. 1984c). The striatal projection areas, globus pallidus, substantia nigra, and subthalamic nucleus showed an enhanced metabolic activity; interestingly, this was also the case for the ventral tegmental area (VTA) and the nucleus accumbens. In grafted animals several of the neuronal cell types removed by the lesion were found in the fetal striatal implants (Dawbarn et al. 1985). Neurochemical studies also demonstrated that the neuronal marker enzyme GAD was increased to normal levels in the grafted striatum. The grafts also affected the CNS metabolic activity, as measured by deoxyglucose utilization.

Ten weeks after transplantation the grafted animals displayed a reduction in the lesion-induced metabolic hyperactivity of several anatomically and functionally linked brain structures. Hence, the projection areas globus pallidus and nucleus subthalamicus showed a normalized glucose utilization, as did the nucleus accumbens and the VTA. The deep layer of the superior colliculus, which is involved in motor behavior, also showed a significant decrease in glucose use compared to the lesioned animals (Isacson et al. 1984c).

Behavioral studies of the animal model have indicated that abnormalities in locomotion, open field activity, and memory occur after striatal excitotoxic KA lesions (Mason and Fibiger 1979, Sanberg and Fibiger 1979, Dunnett and Iversen 1980, 1981, Pisa et al. 1981). Analogously to patients with HD, there is also weight loss and cachexia in the lesioned animals (Sanberg and Fibiger 1979). The lesion-induced locomotor hyperactivity is more pronounced at night, when rats normally express about 90% of their total motor activity (Glick and Cox 1978), and the activity is also increased during food and water deprivation (Dunnett and Iversen, 1980, 1981). In order to characterize the behavioral effects of unilateral and bilateral striatal IA lesions, we tested the animals using a variety of measures. The tests involved maze learning, passive avoidance, sensorimotor integration, catalepsia, motor coordination, spontaneous and drug-induced rotation, and open field activity (Isacson et al. 1984b). Our results demonstrate that the bilateral lesion of the entire caudate-putamen causes impairments in most of the aforementioned tests, while the unilaterally lesioned rats exhibit few deficits and of decreased magnitude. However, a considerable drug-induced side-bias and a spontaneous nocturnal locomotor hyperactivity is clearly present in the latter group. We have recently demonstrated that grafted unilaterally lesioned IA animals show a normalization of the lesion-induced locomotor hyperactivity in overnight open field tests. In addition, another laboratory has reported a functional restitution by striatal grafts in bilaterally lesioned KA rats of behavioral habituation in an open field during the day (Deckel et al. 1983).

Thus, the experimental model of HD induced by KA and IA exhibits many features analogous to the human disease, such as increased motor activity and cognitive impairments. The resemblance of the excitotoxic lesion of the striatum to HD makes it clinically relevant in testing pharmacological and therapeutic strategies. By grafting fetal neurons to lesioned animals, it will perhaps be possible to identify basic cellular mechanisms for growth and recovery in this system. The neuronal replacement and lesion studies, in combination with detailed morphological, neurochemical, metabolic, pharmacological, and behavioral investigations, may cast more light on important characteristics of Huntington's disease as well as providing basic information concerning neostriatal functions.

Animal Models of Parkinsonism

The clinical Parkinsonian syndrome encompasses a variety of different pathological states in humans with differing etiology and pathogenesis, but all of which have in common a dopamine dysfunction in the neostriatum. By far the most common type of Parkinsonism is idiopathic Parkinson's disease (PD), which classically presents a triad of motor symptoms: tremor, rigidity, and akinesia (Yahr 1979). Recent studies have also shown disturbances in cognitive, affective-emotional, and autonomic functions in PD patients (Portin et al. 1984, Mann et al. 1983, Scatton et al. 1983, Lieberman et al. 1979, Alihanka et al. 1983).

PD patients exhibit a more complex pathology than simply a reduction of dopamine-containing cells in the substantia nigra, illustrated by gross depigmentation of these midbrain cells (Marsden 1983). In addition, at the microscopic level the involvement of, for example, the locus coeruleus (Mann and Yates 1983a, 1983b) and nucleus basalis Meynert (Arendt et al. 1983, Candy et al. 1983) is clear, indicating that the condition can involve multifocal cell damage. This is supported by neurochemical findings showing changes in the levels of a variety of different neuropeptides in PD (Taquet et al. 1983, Mauborgne et al. 1983, Studler et al. 1982, Javoy-Agid et al. 1982).

At the cellular level a typical finding in Parkinsonian brains is an eosinophilic intracellular inclusion, the Lewy body, whose origin and significance are unknown (Kimula et al. 1983). However, it has repeatedly been postulated to hold the key to the etiology of idiopathic PD (Marsden 1982, 1983).

The complexity of the symptoms and pathological changes and the fact that, to date, no *naturally* occurring animal homolog of PD has been discovered have made it difficult to establish homologous or even analogous animal models of PD. However, it was the result of early studies with an early animal model that drew attention to the role of dopamine in PD. Carlsson and coworkers found that reserpine-induced akinesia in mice, which shows similarities with clinical Parkinsonism, could be reversed by L-dopa, but not by 5-HTP, leading to the suggestion that dopamine was involved in PD (Carlsson 1959). This finding led to the major breakthroughs in PD research by Birkmayer and Hornykiewicz, who demonstrated the first successful clinical trial with L-dopa (Birkmayer and Hornykiewicz 1961) and who proved that, indeed, in the post-mortem Parkinsonian brain there was a significant dopamine depletion in the striatum (Hornykiewicz 1963).

However, attempts to create a long-term, permanent animal model in primates proved difficult because neither electrolytic substantia nigra lesions (Duvoisin 1976) nor, for example, manganese poisoning (Neff et al. 1969), which can result in Parkinsonism syndrome in humans, could induce reproducible stable changes in dopamine concentrations. The pioneering work with the neurotoxin 6-hydroxydopamine (6-OHDA) by Ungerstedt in 1968 (Ungerstedt 1968) to some degree resolved this problem in research in lower mammals. 6-OHDA, when injected into the brain, destroys catecholamine-containing neurons by a not fully understood mechanism (Cohen 1983, McGeer and McGeer 1981), reproducing the DA-depletion in the striatal complex of PD patients. Bilateral 6-OHDA injections into the ascending dopamine pathways of rats produce an akinetic syndrome with a marked decrease in movement and hunched posture, which is similar to that of the reserpinized rodent (Marsden et al. 1975, Duvoisin

1976). A permanent effect is obtained with an extensive lesion causing over 97% dopamine depletion. However, this results in an induced aphagia and adipsia that makes these animals difficult to keep alive—they have to be maintained by tube feeding. Bilateral 6-OHDA-lesioned rodents can at best be seen as an analog of PD because the model includes the feature of dopamine depletion; however, many aspects of the pathology and clinical symptomatology are lacking.

The unilateral 6-OHDA lesion is a correlative model of PD that has proven versatile in several fields of neuroscience, from neuropharmacology to, more recently, studies of neuronal transplantation. The unilaterally lesioned rat exhibits a marked asymmetrical postural bias towards the side of the lesion (Ungerstedt and Arbuthnott 1970, Duvoisin 1976). There is an extensive sensorimotor impairment illustrated by a neglect of stimuli contralateral to the lesion (Marshall and Gotthelf 1979, Marshall et al. 1980, Schallert et al. 1983). The rats are also unable to turn away from the lesioned side when offered sugarwater reinforcement, a finding that has been interpreted as an inability to initiate contralateral movement (Dunnett and Björklund 1983). Release of dopamine on the intact side of the brain by amphetamine stimulation will make 6-OHDA-lesioned rats actively turn towards the side of the lesion. Conversely, the post-synaptic dopamine agonist apomorphine will act on the denervation-induced supersensitive receptors ipsilateral to the lesion, causing the rat to move in circles in a direction contralateral to the lesion. Similar effects of an extreme side bias during spontaneous and pharmacological stimulation have also been reported in patients with a marked hemiparkinsonism (Trabucchi et al. 1979, Martin 1967).

The unilateral 6-OHDA-lesioned rat can be seen as a correlative model of PD, showing resemblance to hemiparkinsonism. However, there still remain major pathological and behavioral differences between this model and PD.

Several different approaches have been pursued when transplanting neuroectoderm-derived tissue to the brains of 6-OHDA-lesioned rats.

In 1979 Perlow and coworkers used a lumbar puncture needle to inject small pieces of embryonic ventral mesencephalon into the lateral ventricle of unilaterally 6-OHDA denervated rats (Perlow et al. 1979). Their study was the first to report functional effects of intracerebral neuronal grafts characterized by a reduction in apomorphine-induced rotation. Histochemical analysis demonstrated groups of catecholaminergic cells that sent processes out through the ventricular wall into the adjacent striatum. Later studies by the same group showed that the graft-derived reduction of apomorphine-induced rotation is associated with a normalization in spiroperidol binding in the denervated striatum (Freed et al. 1983b).

Using essentially the same technique (for review, cf. Freed 1983) Perlow and Freed have grafted adrenal medullary tissue from different aged donors, even across species barriers (Perlow et al. 1980), into the lateral ventricle of 6-OHDA-lesioned rats. Again some functional effects have been demonstrated (Freed et al. 1981), together with graft survival as indicated by catecholamine fluorescent cells and fibers in the ventricle (Freed et al. 1981, Freed 1983). However, very few fibers actually cross the ependymal lining into the denervated striatum. Thus, it is likely that the functional effects are due to diffusion of catecholamines from the graft. Similar grafts have been shown to contain higher proportions of DA than normal adrenal medulla (Freed et al. 1983a), results that are in agreement with the well-established plasticity of adrenal chromaffin cells *in vitro* (Unsicker et al. 1978).

In our laboratory we have used essentially two different techniques when transplanting embryonic ventral mesencephalic tissue to 6-OHDA-lesioned rats: solid grafts into a cortical cavity or intrastriatal injections of dissociated cell suspensions.

The solid graft procedure involves making a cortical cavity 3–6 weeks prior to placing a piece of embryonic ventral mesencephalon onto the dorsal or lateral aspects of the neostriatum (Björklund and Stenevi 1979a, Stenevi et al. 1976, 1980). Dopaminergic cells in the graft can send out fluorescent processes into the denervated striatum (Björklund and Stenevi 1979a, Stenevi et al. 1980). Occasional cells are seen to migrate from the graft into the host striatum, a finding that is also apparent in cross-species grafts from mouse to rat (Björklund et al. 1982). Behavioral analyses have shown that grafts placed in a dorsal cortical cavity and innervating the dorsal parts of the striatum can reduce both spontaneous and drug-induced rotation to normal levels but have no effect on the sensory neglect syndrome contralateral to the lesion (Björklund et al. 1980a, 1981, Dunnett et al. 1981a). In contrast, grafts placed into a lateral cavity show no effect on rotational behavior but rather ameliorate the sensorimotor deficits (Dunnett et al. 1981b). Thus, transplantation studies can aid in the understanding of the regional specificity of dopaminergic function within the striatum.

The rotational compensation achieved using solid grafts has been shown to be correlated with the degree of reinnervation (Björklund et al. 1980b). Notably, it has been found that reinnervation of approximately 5% of normal DA input is sufficient for compensation of amphetamine-induced rotation (Björklund et al. 1980a, Schmidt et al. 1982). The solid grafts have also been shown to sustain intracranial self-stimulation in the DA-denervated neostriatum (Fray et al. 1983) and have a significant transsynaptic influence on neuronal metabolism, as assessed by ^{14}C-2-deoxy-D-glucose autoradiography, in the host brain (Schmidt et al. 1982).

The behavioral compensation takes 2–6 months to develop after solid graft surgery as opposed to only 3–6 weeks using the alternative procedure of intrastriatal injections of dissociated DA-rich cell suspensions. With this technique pieces of ventral mesencephalon from embryonic day 13–15 rat fetuses are dissociated into a cell suspension as described earlier (Björklund et al. 1983a). These cells show good survival when injected into a variety of sites along the trajectory of the nigrostriatal pathway; however, their fibers remain confined to the graft unless the cells are deposited into or immediately adjacent to their target areas in the striatal complex (Björklund et al. 1983b). Cells injected into the neostriatum can create a dense fluorescent network of up to 1–2 mm radius, restoring DA levels on average to 13–18% of normal levels and, in extreme cases, to 50% of normal (Björklund et al. 1983b, Schmidt et al. 1983). Over half of the animals with 10% restoration of DA levels show not only a full compensation of amphetamine-induced ipsilateral rotation but also exhibit a contralateral turning bias (Schmidt et al. 1983). Approximately 120 surviving catecholaminergic cells (i.e., equivalent to about 1–2% of the normal number of DA neurons constituting the intrinsic nigrostriatal projection system, cf. Björklund and Lindvall 1984) are required to compensate rotational bias when grafts are placed into the dorsal striatum (Brundin et al. 1985). Analysis of DOPAC : DA ratios and DOPA accumulation after DOPA-decarboxylase inhibition indicates that the grafted DA neurons are spontaneously active and have a transmitter turnover 50–100% higher than normal nigrostriatal DA neurons (Schmidt et al. 1983). These findings are of particular interest considering that the few DA neurons that remain in PD patients have been shown to be hyperactive (Scatton et al. 1983).

In more recent studies, using injections of multiple deposits of cells in the neostriatum, reversal of all the behavioral asymmetries, including the sensory neglect, was seen in the unilaterally 6-OHDA-lesioned animals (Dunnett et al. 1983a).

Additionally, both unilateral and bilateral grafts contribute to an amelioration of some aspects of the "bilateral 6-OHDA syndrome," including the sensorimotor and akinetic aspects of the syndrome. However, only marginal effects on aphagia and adipsia were observed, and the rats remained dependent on intragastric feeding (Dunnett et al. 1983b).

The mechanism of function of intracerebral DA-containing grafts may vary according to the technique used. Whereas the intraventricular grafts of Freed and Perlow are likely to exert their major effects via a diffusion of transmitter released into the CSF, we have recently demonstrated at the electron microscopic level that the cells in solid grafts placed in a cortical cavity form synaptic connections with neurons in the host neostriatum. Interestingly, a portion of the synapses exhibited an abnormal arrangement, and a larger than normal proportion of them were found on the somata of giant striatal neurons that possess EM characteristics of cholinergic neurons (Freund et al. 1985). Whether these synaptic contacts are necessary or sufficient for functional recovery is not yet clear.

The performance to date of four clinical trials with autologous transplantations of adrenal medullary tissue to the caudate nucleus of PD patients has drawn particular attention to the research on transplantation of DA-rich CNS tissue. In addition to the significant ethical problems involved, there are major problems facing clinical applications. Until recently transplantation studies on primates have been hampered by the lack of a good primate model of PD. However, the demonstration that intravenous administration of the drug MPTP causes DA depletion in monkeys (Burns et al. 1983) as in humans (Langston et al. 1983) has created an interesting primate homolog of a form of drug-induced Parkinsonism and analog of idiopathic Parkinson's disease, which may be of great importance for developing more selective ameliorative procedures, both pharmacologically and with the aid of neuronal grafting.

Conclusion

Animal models of neurological diseases serve important roles in biomedical research. Correlational models such as the unilateral 6-OHDA lesion of the nigrostriatal bundle and the subsequent drug-induced rotation as a model for Parkinson's disease provide a simple, reproducible, well-characterized system to test new pharmacological and experimental therapies as well as to better understand the functional role that dopamine plays in the mammalian CNS. Analogous models such as the IA-induced destruction of the striatum as a model of Huntington's disease, with its parallel biochemical, anatomical, and behavioral changes, can act as a source of insights into collateral systems affected by striatal damage as well as help to specify structure-function relationships. Potential homologous models such as that provided by taking advantage of the normal pathological changes that occur in subpopulations of aged rats as a model of age-related impairments in humans can, in addition to providing a screening tool for potential therapies, be used to reveal potential etiologies of specific age-related functional deficits.

Intracerebral grafting should be useful in identifying the anatomical structures and transmitter systems that are both necessary and sufficient for the initial deficit or for restoring normal function. As the use of intracerebral grafting expands in this context, we will certainly learn more about its potential and limitations.

Acknowledgments. The skillful technical assistance of Carine Jönsson, Yvette Jönsson, Birgit Haraldsson, Gertrude Stridsberg, Jan Berglund, Ulla Jarl, and Kerstin Fogelström is gratefully acknowledged.

Supported by grants from the National Institute of Aging (AG 06088) and from the Swedish MRC (04X-3874).

References

Alihanka, J., Laihinen, A., Rinne, U.K. (1983). Autonomic nervous activities and motor patterns during sleep in patients with Parkinson's disease. Neurosci. Lett. 14, 55.

Alzheimer, A. (1911). Huntingtoniche chorea und die choreatichen Bewegungen uberhaupt. Z. Neur. Psych. 3, 891.

Arendt, T., Bigl, V., Arendt, A., Tennstedt, A. (1983). Loss of neurons in the nucleus basalis of Meynart in Alzheimer's disease, paralysis agitans and Korsakoff's disease. Acta Neuropathol. 61, 101–108.

Azmitia, E.C., Perlow, M.J., Brennan, M.S., Lauder, S.M. (1981). Fetal raphe and hippocampal transplants into adult and aged C57 BL/6N mice: A preliminary immunocytochemical study. Brain Res. Bull. 7, 703–710.

Barnes, C.A., McNaughton, B.L., O'Keefe, J. (1983). Loss of place specificity in hippocampal complex spike cells of senescent rat. Neurobiol. Aging 4, 113–119.

Bartus, R.T., Dean, R.L., Beer, B., Lippa, A.S. (1982). The cholinergic hypotheses of geriatric memory dysfunction. Science 217, 408–417.

Ben-Ari, Y., Tremblay, E., Ottersen, O.P., Naquet, R. (1979). Evidence suggesting secondary epileptogenic lesions after kainic acid: Pretreatment with diazepam reduces distant but not local brain damage. Brain Res. 165, 362–365.

Bird, E.D. (1980). Chemical pathology of Huntington's disease. Ann. Rev. Pharmacol. Toxicol. 20, 533–551.

Birkmayer, W., Hornykiewicz, O. (1961). Der L-3,4-Dioxyphenylalanin (=DOPA)-Effect bei der Parkinson-Akinese. Wien. Klin. Wochenschr. 73, 787–788.

Björklund, A., Dunnett, S.B., Stenevi, U., Lewis, M.E., Iversen, S.D. (1980a). Functional reinnervation of the neostriatum in the adult rat by use of intraparenchymal grafting of dissociated cell suspensions from the substantia nigra. Cell Tiss. Res. 212, 39–45.

Björklund, A., Dunnett, S.B., Stenevi, U., Lewis, M.E., Iversen, S.D. (1980b). Reinnervation of the denervated striatum by substantia nigra transplants: Functional consequences as revealed by pharmacological and sensorimotor testing. Brain Res. 199, 307–333.

Björklund, A., Lindvall, O. (1984). Dopamine-containing systems in the CNS. In: Handbook of Chemical Neuroanatomy. Vol. 2: Classical transmitters in the CNS. Björklund, A., Hökfelt, T., Kuhar, M.J. (eds.). Amsterdam: Elsevier Science Publishers B.V. In press.

Björklund, A., Stenevi, U. (1977). Reformation of the severed septo hippocampal cholinergic pathway in the adult rat by transplanted septal neurones. Cell Tiss. Res. 185, 289–302.

Björklund, A., Stenevi, U. (1979a). Reconstruction of the nigro striatal dopamine pathway by intracerebral nigral implants. Brain Res. 177, 555–560.

Björklund, A., Stenevi, U. (1979b). Reconstruction of brain circuitries by neural transplants. Trends Neurosci. 2, 301–306.

Björklund, A., Stenevi, U. (1984). Intracerebral neural implants: Neuronal replacement and reconstruction of damaged circuitries. Ann. Rev. Neurosci. 7, 229–308.

Björklund, A., Stenevi, U., Dunnett, S.B., Gage, F.H. (1982). Cross-species neural grafting in a rat model of Parkinson's disease. Nature 298, 652–654.

Björklund, A., Stenevi, U., Dunnett, S.B., Iversen, S.D. (1981). Functional reactivation of the deafferented neostriatum by nigral transplants. Nature 289, 497–499.

Björklund, A., Stenevi, U., Schmidt, R.D., Dunnett, S.B., Gage, F.H. (1983a). Intracerebral grafting of neuronal cell suspensions. I. Introduction and general methods of preparation. Acta Physiol. Scand., Suppl. 522, 1–7.

Björklund, A., Stenevi, U., Schmidt, R.H., Dunnett, S.B., Gage, F.G. (1983b). Intracerebral grafting of neuronal cell suspensions. II. Survival and growth of nigral cell suspensions implanted in different brain sites. Acta Physiol. Scand., Suppl. 522, 9–18.

Björklund, A., Stenevi, U., Svendgaard, N.A. (1976). Growth of tranplanted monoaminergic neurones into the adult hippocampus along the perforant path. Nature 262, 787–790.

Brundin, P., Isacson, O., Björklund, A. (1985). Monitoring of cell viability in suspensions of embryonic CNS tissue and its criterion for intracerebral graft survival. Brain Res, 331, 251–259.

Bruyn, G.W. (1968). Huntington's disease chorea. Historical, clinical and laboratory synopsis. In: Handbook of Clinical Neurology, Vol. 6. Vinkers, P.J., Bruyn, P.J. (eds).

Bruyn, G.W. (1982). Neurotransmitters in Huntington's chorea—a clinician's view. Prog. Brain Res. 55, 445–464.

Burns, R.S. Chiuch, C.C., Markey, S.P., Ebert, M.H., Jacobowitz, D.M., Kopin, I.J.

(1983). A primate model of parkinsonism: Selective destruction of dopaminergic neurons in the pars compacta of the substantia nigra by N-methyl-4-phenyl-1,2,3,6-tetrahydropyridine. Proc. Natl. Acad. Sci. USA 80, 4546–4550.

Campbell, B.A., Krauter, E.E., Wallace, J.E. (1980). Animal models of aging: Sensory-motor and cognitive function in the aging rat. In: Psychology of Aging: Problems and Prospectives. Stein, D.G. (ed.). Amsterdam: Elsevier North-Holland Inc., pp. 201–226.

Candy, J.M., Perry, R.H., Perry, E.K. (1983). Pathological changes in the nucleus of Meynert in Alzheimer's and Parkinson's diseases. J. Neurol. Sci. 54, 59, 277–289.

Carlsson, A. (1959). The occurrences, distribution and physiological role of catecholamines in the nervous system. Pharm. Rev. 11, 490–493.

Cohen, G. (1983). The pathobiology of Parkinson's disease: Biochemical aspects of dopamine neuron senescence. J. Neural Transm. Suppl. 19, 89–103.

Coyle, J., Price, D., DeLong, M. (1983). Alzheimer's disease: A disorder of cortical cholinergic innervation. Science 219, 1184–1190.

Coyle, J.T., Schwarcz, R. (1976). Lesion of striatal neurones with kainic acid provides a model for Huntington's chorea. Nature 263, 244–246.

Cubells, J.F., Joseph, J.A. (1981). Neostriatal dopamine receptor loss and behavioural deficits in the senescent rat. Life Sci. 28, 1215–1218.

Das, G.D., Hallas, B.H., Das, K.G. (1980). Transplantation of brain tissue in the brain of rat. I. Growth characteristics of neocortical transplants from embryos of different ages. Am. J. Anat. 158, 135–145.

Dawbarn, D., Brundin, P., Isacson, O., Gage, F.H., Emson, P.C., Björklund, A. (1985). Striatal transplants in ibotenic acid lesioned rats: Survival of neurones and development of peptide immunoreactivity. In preparation.

Deckel, A.W., Robinson, R.G., Coyle, J.T., Sandberg, P.R. Reversal of long-term locomotor abnormalities in the kainic acid model of Huntington's disease by day 18 fetal striatal implants. Europ. J. Pharmacol. 93, 287.

Del Conte, G. (1907). Einpflanzungen von embryonalem Gewebe ins Gehirn. Beitr. Pathol. Anat. Allg. Pathol. 42, 193–202.

Divac, I., Rosvold, H.E., Schwarcbart, M.K. (1967). Behavioural effects of selective ablation of the caudate nucleus. J. Comp. Phys. Psychol. 63, 184–190.

Dunn, E.H. (1917). Primary and secondary findings in a series of attempts to transplant cerebral cortex in albino rat. J. Comp. Neurol. 27, 565–582.

Dunnett, S.B., Björklund, A. (1983). Conditioned turning in rats: Dopmainergic involvement in the initiation of movement rather then the movement itself. Neurosci. Lett. 41, 173–178.

Dunnett, S.B., Björkiund, A., Schmidt, R.H., Stenevi, U., Iversen, S.D. (1983a). Intracerebral grafting of neuronal cell suspensions. IV. Behavioural recovery in rats with unilateral 6-OHDA lesions following implantation of nigral cell suspensions in different brain sites. Acta Physiol. Scand. Suppl. 522, 29–37.

Dunnett, S.B., Björklund, A., Schmidt, R.H., Stenevi, U., Iversen, S.D. (1983b). Intracerebral grafting of neuronal cell suspensions. V. Behavioral recovery in rats with bilateral 6-OHDA lesions following implantation of nigral cell suspensions. Acta Physiol. Scand. Suppl. 522, 39–47.

Dunnett, S.B., Björklund, A., Stenevi, U. (1983c). Dopamine-rich transplants in experimental Parkinsonism. Trends Neurosci. 6, 266–270.

Dunnett, S.B., Björklund, A., Stenevi, U., Iversen, S.D. (1981a). Behavioral recovery following transplantation of substantia nigra in rats subjected to 60HDA lesions of the nigrostriatal pathway. I. Unilateral lesions. Brain Res. 215, 147–161.

Dunnett, S.B., Björklund, A., Stenevi, U., Iversen, S.D. (1981b). Grafts of embryonic substantia nigra reinnervating the ventrolateral striatum ameliorate sensorimotor impairments and akinesia in rats with 6-OHDA lesions of the nigrostriatal pathway. Brain Res. 229, 209–217.

Dunnett, S.B., Björklund, A., Stenevi, U., Iversen, S.D. (1981c). Behavioural recovery following transplantation of substantia nigra in rats subjeced to 60HDA lesions of the nigrostriatal pathway. II. Bilateral lesions. Brain Res. 229, 457–470.

Dunnett, S.B., Iversen, S.D. (1980). Regulatory impairments following selective kainic acid lesions of the neostriatum. Beh. Brain Res. 1, 497–506.

Dunnett, S.B., Iversen, S.D. (1981). Learning impairments following selective kainic acid-induced lesions within the neostriatum of rats. Beh. Brain Res. 2, 189–209.

Dunnett, S.B., Low, W.C., Iversen, S.D., Stenevi, U., Björklund, A. (1982). Septal transplants restore maze learning in rats with fornix-fimbria lesions. Brain Res. 251, 335–348.

Duvoisin, R.C. (1976). Parkinsonism: Animal analogues of the human disorder. In: The Basal Ganglia. Yahr, M.D. (ed.). New York: Raven Press, pp. 293–303.

Earle, K.M. (1973). Pathology and experimental models of Huntington's chorea. Adv. Neurol. 1, 341–351.

Fray, P.J., Dunnett, S.B., Iversen, S.D., Björklund, A., Stenevi, U. (1983). Nigral transplants reinnervating the dopamine-depleted neostriatum can sustain intracranial self-stimulation. Science 219, 416–419.

Freed, W.J. (1983). Functional brain tissue transplantation: Reversal of lesion-induced rotation by intraventricular substantia nigra and adrenal medulla grafts, with a note on intracranial retinal grafts. Biol. Psych. 18, 1205–1267.

Freed, W.J., Karoum, F., Spoor, H.E., Morihisa, J.M., Olson, L., Wyatt, R.J. (1983a). Catecholamine content of intracerebral adrenal medulla grafts. Brain Res. 269, 184–189.

Freed, W.J., Ko, G.N., Niehoff, D.L. (1983b). Normalization of spiroperidol binding in the denervated rat striatum by homologous grafts of substantia nigra. Science 222, 937–939.

Freed, W.J., Morihisa, J.M., Spoor, E. (1981). Transplanted adrenal chromaffin cells in rat brain reduce lesion-induced rotational behavior. Nature 292, 351–352.

Freed, W.J., Perlow, M.J., Karoum, M.J., Seiger, Å., Olson, L., Hoffer, B.J., Wyatt, R.J. (1980). Restoration of dopaminergic function by grafting of fetal rat substantia nigra to the caudate-nucleus: Long-term behavioural, biochemical, and histochemical studies. Ann. Neurol. 8, 510–519.

Freund, T., Bolam, P., Björklund, A., Stenevi, U., Dunnett, S.B., Smith, A.D. (1985). Synaptic connections of nigral transplants reinnervating the host neostriatum: A TH-immuocytochemical study. J. Neurosci. In press.

Frey, K.A., Agranoff, B.W. (1983). Barbiturate-enhanced detection of brain lesions by carbon-14-labelled 2-deoxyglucose autoradiography. Science 219, 889–891.

Gage, F.H., Björklund, A., Stenevi, U., Dunnett, S.B. (1983a). Intracerebral grafting in the aging brain. In: Aging of the Brain. Gaspar, W.H., Traber, J. (eds.). Amsterdam: Elsevier Science Publishers B.V.

Gage, F.H., Björklund, A., Stenevi, U., Dunnett, S.B. (1983b). Intracerebral grafting of neuronal cell suspensions. VII. Cell survival and axonal outgrowth of dopaminergic and cholinergic cells in the aged brain. Acta Physiol. Scand. Suppl. 522, 67–75.

Gage, F.H., Björklund, A., Stenevi, U., Dunnett, S.B., Kelly, P.A.T. (1984a). Intrahippocampal septal grafts ameliorate learning impairments in aged rats. Science. 225, 533–535.

Gage, F.H., Dunnett, S.B., Björklund, A. (1984b). Spatial learning and motor deficits in aged rats. Neurobiol. Aging. 5, 45–48.

Gage, F.H., Dunnett, S.B., Stenevi, U., Björklund, A., (1983c). Aged rats: Recovery of motor impairments by intrastriatal nigral grafts. Science 221, 966–969.

Gage, F.H., Kelly, P.A.T., Björklund, A. (1984c). Regional changes in brain glucose metabolism reflect cognitive impairments in aged rats. J. Neurosci. 4, 2856–2865.

Garron, D.C. (1973). Huntington's chorea and schizophrenia. Adv. in Neurol. 1, 729–734.

Gash, D., Sladek, J.R., Sladek, C.D. (1980). Functional development of grafted vasopressin neurons. Science 210, 1367–1369.

Geinisman, Y., Bondareff, W., Dodge, J.T. (1977). Partial deafferentation of neurons in the dentate gyrus of the senescent rat. Brain Res. 134, 541–545.

Gusella, J.F., et al. (1983). A polymorphic DNA marker genetically linked to Huntington's disease. Nature 306, 234–238.

Glick, S.D., Cox, R.D. (1978). Nocturnal rotation in normal rats: Correlation with an amphetamine-induced rotation and effects of nigrostriatal lesions. Brain Res. 150, 149–161.

Guldin, W.O., Markowitsch, H.J. (1981). No detectable remote lesions following massive intrastriatal injections of ibotenic acid. Brain Res. 225, 446–451.

Gebbink, T.B. (1968). Huntington's chorea. Fibre changes in the basal ganglia. In: Handbook of Clinical Neurology, Vol. 6. Vinken, P.J., Bruyn, G.W. (eds.). pp. 399–408.

Hallas, B.H., Das, G.D., Das. K.G. (1980). Transplantation of brain tissue in the brain of rat. II. Growth characteristics of neocortical transplants in hosts of different ages. Am. J. Anat., 158, 147–159.

Hornykiewicz, O. (1963). Die topische Lokalisation und das Verhalten von Noradrenalin und Dopamin (3-Hydroxytyramin) in der Substanti nigra des normalen und Parkinsonkranken Menschen. Wien. Klin. Wochensch. 18, 309–312.

Isacson, O., Brundin, P., Gage, F.H., Björklund, A. (1985a). Neural grafting in a rat model of Huntington's disease: Progressive neurochemical changes after neostriatal ibotenate lesions and striatal tissue grafting. J. Neurosci. In press.

Isacson, O., Brundin, P., Gage, F.H., Björklund, A. (1985b). A behavioural characterization of rats with neostriatal ibotenic acid lesions and striatal neuronal transplants. In preparation.

Isacson, O., Brundin, P., Kelly, P.A.T., Gage, F.H., Björklund, A. (1984c). Functional neuronal replacement by grafted striatal neurones in the ibotenic acid-lesioned rat striatum. Nature, 311, 458–460.

Jaeger, C.B., Lund, R.D. (1980). Transplantation of embryonic occipital cortex to the brain of newborn rats. An autoradiographic study of transplant histogenesis. Exp. Brain Res. 40, 265–272.

Jaeger, C.B., Lund, R.D. (1981). Transplantation of embryonic occipital cortex to the brain of newborn rats: A Golgi study of mature and developing transplants. J. Comp. Neurol. 200, 213–230.

Javoy-Agid, F., Ruberg, M., Taquet, H. (1982). Biochemical neuropathology of Parkinson's disease. Proceedings of the VIIth International Symposium on Parkinson's Disease, June 1982, Frankfurt, Adv. Neurol. New York: Raven Press.

Joseph, J.A., Bartus, R.T., Clody, D., Morgan, D., Finch, C., Beer, B., Sesack, S. (1983). Psychomotor performance in the senescent rodent: Reduction of deficits via striatal dopamine receptor up-regulation. Neurobiol. Aging 4, 313–319.

Kelly, P.A.T., Graham, D.I., McCulloch, J. (1982). Specific alterations in local cerebral glucose utilization following striatal lesions. Brain Res. 201, 173–184.

Kelly, P.A.T., McCulloch, J. (1982). Gaba-ergic and dopaminergic influences on glucose utilization in the extrapyramidal system. Brit. J. Pharmacol. 76, 290.

Kelly, P.H., Seviour, P.W., Iversen, S.D. (1975). Amphetamine and apomorphine responses in the rat following 6-OHDA lesions of the nucleus accumbens septi and corpus striatum. Brain Res. 94, 507–522.

Kimula, Y., Utsuyama, M., Yoshimura, M., Tomonaga, M. (1983). Element analysis of Lewy and adrenal bodies in Parkinson's disease by electron probe microanalysis. Acta. Neuropathol. (Berl.) 59, 233–236.

Kimura, H., McGeer, E.G., McGeer, P.L. (1980). Metabolic alterations in an animal model of Huntington's disease using the ^{14}C-deoxyglucose method. J. Neural Transm. Suppl. 16, 103–109.

Koestner, A. (1973). Animal models for dyskinetic disorders. Adv. Neurol. 1, 625–645.

Krammer, E.B. (1980). Anterograde and transsynaptic degeneration 'en cascade' in basal ganglia induced by intrastriatal injection of kainic acid: An animal analogue of Huntington's disease. Brain Res. 196, 209–219.

Krieger, D., Perlow, M.J., Gibson, M.J., Dames, T.F., Zimmerman, E.A., Ferin, M., Charlton, H.M. (1982). Brain grafts reverse hypogonadism of gonadotropin-releasing hormone deficiency. Nature 298, 468–471.

Kromer, L.F., Björklund, A., Stenevi, U. (1983). Intracephalic neural implants in the adult rat brain. I. Growth and mature organization of brain stem, cerebellar and hippocampal implants. J. Comp. Neurol. 218, 433–459.

Labbe, R., Firl, A., Mufson, E.J., Stein, D.G. (1983). Fetal brain transplants: Reduction of cognitive deficits in rats with frontal cortex lesions. Science 221, 470–472.

Langston, J.W., Ballard. P., Tetrud, J.W., Irwin, I. (1983). Chronic Parkinsonism in humans due to a product of mepiridine analog synthesis. Science 219, 979–980.

Lieberman, A., Dziatolowski, M., Kupersmith, M. (1979). Dementia in Parkinson's disease. Ann. Neurol. 6, 355–359.

Low, W.C., Lewis, P.R., Bunch, S.T. (1983). Embryonic neuronal transplants across a major histocompatibility barrier: Survival and specificity of innervation. Brain Res. 262, 228–234.

Low, W.C., Lewis, P.R., Bunch, S.T., Dunnett, S.B., Thomas, S.R., Iversen, S.D., Björklund, A., Stenevi, U. (1982). Functional recovery following neural transplantation of embryonic septal nuclei in adult rats with septohippocampal lesions. Nature 300, 260–262.

Lund, R.D., Harvey, A.R., Jaeger, C.B., McLoon, S.C. (1982). Transplantation of embryonic neural tissue to the tectal region of newborn rats. In: Changing Concepts of the Nervous System. Morrison, A.R., Strick, P.I., (eds.). New York: Academic Press.

Mann, D.M.A., Yates, P.O. (1983a). Possible role of neuromelanin in the pathogenesis of Parkinson's disease. Mech. Aging Develop. 21, 193–203.

Mann, D.M.A., Yates, P.O. (1983b). Pathological basis for neurotransmitter changes in Parkinson's disease. Neuropath. Appl. Neurobio. 9, 3–19.

Mann, J.J., Stanley, M., Kaplan, R.D., Sweeney, J., Neophytides, A. (1983). Central catecholamine metabolism in vivo and the cognitive and motor deficits in Parkinson's disease. J. Neurol. Neurosurg. Psychiat. 46, 905–910.

Marsden, C.D. (1982). Basal ganglia disease. The Lancet No. 8308, Vol. 2, 1141.

Marsden, C.D. (1983) Neuromelanin and Parkinson's disease. J. Neural Transm. 19, 121–141.

Marsden, C.D., Duvoisin, R.C., Jenner, P., Parkes, J.D., Pycock, C., Tarsy, D. (1975). Relationship between animal models and clinical parkinsonism. Adv. Neurol. 9, 165–175.

Marshall, J.F., Berrios, N. (1979). Movement disorders of aged rats: Reversal by dopamine receptor stimulation. Science 206, 477–479.

Marshall, J.F., Berrios, N., Sawyer, S. (1980). Neostriatal dopamine and sensory inattention. J. Comp. Phys. Psych. 94, 833–846.

Marshall, J.F., Gotthelf, T. (1979). Sensory inattention in rats with 6-hydroxydopamine-induced degeneration of ascending dopaminergic neurons: Apomorphine-induced reversal of deficits. Exp. Neurol. 65, 398–411.

Martin, J.P. (1967). Curvature of the spine in postencephalitic parkinsonism. In: The Basal Ganglia and Posture. London: Pittman, pp. 100–105.

Mason, S.T., Fibiger, H.C. (1978). Kainic acid lesions of the striatum: Behavioural sequelae similar to Huntington's chorea. Brain Res. 155, 313–329.

Mason, S.T., Fibiger, H.C. (1979). Kainic lesions of the striatum in rats mimic the spontaneous motor abnormalities of Huntington's disease Neuropharmacol. 18, 403–407.

Mauborgne, A., Javoy-Agid, F., Legrand, J.C., Agid, Y., Cesselin, F. (1983). Decrease of Substance P-like immunoreactivity in the substantia nigra and pallidum of parkinsonian brains. Brain Res. 268, 167–170.

McGeer, E.G., McGeer, P.L. (1976). Duplication of biochemical changes of Huntington's chorea by intrastriatal injection of glutamic and kainic acids. Nature 263, 517–519.

McGeer, E.G., McGeer, P.L. (1981). Neurotoxins as tools in neurobiology. Int. Rev. Neurol. 22, 173–204.

McLoon, S.C., Lund, R.D., (1980a). Identification of cells in retinal transplants which project to host visual centers: A horseradish perioxidase study in rats. Brain Res., 197, 431–495.

McLoon, S.C., Lund, R.D. (1980b). Specific projections of retina transplanted to rat brain. Exp. Brain Res. 40, 273–282.

Metter, E.J., Riege, W.H., Kameyama, M., Phelps, M.E., Kuhl, D.E. (1982). Correlational differences of regional glucose metabolism in Huntington, Parkinson, and Alzheimer diseases. Annals Neurol. 12, 88.

Morris, R.G.M. (1981). Spatial localization does not require the presence of locus cues. Learn. Motiv. 12, 239–260.

Mountjoy, C., Roth, M., Evans, N., Evans, H. (1983). Cortical neuronal counts in normal elderly control and demented patients. Neurobiol. Aging 4, 1–11.

Nachtsheim, H. (1934). Schuttelähmung–ein Beispiel fur ein einfach mendelndes rezessives Nervenleiden beim Kaninchen. Erbarzt 1, 36–38.

Nadler, J.V., Perry, B.W., Cotman, C.W. (1978). Intraventricular kainic acid preferentially destroys hippocampal pyramidal cells. Nature 271, 676–677.

Neff, N.H., Barrett, R.E., Costa, E. (1969). Selective depletion of caudate nucleus dopamine and serotonin during chronic manganese dioxide administration to squirrel monkey. Experientia 25, 1140–1141.

Olson, L., Seiger, Å., Strömberg, I. (1982). Intraocular transplantation in rodents. A detailed account of procedure and example of its use in neurobiology with special reference to brain tissue grafting. In: Advances in Cellular Neurobiology, Vol. 4. Fed, S. (ed.). New York: Academic Press.

Perlow, M.J. (1980). The brain and subarachnoid space as possible sites for endocrine tissue transplantation. Res. Bull. 6, 171–176.

Perlow, M.J., Freed, W.J., Hoffer, B.J., Seiger, Å., Olson, L., Wyatt, R.J. (1979). Brain grafts reduce motor abnormalities produced by destruction of nigrostriatal dopamine system. Science 204, 643–647.

Perlow, M.J., Kumakura, K., Guidotti, A. (1980). Prolonged survival of bovine adrenal chromaffin cells in rat cerebral ventricles. Proc. Natl. Acad. Sci. USA 77, 5278–5281.

Pijnenberg, A.J.J., Van Rossum, J.M. (1973). Stimulation of locomotor activity following injection of dopamine into the nucleus accumbens. J. Pharm. Pharmac. 25, 1003–1005.

Pisa, M., Sanberg, P.R., Fibiger, H.C. (1981). Striatal injections of kainic acid selectively impair serial memory performance in the rat. Exp. Neurol. 74, 633–653.

Plaitakis, A., Berl, S., Yahr, M.D. (1982). Abnormal glutamate metabolism in adult-onset degenerative neurological disorders. Science 216, 193–196.

Portin, R., Reininko, R., Rinne, U.K., (1984). Neurophysiological disturbances and cerebral atrophy determined by computerized tomography in Parkinsonian patients with long-term levodopa treatment. In: Advances in Neurology 40. Hassler, R.G., Christ, J.F. (eds.). New York: Raven Press, pp. 219–227.

Sabel, B.A., Stein, D.G., (1981). Extensive loss of subcortical neurons in the aging rat brain. Exp. Neurol. 73, 507–516.

Saltykow, S. (1907). Versuche uber Gehirplantation zugleich ein Betrag zur Kentriss der Vorgänge an den zelligen Gehirne-elementen. Arch. Psychiatr. Nervenkr. 40, 329–388.

Sanberg, P.R., Fibiger, H.C. (1979). Body weight, feeding and drinking behaviours in rats with kainic acid-induced lesions of striatal neurons—with a note on body weight symptomatology in Huntington's disease. Exp. Neurol. 66, 444–466.

Scatton, B., Javoy-Agid, F., Rouquier, L., Dubois, B., Agid, Y. (1983). Reduction of cortical dopamine, noradrenaline, serotonin and their metabolites in Parkinson's disease. Brain Res. 275, 321–328.

Schallert, T., Upchurch, M., Wilcox, R.E., Vaughn, D.M. (1983). Posture-independent sensorimotor analysis of inter hemispheric receptor asymmetry in neostriatum. Pharmacol. Biochem. Behav. 18, 753–759.

Schmidt, R.H., Björklund, A., Stenevi, U. (1981). Intracerebral grafting of dissociated CNS tissue suspensions: A new approach for neuronal transplantation to deep brain sites. Brain Res. 218, 347–356.

Schmidt, R.H., Björklund, A., Stenevi, U., Dunnett, S.B., Gage, F.H. (1983). Intracerebral grafting of neuronal cell suspension. III. Activity of intrastriatal nigral suspension implants as assessed by measurements of dopamine synthesis and metabolism. Acta Physiol. Scand. Suppl. 522, 19–28.

Schmidt, R.H., Ingvar, M., Lindvall, O., Stenevi, U., Björklund, A. (1982). Functional activity of substantia nigra grafts reinnervating the striatum: Neurotransmitter metabolism and (^{14}C)2-deoxy-D-glucose autoradiography. J. Neurochem 38, 737–748.

Schwarcz, R., Coyle, J.T. (1977). Striatal lesions with kainic acid: Neurochemical characteristics. Brain Res. 127, 235–249.

Schwarcz, R., Hökfelt, T., Fuxe, K., Jonsson, G., Goldstein, M., Terenius, L. (1979). Ibotenic acid-induced neuronal degeneration: A morphological and neurochemical study. Exp. Brain Res. 37, 199–216.

Sims, N.R., Marek, K.L., Bowen, D.M., Davison, A.N. (1982). Production of (^{14}C)acetylcholine and (^{14}C)carbon dioxide from $(U^{14}C)$glucose in tissue prisms from aging rat brain. J. Neurochem. 38, 488–492.

Sokoloff, L. (1977). Relation between physiological function and energy metabolism in the central nervous system. J. Neurochem. 29, 13–26.

Spokes, E.G.S. (1980). Neurochemical alterations in Huntington's chorea. Brain 103, 179–210.

Stenevi, U., Björklund, A., Dunnett, S.B. (1980). Functional reinnervation of the denervated neostriatum by nigral transplants. Peptides 1 Suppl. 1, 111–116.

Stenevi, U., Björklund, A., Svendgaard, N.A. (1976). Transplantations of central and peripheral monoamine neurons to the adult rat brain: Techniques and conditions for survival. Brain Res. 114, 1–20.

Studler, J.M., Javoy-Agid, F., Cesselin, F., Legrand, J.C., Agid, Y. (1982). CCK-8 immunoreactivity distribution in the human brain: Selective decrease in the substantia nigra from parkinsonian patients. Brain Res. 243, 176–179.

Taquet, H., Javoy-Agid, F., Cesselin, F., Agid, Y. (1981). Methionine-enkephalin deficiency in brains of patients with Parkinson's disease. The Lancet 1, 1367–1368.

Taquet, H., Javoy-Agid, F., Haman, M., Legrand, J.C., Agid, Y., Cesselin, F. (1983). Parkinson's disease affects differently Met^5-and Leu^5-enkephalin in the human brain. Brain Res. 280, 379–382.

Terry, R., Katzman, R. (1983). Senile dementia of the Alzheimer type. Ann. Neurol. 5, 497–506.

Thompson, W.G. (1890). Successful brain grafting. N.Y. Med. J. 51, 701–702.

Trabucchi, M., Albizzati, M.G., Frattola, L., Scarlato, G. (1979). Hemiparkinsonism. A human model for studying dopaminergic supersensitivity. Arch. Neurol. 36, 246–248.

Ungerstedt, U. (1968). 6-hydroxydopamine induced degeneration of central monoamine neurons. Europ. J. Pharmacol. 5, 107–110.

Ungerstedt, U., Arbuthnott, G.W. (1970). Quantitative recording of rotational behavior in rats after 6-hydroxydopamine lesions of the nigrostriatal dopamine system. Brain Res. 24, 485–493.

Unsicker, K., Krisch, B., Otten, U., Thoenen, H. (1978). Nerve growth factor-induced fiber outgrowth for isolated rat adrenal chromaffin cells: Impairment by glucocorticoids. Proc. Natl. Acad. Sci. USA 75, 3498–3502.

Wallace, J.E., Krauter, E.E., Campbell, B.A. (1980). Animal models of declining memory in the aged: Short-term and spatial memory in the aged rat. J. Gerontol. 35, 355–363.

Wells, J., McAllister, J.P. (1982). The development of cerebellar primordia transplanted to the neocortex of the rat. Devel. Brain Res. 4, 167–179.

Whittier, J.R., Orr, A. (1962). Hyperkinesis and other physiologic effects of caudate deficits in the adult albino rat. Neurology 12, 529–539.

Wooten, G.F., Collins, R.C. (1980). Regional brain glucose utilization following intrastriatal injections of kainic acid. Brain Res. 201, 173–184.

Yahr, M.D. (1979). The Parkinsonian syndrome. In: A Textbook of Neurology, Merritt, H. (ed.). Lee & Fibiger, pp. 508–529.

Zaczek, R., Simonton, S., Coyle, J.T. (1980). Local and distant neuronal degeneration following intrastriatal injections of kainic acid. J. Neuropathol. Exp. Neurol. 39, 245–264.

Chapter 5

Differentiation of Rat Fetal Retina Transplanted to the Occipital Cortex either in Isolation or Together with a Second Transplant of Superior Colliculus to Induce Sprouting of Optic Fibers

Murray A. Matthews*

Background

The coordinated development of neurons within the central nervous system is considered to follow an intrinsic, genetically coded series of morphological and biochemical changes during initial phases of growth, but the process of maturation and differentiation seems to be controlled, to some extent, by extrinsic determinants, including precise temporal and spatial interactions with the neurons of other, functionally related, centers (Jacobson 1978). Such interactions involve the establishment of an appropriate complement of afferent fiber inputs that appear to influence the modeling of the dendritic arbor of the postsynaptic cell (Cowan 1970). Similarly, axons arising from these cells must be guided to, and form a functional synaptic contact with, their proper targets (other neurons, muscles, etc.), in order for the cell to completely mature or even survive (Sperry 1963, Gaze, 1970, Cowan 1978).

Guidance mechanisms have also been postulated and are considered to consist of tissue gradients or substrate pathways established during the earliest stages of CNS development that direct the pattern of axonal growth (Hibbard 1965, Katz and Lasek 1981). However, if the position or orientation of the target cells is changed, as, for example, in the optic tectum, axons destined to grow into this area (from the retina) will reorient their direction of growth to reach appropriate tectal neurons, despite the fact that the experimental procedure destroyed possible mechanical cues (Crossland et al. 1974, Yoon 1975, Jacobson and Levine 1975). Such findings tend to favor the chemoaffinity theory of axonal growth and guidance (Sperry 1963), but more importantly suggest that if neurons can be induced to regenerate their injured axonal processes, the

* Department of Anatomy, Louisiana State University Medical Center, New Orleans, Louisiana 70119 U.S.A.

capability might exist to reestablish their connections with proper target centers.

One approach toward examining and understanding mechanisms of neuronal differentiation, plasticity, and axonal growth and guidance, as well as assessing regenerative capacity, has been the removal and transplantation of different components of the CNS of nonmammalian vertebrates from one animal to the brain of a host animal to isolate these components at various stages of development and determine the extent to which they are capable of continuing the process of growth, differentiation, and formation of appropriate connections. Such transplants were found to mature, become histotypically organized, and form reciprocal connections with the brain of the host (Das 1974, Jacobson 1978, Lund 1978). However, many of the nonmammalian forms can almost completely regenerate injured components of their central nervous system, an inherent capacity not enjoyed by mammals to any significant extent. The success of transplantation experiments using these types of animal models would therefore come as no surprise. An obvious progression from these investigations would be to determine the efficacy of performing similar transplantation experiments using the mammalian CNS.

Initial attempts to transplant portions of mammalian CNS tissues were only minimally successful (see review by Das 1974), and these results seemed to emphasize the apparent lack of regenerative ability in such animals. If, however, fetal mammalian CNS components are transplanted to a host animal, a significant proportion of these will continue to grow and mature, with many of the neurons characteristic of the tissue becoming recognizable (Das et al. 1979). Additionally, transplants of fetal tissue have more recently been used to replace CNS components removed from, or congenitally lacking in, the host (Björklund and Stenevi 1979, Perlow et al. 1979, Gash et al. 1979) and to explore the types of connections that are formed between the transplant and the host CNS (Harvey and Lund 1979, Jaeger and Lund 1979, 1980a, Lewis and Cotman 1980, Björklund et al. 1976, Hallas et al. 1980, Oblinger et al. 1980). It has also been shown that such tissues can be transplanted to other ectopic sites such as the anterior chamber of the eye and grow quite well, especially if they are placed in the chamber in tandem with a second CNS transplant, suggesting the presence of some form of trophic interaction (Olson et al. 1979, Björklund et al. 1983).

Our studies were initiated in order to analyze the development of such fetal transplants at the ultrastructural level, principally to document neuronal differentiation and synaptic development under conditions in which normal appropriate connections with the proper target cannot form. The retina was chosen for these studies because of its laminar organization and well-characterized neuronal and synaptic populations, both *in situ* (Weidman and Kuwabara 1969, Sosula and Glow 1970) and in culture, wherein a highly histotypic organization is retained (LaVail and Hild 1971, Smalheiser et al. 1981). We were particularly interested in determining if the normal complement of ganglion cells and synapses differentiates in transplanted retina lacking retino-recipient target cells for the optic projection and if photoreceptor elements form in the absence of pigment cells that would have been removed during the process of transplantation (Matthews 1981, Matthews et al. 1982d).

These studies provided the basis for a second set of experiments in which dual transplants of retina and superior colliculus were placed adjacent to one another in the occipital cortex. This was calculated to provide the isolated retina with the correct target tissue and thereby stimulate the vigorous development of an optic projection (Matthews and West 1982).

Techniques

Timed pregnant Holtzman albino rats were given an injection of [^{3}H] thymidine (10μCi/g body weight) at gestation days 13 and 14 in order to label fetal neurons in the transplant tissue and thereby facilitate their identification after having been allowed to develop in the host. The pregnant rats were then laparotomized on gestation day 15 and the fetuses exteriorized one by one from the uterus, as needed to obtain tissue for transplantation. The eyes were removed, placed in Hams F-10 culture medium, and the retina exposed by cutting away the cornea and lens. The dorsal half of the neural retina was freed of the pigment cell layer as well as surrounding adventitial tissues and set aside until it was ready for placement into the host. The lateral half of the contralateral superior colliculus was also removed from the fetus and used as the correct target tissue for those animals receiving a dual transplant. As a control, non-retino-recipient tissue, medial thalamus, was removed and used for some dual transplants to assess the specificity of orientation of the optic fiber outgrowth.

Neonatal rates were used as host animals and were prepared for the transplantation procedure by cutting a small flap into the skull over the motor cortex. The donor tissue was drawn up into a small glass cannula whose tip was inserted into the skull flap and guided into position over the occipital cortex. The transplant was then extruded and the cannula slowly removed while releasing a small amount of the culture medium in order to inhibit excessive movement of the transplant. These procedures generally followed those given by Das (1974).

Host animals were sacrificed at intervals ranging from 5 to 30 days after transplantation and their brains processed for light or electron microscopic study by methods described in detail elsewhere (Matthews 1973, Matthews et al. 1982a, Matthews and West 1982). Autoradiographs were prepared from alternate slides of light microscopic serial sections (Matthews et al. 1982b) at 2 in order to clearly delineate the borders of the tectal and thalamic transplants and determine if migration of cells out of the transplant had taken place.

A quantitative analysis was also performed to determine the numbers of sensory cells, as well as cells of the inner nuclear layer and ganglion cell layer at 15, 20, and 30 days after transplantation. For this analysis, sets of 20 semithin sections from each block were cut at regular intervals, stained, and photographed at constant magnification.

Results

Isolated Retina

During the early stages of development, retinal transplants tend to curl up and become radially oriented with their scleral or outer surface directed centrally and the vitreal or inner surface occupying the periphery (Figure 5-1). Large numbers of mitotic figures occur at the center of the transplant, and layers of

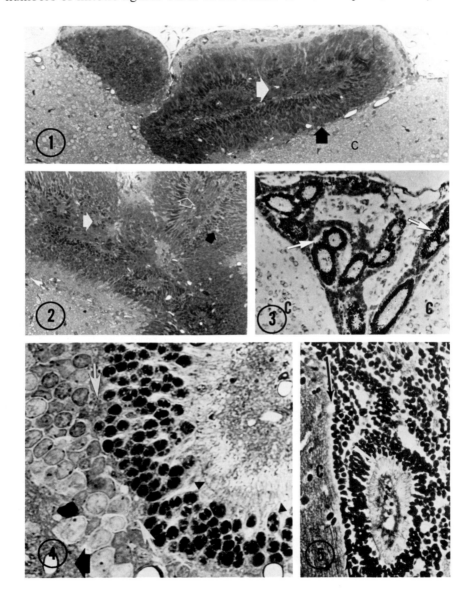

presumptive neuroblasts extend out to the edge. After 10–15 days, the retinal transplants become subdivided into varying numbers of rosettes and the relatively primitive neural elements seen at earlier stages have transformed into cellular categories seen in the normal retina at this stage of development (Figures 5-2 and 5-3). Each rosette displays a lightly stained center surrounded by a cell-rich zone, and these are separated and delineated by a rudimentary outer limiting membrane. The outer zone can be further subdivided into an outer and inner nuclear layer.

At 20–30 days following transplantation (Figure 5-4), examination of rosettes reveals the presence of photoreceptor elements, a definitive outer limiting membrane, sensory cells, recognizable by their small, dark, multilobate nuclei and arrangement into a typical layer of columns of 5–8 cells. The inner nuclear layer contained large numbers of bipolar cells with nuclei of moderate density, and scattered among these were more lightly stained cells suggestive of horizontal or amacrine neurons. The inner and outer plexiform layers could also be distinguished, as well as the ganglion cell layer, but this latter zone

---

Figure 5-1. A typical example of transplanted retina allowed to develop for 5 days. A 2-μm section is shown stained with toluidine blue. The white arrow indicates the original, scleral side of the retina, and the black arrow points to the vitreal surface that is apposed to the host cortex (C). 93×. From Matthews et al. (1982c).

Figure 5-2. A transplant is shown at 15 days and exhibits several rosettes. The white arrow points to a mitotic figure near the center of a rosette while the black arrow depicts the junction between the more centrally located layer of primitive sensory cells and the more lightly stained inner nuclear layer. The open white arrow points to a poorly developed outer limiting membrane. 222×. From Matthews et al. (1982c).

Figure 5-3. A paraffin section stained with cresyl violet and photographed at low magnification illustrates numerous rosettes within a retinal transplant after 15 days. The deeply stained elements are the nuclei of sensory cells that surround a relatively cell-free zone. The moderately stained cells represent the inner nuclear layer that is separated from the sensory cells in a thin outer plexiform layer (arrows). This transplant is deeply embedded into the cortical plate (C). 74×. From Matthews et al. (1982c).

Figure 5-4. An Epon-embedded 2-μm section best illustrates the details of cellular patterns within a rosette at 30 days postoperative. A distinctive outer limiting membrane (arrowheads) separates prominent outer segments from the inner segments and perikarya of the sensory cells. Note the dark, bilobate nuclei of these neurons. Neurons of the inner nuclear layer vary in staining intensity and are separated from the sensory cell layer by a thin outer plexiform layer (white arrows). The inner plexiform zone is indicated by a large black arrow and a ganglion cell can be seen at the lower left corner of the micrograph. 481×. From Matthews et al. (1982c).

Figure 5-5. A section stained with the Bodian silver method shows the host cortex (C) adjacent to a portion of the retina after 20 days. Numerous axons occur within the cortex but none appear to course between the host-transplant interface (large arrows). Note the outer limiting membrane and developing outer segments at the center of the rosette (white arrow). 222×. From Matthews et al. (1982c).

appeared to contain fewer cells than normal retina at the same stage of development.

Sets of serial sections encompassing the transplant and surrounding host cortex were stained with the Bodian silver method, and these revealed that only a minimal number of axons coursed through the interface between host and transplant (Figure 5-5). The small size of the retinal transplants prevented the use of tracer injections to completely confirm these findings; however, the Bodian method stains a wide range of fiber sizes, both within the transplanted retina as well as the host cortex. It seems reasonable to conclude that all but the tiniest axons crossing the interface would be demonstrated by this method.

Electron microscopic analysis of normal retinal development has shown that photoreceptor elements begin to form and protrude beyond the outer limiting membrane by 3–5 days postnatal. Further differentiation of the element quickly ensues, with the appearance of the outer segments and synthesis of lamellar membranes of the photoreceptor segment (Weidman and Kuwabara 1968, 1969, McArdle et al. 1977). Ultrastructural examination of the central portion of rosettes within the retinal transplants at 5 days postoperative showed that photoreceptor development is restricted to a series of closely adjacent cellular processes containing a few ribosomes and filaments, scattered centrioles, and basal bodies typical of inner segments (Figure 5-6). The electron microscope also confirmed the complete absence of pigment cells within this region and throughout the transplant.

Transplants studied at longer postoperative intervals showed that photoreceptor cells remained at this primitive phase of development until 20 days after surgery. However, between 20 and 30 days postoperative, the inner segments enlarged and began to display hypertrophied mitochondria, and a ciliary apparatus appeared and displayed prominent basal bodies and ciliary rootlets. Outer segments also became evident with multiple invaginations of the plasma membrane forming the photoreceptor lamellae. However, these were contorted in appearance and showed scattered areas of lamellar vesiculation, particularly at the distal end of the segment (Figures 5-7 and 5-8).

The original outer layer of the transplant contains concentrations of moderately dense, elongate cells with oval heterochromatin nuclei at 5 days. These are soon replaced by more definitive neuronal categories, including sensory cells (Figure 5-9), typical bipolar cells, and a contingent of pale neurons with euchromatic nuclei, found most often at the edges of the bipolar cell layer (Figure 5-10). An outer plexiform layer could be distinguished by 5 days postoperative and contained a mixture of both pale and dense cytoplasmic processes extending into the zone from the adjacent cell neuronal layers (Figure 5-11). However, the differentiation of these processes into synapses did not take place until between 20 and 30 days of development, during which time vesicles appeared in the enlarged processes, followed by the formation of synaptic ribbons and transformation into the characteristic dyad pattern (Figures 5-12 and 5-13).

The inner plexiform layer also becomes evident during the earliest stages of transplant maturation but only displays large numbers of intertwined cellular processes without any signs of membrane thickening or vesicle formation (Fig-

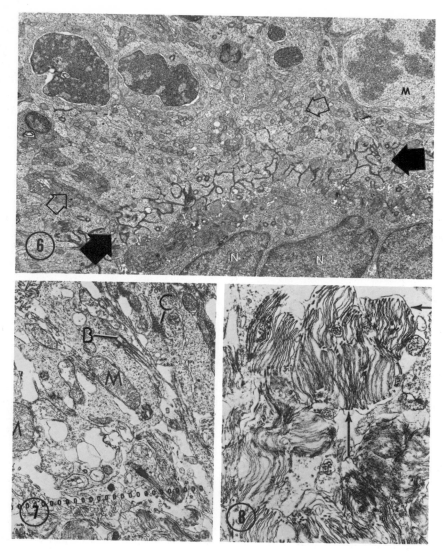

Figure 5-6. Solid black arrows indicate the apico-lateral junctions of immature retinal neural elements forming a portion of a rosette at 5 days following transplantation. Primitive neuroepithelial cells (N) within the center of a rosette are shown in the lower right. The mitotic fugure (M) lies adjacent to the line of junctions that make up a primitive outer limiting membrane. Open arrows delineate the developing cytoplasmic processes from which the inner and outer segments will arise. 2,590×. From Matthews et al. (1982c).

Figure 5-7. Transplanted retina after 30 days. Inner segments of sensory cells are shown above the dotted line. These display large mitochondria (M), basal bodies (B), and ciliary rootlets (C). The arrow indicates a connecting piece of an outer segment within which a few photoreceptor lamellae can be seen. More of these can be seen below the dotted line. 7,030×. From Matthews et al. (1982c).

Figure 5-8. Profiles of photoreceptor outer segments reveal contorted lamellae (arrow). 11,470×. From Matthews et al. (1982c).

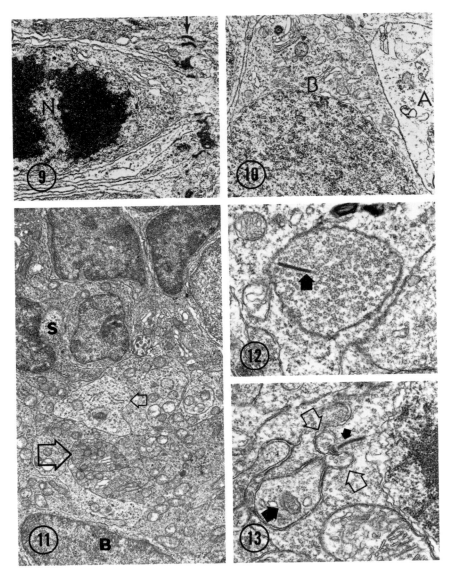

Figure 5-9. The perikaryon of a sensory cell is shown after 15 days of development in the host cortex. This cell displays a multilobate heterochromatin pattern within its nucleus (N). Note the line of zonulae adherentes forming the outer limiting membrane (arrow). 7,400×. From Matthews et al. (1982c).

Figure 5-10. A moderately dense bipolar cell (B) lies next to a presumptive amacrine cell (A), which displays a pale cytoplasm. 7,548×. From Matthews et al. (1982c).

Figure 5-11. Sensory cells (S) and bipolar cells (B) are shown. The poorly developed outer plexiform layer occupies the center of this micrograph. Processes of bipolar (small arrow) and sensory (large arrow) cells fill this region but synaptogenesis has not taken place by 15 days after transplantation. 7,400×. From Matthews et al. (1982c).

ure 5-14) until 20–30 days after implantation. At this time synaptic vesicles began to appear, and most complexes were seen to consist of a junction between two vesicle-filled processes, which often formed another junction with a third process (Figure 5-15). Based upon criteria established by Sosula and Glow (1970), most of these were classified as amacrine to amacrine junctions. Other complexes displayed a small synaptic ribbon adjacent to the presynaptic membrane at the point of contact with two postsynaptic elements to form a dyad characteristics of some bipolar cell terminals (Figure 5-16). Other complexes consisted of multiple amacrine junctions, amacrine to bipolar contacts, and rare instances of amacrine processes synapsing on ganglion cell soma. Criteria for these categories are presented elsewhere (Matthews et al. 1982a).

A quantitative assessment of synaptic categories showed that the percentage of presumptive amacrine to amacrine synapses was increased when compared with the number of similar complexes in normal retina at the same stage of development (Table 5-1). This finding was based on the figures given by Sosula and Glow (1970) together with the information derived from our studies of normal retinal development in the rat (Matthews et al. 1982a,b).

Along the periphery of rosettes a rudimentary ganglion cell layer could be distinguished, but the cells within it were small when compared to ganglion cells of normal retina. Most displayed a large, euchromatic nucleus and a small rim of cytoplasm containing ribosomal rosettes and a few short profiles of granular endoplasmic reticulum (Figure 5-17). Unmyelinated axons (0.2–0.5μm in diameter) could be found in this zone during the period of 15–30 days after transplantation. None became myelinated within the period examined, and no evidence suggested that such fibers projected out into the adjacent host cortex. It is assumed that many of these axons may represent a poorly developed optic projection, but other sources, such as bipolar cells, cannot be eliminated. In any event, their failure to myelinate suggests a minimal functional significance, and it is likely that this finding is related to the lack of appropriate target cells in the vicinity of the transplant.

Dual Transplants

Care was taken during the placement of dual transplants and subsequent closure of the host's skull to insure that the transplant tissues remained apposed.

Figure 5-12. A sensory cell terminal is shown at 20 days of development. This vesicle-filled process displays a synaptic ribbon (arrow) but no other specializations. 18,722×. From Matthews et al. (1982c).

Figure 5-13. A mature sensory cell terminal is illustrated after 30 days of development. The complex consists of a synaptic ribbon (small solid black arrow) adjacent to an arciform density of the presynaptic membrane. Two vesicle-filled, horizontal cell processes (open arrows) invaginate the sensory terminal from the lateral aspect, and a central bipolar cell dendrite is shown on the left (large solid arrow). 18,722×. From Matthews et al. (1982c).

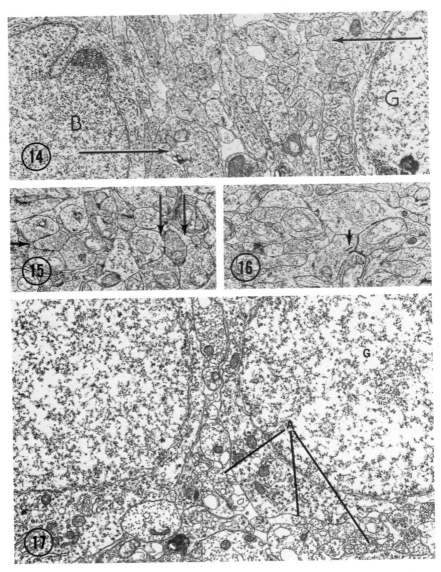

Figure 5-14. Arrows indicate the inner plexiform layer in which processes of bipolar cells (B) and ganglion cells (G) intermingle. At 10 days, evidence of synaptogenesis is lacking. 8,140×. From Matthews et al. (1982c).

Figure 5-15. Arrows indicate clusters of amacrine to amacrine terminals forming multiple junctions involving 3 to 4 terminals. 7,030×. From Matthews et al. (1982).

Figure 5-16. Arrow points to a synaptic ribbon within a bipolar cell terminal at 20 days of development. 7,030×. From Matthews et al. (1982c).

Figure 5-17. Two large ganglion cells are shown (G). Numerous axons (A) of varying diameters are present among these cells and are presumed to represent the rudimentary optic fiber layer. 11,544×. From Matthews et al. (1982c).

Table 5-1. Relative Proportion of Neurons in Transplanted and Normal Retina

Time after transplanting (days)	Transplant	Normal	Postnatal age (days)
15	A[a] 0.574	0.384	
	B[b] 0.074[c]	0.256	10
	C[d] 0.042[e]	0.098	
20	A 0.625	0.476	
	B 0.114[f]	0.163	15
	C 0.071[f]	0.078	
30	A 0.464	0.492	
	B 0.103[e]	0.148	25
	C 0.048[f]	0.073	

[a] Ratio of bipolar, horizontal, and amacrine cells to sensory cells.
[b] Ratio by ganglion cells to bipolar, horizontal, and amacrine cells.
[c] Differences from normal retina significant at $P < 0.001$.
[d] Ratio of ganglion cells to sensory cells.
[e] Difference from normal retina significant at $P < 0.01$.
[f] Differences from normal retina significant at $P < 0.05$.

This was verified by gross observation together with the use of autoradiographic analysis to delineate the position and boundaries of the sample of superior colliculus or medial thalamus (Figures 5-18 and 5-19).

Thalamic tissue transplants displayed large robust neurons by 10–20 days, together with a dense network of axons coursing about the transplant and, infrequently, extending into the host cortex (Figure 5-20). Adjacent retinal transplants were also well developed, following a time course similar to that of isolated retina. Examination of the interface between the two transplants revealed few axons coursing across this border nor were fibers seen to sprout from the retina into the cortex.

Dual transplants of superior colliculus and retina grew successfully and contained large numbers of well-developed neurons together with a network of intensely stained axons in the superior colliculus (Figures 5-21 and 5-22). The interface between the retina and superior colliculus was uniquely distinguished by heavy concentrations of fibers that appeared to begin in the peripheral layer of retinal neurons, assume a perpendicular orientation to the surface of the transplant, and extend deep into the tissue of the adjacent superior colliculus. Again, it must be emphasized that no such vigorous outgrowth occurred along those surfaces of the retinal transplants in contact with the host cortex.

The examination of these transplants with the electron microscope was principally confined to the interface between the two transplants. In the early stages of development, unmyelinated fibers were found within the retinal transplant, but these remained small in size and numbers in those cases in which retina was implanted in tandem with pieces of medial thalamus. However, the

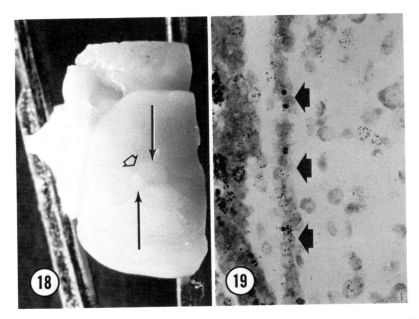

Figure 5-18. A dual transplant of fetal retina and superior colliculus is shown after 20 days of development in the occipital cortex of the host brain. The black and white arrow points to the retinal transplant while the black arrow indicates the tectal transplant. A distinct border (open arrow) is evident between these two types of tissue. From Matthews and West (1982).

Figure 5-19. An autoradiograph demonstrates labeled neurons in the transplanted retina, at the left, and the adjacent transplanted tectum, at the right. Arrows indicate the zone of apposition between them. 319×. From Matthews and West (1982).

dual transplants of retina and superior colliculus displayed a progression of development of such fibers characterized by growth of fascicles of three or more fibers across the interface between the two transplants and the appearance of increasing numbers of myelinated axons. Sections cut through the tectal or thalamic transplants parallel to the line of transplant apposition revealed collections of myelinated axons 1–5 μm in diameter, most of which were cut in cross section, suggestive of a directed growth (Figures 5-23 and 5-24). While axons were seen at a similar site in the thalamic transplant, few were myelinated and none appeared to be oriented in a specific plane of growth.

Quantitative Analysis

The numbers of cells with the ganglion cell layer was determined and expressed in proportion to sensory cells and neurons of the inner nuclear layer and found to be reduced in those regions of the retinal transplant next to the host cortex or

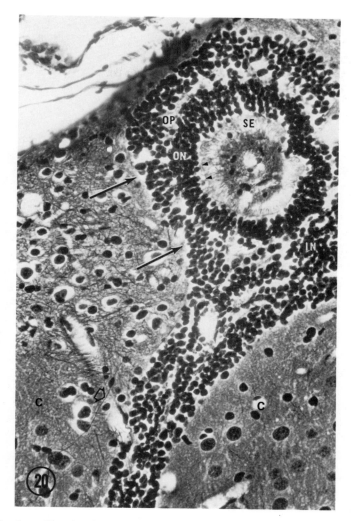

Figure 5-20. A profile of retina is shown adjacent to a second transplant taken from the medial thalamus of the donor fetus. A large rosette occupies much of the upper part of the retinal transplant and displays, from center to periphery, a layer of sensory elements (SE), the outer limiting membrane (arrowheads), an outer nuclear layer (ON), an outer plexiform layer (OP), and an inner nuclear layer (IN). Arrows delineate the zone of apposition between the retina and thalamic transplant. From Matthews and West (1982).

a second transplant of thalamic tissue. Alternatively, those areas of the retinal transplant located adjacent to a transplant of superior colliculus displayed both larger and significantly greater numbers of neurons in the ganglion cell layer during the period from 10 to 20 days following placement in the cortex. By 30 days of development, the difference was somewhat less significant, suggesting that the period of viability of some of these cells is limited (Table 5-2).

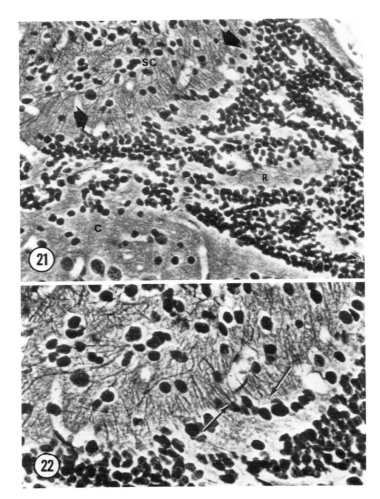

Figure 5-21. A dual transplant of retina (R) and superior colliculus (SC) is shown. The host cortex (C) can be seen below the retina. Large numbers of fibers (arrows) extend from the outer border of the retinal tissue and penetrate the adjacent superior colliculus, whereas no fibers course between the retina and surrounding host cortex. 228×. From Matthews and West (1982).

Figure 5-22. A portion of Figure 5-4 at higher magnification to show that may of the axons extending from the retina into the superior colliculus are in direct contact with the outer layer of neurons in the retinal transplant (arrows). From Matthews and West (1982).

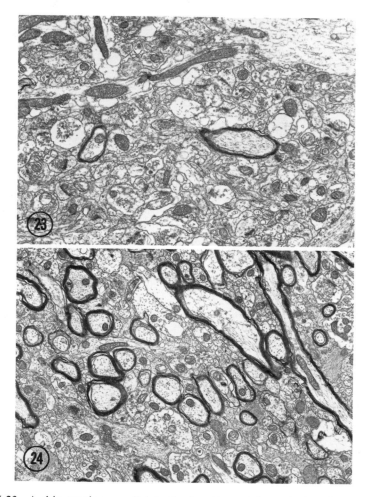

Figure 5-23. A thin section parallel to the junction of the retinal and thalamic transplants and approximately 50 μm into the thalamic neuropil. Note the numerous mature synapses in this region. After 30 days of development in the host, a few myelinated axons can be found in this tissue. 4,455×. From Matthews and West (1982).

Figure 5-24. A similarly oriented section in a dual transplant of retina and superior colliculus reveals numerous myelinated axons coursing together in a similar direction. 4,455×. From Matthews and West (1982).

Table 5-2. Neuron Ratios in Transplants of Fetal Retina Placed
Adjacent to Host Occipital Cortex or to a Second Transplant of either
Medial Thalamus or Visual Tectum

Survival period (days)	Retinal-cortical interface	Retinal-thalamic interface	Retinal-tectal interface
	A[a] 0.602	0.583	0.447
15	B[b] 0.059	0.071	0.288[c]
	C[d] 0.035	0.052	0.101[c]
	A 0.713	0.541	0.517
20	B 0.082	0.069	0.212[e]
	C 0.068	0.052	0.145[c]
	A 0.466	0.530	0.538
30	B 0.086	0.104	0.127
	C 0.029	0.032	0.092[e]

[a] Ratio of inner nuclear cells to sensory cells.
[b] Ratio of ganglion cells to inner nuclear cells.
[c] Significant difference at $P<0.01$.
[d] Ratio of ganglion cells to sensory cells.
[e] Significant difference at $P< 0.05$.

Discussion

Development of the Transplant and Formation of Optic Fibers

Our studies have shown that fetal retina can be successfully transplanted to the occipital cortex of a host neonatal rat wherein it will remain viable for periods of at least 30 days. Light and electron microscopic analysis demonstrated the presence of all major types of retinal neurons. However, the tissue becomes distorted, exhibiting varying numbers of rosette formations within which the different layers of retinal neurons become positioned in a series of roughly concentric circles. Sensory cells occupy the innermost ring of each rosette, and their developing photoreceptor elements project centrally. The inner and outer plexiform layers, inner nuclear layer, and ganglion cell layer form the progressively wider circles such that within each rosette the histotypic organization of the retina is retained. This form of reorganization has been described in retinal explant cultures (LaVail and Hild 1971) and seen in cultured embryonic retinae transplanted to the superior colliculus after periods ranging from 2 to 14 days *in vitro* (McLoon et al. 1981).

Our quantitative analyses revealed that the number of neurons in the ganglion cell layer was reduced in proportion to other neuronal categories and that optic fibers remained small and failed to become myelinated. The best explanation for this finding appears to be the lack of appropriate target neurons in the vicinity of the transplant to selectively stimulate the development of optic fibers. Other factors, such as the retrograde degeneration of optic fibers or the placement of the retinal tissue in an abnormal milieu, might have a small effect on transplant differentiation, as considered in detail elsewhere (Matthews et al. 1982c), but a number of reasons exist to strongly support the first alternative. For example, specific glycoproteins have been extracted from sciatic nerve and been shown to exhibit potent trophic effects upon muscle tissue culture preparations (Oh 1976, Oh et al. 1980). Similarly, nerve growth factor is well known to have a potentiating effect upon the development and survival of dorsal root and superior cervical ganglion neurons (Smith and Kreutzberg 1977, Hendry and Campbell 1976). More direct lines of evidence to support this concept come from tissue culture studies of retina. LaVail and Hild (1971) examined the differentiation of retina in culture using electron microscopy and were able to document many types of retinal neurons and synapses. Later studies indicated that the growth of such explants was particularly successful when they were placed in culture with pieces of superior colliculus. Neurite production and elongation was preferentially stimulated (Smalheiser et al. 1981). Neurites growing from retinae isolated in culture were much smaller in size and often degenerated after approximately 10 days *in vitro*.

A quantitative analysis of ganglion cell populations in dissociated retinal cultures showed a 50% loss of ganglion cells within 24 hours after plating (McCaffery et al. 1982). Co-culturing the retina with either thalamus or midbrain that contains retino-recipient nuclei enhanced the survival of ganglion cells to 100%. Co-culturing with cerebellum failed to enhance their survival.

Such studies correlate with *in vivo* analyses which have shown that the normal amount of ganglion cell death occurring with development can be greatly exaggerated by the partial or total removal of the optic tectum (Hughes and McLoon 1979). Alternatively, enlargement of the amount of available target tissue has been shown in various model systems to preserve a larger than normal number of those neurons that project to this area (Hollyday and Hamberger 1976, Narayanan and Narayanan 1978). These kinds of studies further support the concept of competition among developing neurons for the trophic factors contained within target tissues (Cowan 1979).

Based on the assumption that the complete maturation of ganglion cells requires an interplay between the intrinsic programming of retinal development and the stimulation provided by the proximity of appropriate target tissue recipient to optic fibers, portions of fetal superior colliculus were transplanted adjacent to the retina to determine if the presence of this tissue would stimulate the growth of axons from the transplanted retina. A vigorous and directed outgrowth of fibers from the retina into the tectal tissue was observed, and this outgrowth was restricted only to those portions of the retinal transplant in direct apposition to the second transplant. Neurons within the ganglion cell layer were also preserved in the zone along the interface with the tectal tissue. A transplant of tissue removed from the medial thalamus failed to result in an outgrowth of axons from the adjacent retinal transplant, nor were significant numbers of axons found to course between the retinal transplant and the host cortex. This suggested a considerable degree of specificity in the process of sprouting and elongation and correlates well with those studies which have shown that transplants of retina placed adjacent to the superior colliculus of neonatal host rats will develop a projection to the stratum zonale, griseum superficiale, and upper portions of stratum opticum. The density of this projection could be increased somewhat by the prior removal of the contralateral eye, which eliminated most of the normal retino-tectal input thus serving to increase available synaptic space (McLoon and Lund, 1980a,b). This study also showed evidence of a projection from the transplant to the dorsal lateral geniculate nucleus and pre-tectal complex. The authors interpreted their findings as being supportive of a special affinity between axons arising in the transplant and retino-recipient nuclei in the host. Mechanical factors (Silver and Sidman 1980) or organizational gradients (Hibbard 1965, Constantine-Paton and Capranica 1976) would not be a major factor because transplant axons reached their targets by growing in a direction opposite to that of the host's optic fiber projection. The presence of a special affinity is further emphasized by the fact that retinal transplants found lying between the inferior colliculi and cerebellum exhibited a projection that extended to the superior colliculus without innervating any of the adjacent tissues.

Synaptic Development

Synaptogenesis occurs in the retinal transplants and produces arrays of dyads and conventional synapses, but the process is delayed until the period between 20 and 30 days following transplantation. This corresponds to a postnatal age of 15–25 days and represents a delay of 5–7 days when compared with synaptogenesis in normal retina (Matthews et al. 1982c). The reasons for such a delay are not clear. Although the transplanted retina shows a high degree of differentiation, the unique form of sensory deprivation imposed upon the retinal photoreceptors and neurons as a result of removal of the retina from the eye and placement in an ectopic site within the CNS must precipitate an abnormal form of electrophysiological activity among this complex of neurons. However, the effect of impulse activity upon the developing CNS remains a controversial issue. Synapses have been shown to form in culture in the presence of toxins that block impulse activity (Crain 1977, Obata 1977), and the retino-tectal projection has been shown to grow successfully and establish proper connection under similar conditions (Harris 1980a). Nonetheless, other studies have demonstrated a significant effect of impulse blockade on neurotransmitters, receptor distribution and pharmacology and several enzymes in the visual and other model systems (Black and Green 1974, Berg and Hall 1975, Rubin et al. 1979). Morphological studies have shown a small reduction in the normal arborization of geniculo-striate axons following monocular deprivation (Thorpe and Blakemore 1975). Similarly, impulse blockade induced by tetrodotoxin has been shown to hinder goldfish optic nerve regeneration and branching within the tectum (Edwards and Grafstein 1983, Schmidt et al. 1983, Schmidt and Edwards 1983).

Examination of the effects of sensory deprivation on the retina has revealed minimal changes in neuronal morphology. A mild degree of synaptic reorganization does, however, take place and may be relevant to our studies. Thus, Fifkova (1972) reported that the incidence of amacrine to amacrine junctions increased by 41% and amacrine to bipolar contacts decreased by 5.3% following perinatal lid suture. A lack of patterned input has also been associated with alterations in the development of amacrine synaptic patterns in the retina of *Necturus* (Werblin and Dowling 1969). It must be emphasized, however, that ganglion cells and their axons are not substantially affected by lid suture (Globus 1975). Moreover, these *in vivo* deprivation models did not result in a significant delay in synapse formation. It therefore seems likely that the reduction in the number of ganglion cells and the resulting available postsynaptic space within the inner plexiform layer induced a form of synaptic reorganization manifested by an increase in amacrine to amacrine contacts. This would be somewhat comparable to the synaptic reorganization shown to take place in the lateral geniculate nucleus after cortical ablation. This phenomenon was clearly related to a loss of dendritic surface (Ralston and Chow 1973).

In conclusion, our studies of fetal retina transplanted in isolation and with portions of the superior colliculus have emphasized the interdependency of functionally related neurons. The use of these dual transplantation experiments serves not only to demonstrate the presence of a special affinity between developing axons and their target cells but also to indicate that such an affinity is operational in the absence of aligned guidance cues to form a substrate pathway (Katz and Lasek 1981).

Acknowledgment. Supported in part by grant NS 14699 from the NINCDS.

References

Berg, D.K., Hall, Z. (1975). Increased extrajunctional acetylcholine sensitivity produced by chronic postsynaptic neuromuscular blockade. J. Physiol. 244, 659–666.

Björklund, H., Seiger, A., Hoffer, B., Olson, L. (1983). Trophic effects of brain areas on the developing cerebral cortex. I. Growth and histological organization of intraocular grafts. Dev. Brain Res. 6, 131–140.

Björklund, A., Stenevi, U. (1979). Reconstruction of nigrostriatal dopamine pathway by intracerebral nigral transplants. Brain Res. 177, 555–560

Björklund, A., Stenevi, U., Svendgaard, N.A. (1976). Growth of transplanted monoaminergic neurons into the adult hippocampus along the perforant path. Nature 262, 787–790.

Black, I.B., Green, S.C. (1974). Inhibition of the biochemical and morphological maturation of adrenergic neurons by nicotine receptor blockade. J. Neurochem. 22, 301–306.

Constantine-Paton M., Capranica, R.P. (1976). Axonal guidance of developing optic nerves in frog. I. Anatomy of the projection from transplanted eye primordia. J. Comp. Neur. 170, 17–31.

Cowan, W.M. (1970). Anterograde and retrograde transneuronal degeneration in the central and peripheral nervous system. In: Contemporary Research Methods in

Neuroanatomy. Nauta, W., Ebkesson, S. (eds.). Berlin: Springer-Verlag, pp. 271–251.

Cowan, W.M. (1978). Aspects of neural development. In: International Review of Physiology Neurophysiology. III. Porter, R. (ed.). Baltimore: University Press, pp. 149–189.

Cowan, W.M. (1979). Selection and control in neurogenesis. In: The Neurosciences Fourth Study Program. Schmitt, F.O., Worden, F.6. (eds.). Cambridge, MA: MIT Press pp. 59–79.

Crain, S. (1977). Synapse formation in neural tissue cultures. In: Cell, Tissue and Organ Cultures in Neurobiology. S, Hertz, L. (eds.). New York: Academic Press, pp. 147–190.

Crossland, W.J., Cowan, W.M., Rogers, L.A., Kelly, J.P. (1974). The specification of the retino-tectal projection in the chick. J. Comp. Neur. 155, 127–164.

Das, G.D. (1974). Transplantation of embryonic tissue in the mammalian brain. I. Growth and differentiation of neuroblasts from various regions of the embryonic brain in the cerebellum of neonate rats. TIT J. Life Sci. 4, 93–124.

Das, G.D., Hallas, B.H., Das, K.G. (1979). Transplantation of neural tissues in the brains of laboratory mammals. Technical details and comments. Experientia 35, 143–153.

Das, G.D., Hallas, B.H., Das, K.G. (1980). Transplantation of brain tissue in the brain of rat. I. Growth characteristics of neocortical transplants from embryos of different ages. Am. J. Anat. 158, 135–145.

Edwards, D.L., Grafstein, B. (1983). Intraocular tetrodotoxin hinders optic nerve regeneration. Brain Res. 269, 1–14.

Fifkova, E. (1972). Effect of visual deprivation and light on synapses of the inner plexiform layer. Exp. Neurol. 35, 458–469.

Gash, D., Sladek, J.R., Sladek, C. (1979). Development of normal fetal supraoptic neurons grafted into adult hosts with a congenital lack of vasopressin producing neurons. Soc. Neurosci. Abst. 5, 445.

Gaze, R.M. (1970). The Formation of Nerve Connections. London/New York: Academic Press, pp. 1–28.

Globus, A. (1975). Brain morphology as a function of presynaptic morphology and activity. In: Developmental Neuropsychology of Sensory Deprivation, Riesen, A.H. (ed.). New York: Academic Press, pp. 9–91.

Hallas, B.H., Oblinger, M.M., Das, G.D. (1980). Heterotopic neural transplants in the cerebellum of the rat: Their afferents. Brain Res. 196, 242–246.

Harris, W.A. (1980a). The effects of eliminating impulse activity on the development of the retino-tectal projection in salamanders. J. Comp. Neur. 194, 303–317.

Harris, W.A. (1980b). Regions of the brain influencing the projection of developing optic tracts in the salamander. J. Comp. Neur. 194, 319–333.

Harvey, A.R., Lund, R.D. (1979). Neurons in host rat brains which project to tectal transplants. Neurosci. Abst. 5, 627.

Hendry, I.A., Campbell, J. (1976). Morphometric analysis of rat superior cervical ganglion after axotomy and nerve growth factor treatment. J. Neurocytol. 5, 351–360.

Hibbard, E. (1965). Orientation and directed growth of Mauthner's cell axons from duplicated vestibular nerve roots. Exp. Neurol. 13, 289–301.

Hollyday, M., Hamburger, V. (1976). Reduction of the naturally occurring motor neuron loss by enlargement of the periphery. J. Comp. Neur. 170, 311–320.

Hughes, W.F., McLoon, S.C. (1979). Ganglion cell death during normal retinal development in the chick: Comparisons with cell death induced by early target field destruction. Exp. Neurol. 66, 587–601.

Jacobson, M. (1978). Developmental Neurobiology, 2nd ed. New York/London: Plenum Press.

Jacobson, M., Levine, R.L. (1975). Stability of implanted duplicate tectal positional markers serving as target for optic axons in adult frogs. Brain Res. 92, 468–471.

Jaeger, C.B., Lund, R.D. (1979). Efferent fibers from transplanted cerebral cortex of rats. Brain Res. 165, 338–342.

Jaeger, C.B., Lund, R.D. (1980). Transplantation of embryonic occipital cortex to the brain of newborn rats. Exp. Brain Res. 40, 265–272.

Katz, M.J., Lasek, R.J. (1981). Substrate pathway demonstrated by transplanted Mauthner axons. J. Comp. Neurol. 195, 627–641.

Lavail, M.M., Hild, W. (1971). Histotypic organization of the rat retina in vitro. Z. Zellforsch. 114, 557–579.

Lewis, E.R., Cotman, C.W. (1980). Mechanisms of septal lamination in the developing hippocampus revealed by outgrowth of fibers from septal implants. I. Positional and temporal factors. Brain Res. 196, 307–330.

Lund, R.D. (1978). Developmental and plasticity of the brain: An introduction. New York: Oxford University Press.

Matthews, M.A. (1973). Death of the central neuron: An electron microscopic study of thalamic retrograde degeneration following cortical ablation. J. Neurocytol. 2, 265–288.

Matthews, M.A. (1981). Transplantation of fetal retina, superior colliculus and lateral geniculate nucleus to host visual cortex. A light and electron microscopic analysis. Soc. Neurosci. ABS. 11th Annual Meeting, p. 466.

Matthews, M.A., Cornell, W.J., Alchediak, T. (1982a). Axoplasmic transport inhibition in the developing visual system of the rat. I. Structural changes in the retina and optic nerve with graded doses of intraocular colchicine. Neuroscience 7, 365–384.

Matthews, M.A., West, L.C. (1982). Optic fiber development between dual transplants of retina and superior colliculus placed in the occipital cortex. Anat. Embryol. 163, 417–433.

Matthews, M.A., West, L., Clarkson, D.B. (1982b). Axoplasmic transport inhibition in the developing visual system of the rat. II. Quantitative analysis of alterations in transport of tritiated Proline or Fucose. Neuroscience 7, 385–404.

Matthews, M.A., West, L.C., Riccio, R.V. (1982c). An ultrastructural analysis of the development of fetal rat retina transplanted to the occipital cortex, a site lacking appropriate target neurons for optic fibers. J. Neurocytol. 11, 533–557.

McArdle, C.B., Dowling, J.E., Masland, R.H. (1977). Development of outer segments and synapses in the rabbit retina. J. Comp. Neur. 175, 253–274.

McCaffery, C.A., Bennett, M.R., Dreher, B. (1982). The survival of neonatal rat retinal ganglion cells in vitro is enhanced in the presence of appropriate parts of the brain. Exp. Brain Res. 48, 377–386.

McLoon, S.C., Lund, R.D. (1980a). Identification of cells in retinal transplants which project to host visual centers: A horseradish peroxidase study in rats. Brain Res. 197, 491–495.

McLoon, S.C., Lund, R.D. (1980b). Specific projections of retina transplanted to rat brain. Exp. Brain Res. 40, 273–282.

McLoon, L.K., McLoon, S.C., Lund, R.D. (1981). Cultured embyronic retinae transplanted to rat brain: Differentiation and formation of projections to host superior colliculus. Brain Res. 226, 15–31.

Narayanan, C.H., Narayanan, Y. (1978). Neuronal adjustments in developing nuclear centers of the chick embryo fellowing transplantation of an additional optic primordium. J. Embryol. Exp. Morphol. 44, 53–70.

Obata, K. (1977). Development of neuromuscular transmission in culture with a variety of neurons and in the presence of cholinergic substances and tetrodotoxin. Brain Res. 119, 141–153.

Oblinger, M.M., Hallas, B.H., Das, G.D. (1980). Neocortical transplants in the cerebellum of the rat: Their afferents and efferents. Brain Res. 189, 228–232.

Oh, T.H. (1976). Neurotrophic effects of sciatic nerve extracts on muscle development in culture. Exp. Neurol. 50, 376–386.

Oh, T.H., Markelonis, C.J., Reier, P.J., Zalewski, A.A. (1980). Persistence in degenerating sciatic nerve of substances having a trophic influence upon cultured muscle. Exp. Neurol. 67, 646–654.

Olson, L., Seiger, A., Hoffer, B., Taylor, D. (1979). Isolated catecholaminergic projections from substantia nigra and locus coeruleus to caudate, hippocampus and cerebral cortex formed by intraocular sequential double brain grafts. Exp. Brain Res. 35, 47–67.

Perlow, M.J., Freed, W.J., Hoffer, B.J., Seiger, A., Olson, L., Wyatt, R.J. (1979). Brain grafts reduce motor abnormalities produced by destruction of the nigrostriatal dopamine system. Science 204, 643–646.

Ralston, H.J., Chow, K.L. (1973). Synaptic reorganization in the degeneration lateral geniculate nucleus of the rabbit. J. Comp. Neur. 147, 321–350.

Ranson, S.W. (1914). Transplantation of the spinal ganglion cells. J. Comp. Neur. 24, 547–558.

Rubin, L., Scheutz, S.M., Fischbach, G.D. (1979). Accumulation of acetylcholinesterase at newly formed nerve-muscle synapses. Dev. Biol. 69, 46–58.

Saltykow, S. (1905). Versuche über gehirnplantation zugleich einbeitrag zur Kenntniss der Borgange an den zelligen gehirnelementen. Arch. Psych. 40, 320.

Schmidt, J.T., Edwards, D.L. (1983). Activity sharpens the map during the regeneration of the retino-tectal projection in goldfish. Brain Res. 269, 29–39.

Schmidt, J.T.M., Edwards, D.L., Stuermer, C. (1983). The reestablishment of synaptic transmission by regenerating optic axons in goldfish: Time course and effects of blocking activity by intraocular injection of tetrodotoxin. Brain Res. 269, 15–27.

Silver, J., Sidman, R.L. (1980). A mechanism for the guidance and topographic patterning of retinal ganglion cell axons. J. Comp. Neur. 189, 101–111.

Smalheiser, N.R., Crain, S.M., Bornstein, M.B. (1981). Development of ganglion cells and their axons in organized cultures of fetal mouse retinal explants. Brain Res. 204, 159–178.

Smith, B.H., Kreutzberg, G.W. (1977). Neuron-target cell interactions. NRP Bull. 14, 209–453.

Sosula, L., Glow, P.H. (1970). A quantitative ultrastructural study of the inner plexiform layer of the rat retina. J. Comp. Neur. 140, 439–478.

Sperry, R.W. (1963). Chemoaffinity in the orderly growth of nerve fiber patterns and connections. Proc. Natl. Acad. Sci. USA 50, 703–710.

Thorpe, P.A., Blakemore, C. (1975). Evidence for a loss of afferent axons in the visual cortex of monocularly deprived cats. Neurosci. Let. 1, 271–276.

Weidman, T.A., Kuwabara, T. (1968). Postnatal development of the rat retina. Arch. Ophthalmol. 79, 470–484.

Weidman, T.A., Kuwabara, T. (1969). Development of the rat retina. Invest. Ophthalmol. 8, 60–69.

Werblin, F.S., Dowling, J.E. (1969). Organization of the retina of the mudpuppy, *Necturus maculosus*. II. Intracellular recording. J. Neurophysiol. 32, 339–355.

Woodward, D.J., Seiger, A., Olson, L., Hoffer, B.J. (1977). Intrinsic and extrinsic determinants of dendritic development as revealed by Golgi studies of cerebellar and hippocampal transplants in oculo. Exp. Neurol. 57, 984–998.

Yoon, M.G., (1975). Topographic polarity of the optic tectum studied by reimplantation of the tectal tissue in adult goldfish. Cold Spring Harbor Symp. Quant. Biol. 40, 503–519.

Chapter 6

Quantitative Studies of Reactive Events in the Site of Injury Following Transection of the Spinal Cord in the Rat

MURRAY A. MATTHEWS* and JOHN B. GELDERD†

Background

Transection of the mammalian spinal cord results in a complete and permanent loss of voluntary motor function below the level of the lesion accompanied by an equally profound sensory loss. In many phylogenetically lower animals, massive axonal regeneration occurs and often results in some degree of functional restitution, despite the presence of scar formation within the site of injury (Bernstein and Bernstein 1967), but in mammalian forms regeneration of CNS axons is considered to be minimal and abortive (Ramon v Cajal 1928). A variety of treatment methods have been employed in an attempt to promote the regeneration of axons across the transection site (Puchala and Windle 1977). These have included the implanting of grafts of fetal brain tissue, degenerated sciatic nerve or muscle into the lesion site in order to improve the environment for optimal axonal growth (Sugar and Gerard 1940), administration of adreno-corticotrophic hormones (McMasters 1962), millipore cylinders (Campbell and Windle 1960), or Piromen, a pyrogenic bacterial polysaccharide thought to enhance regeneration by preventing the formation of a dense fibrous scar following injury (Clemente and Windle 1954, Littrell 1955). Application of Piromen seemed to increase the number of regenerating fibers as shown by morphological and electrophysiological techniques, but the animals failed to demonstrate an improvement in their sensorimotor function.

Feringa et al. (1973, 1974, 1975, 1976, 1977, 1980) approached the problem based on the concept that an autoallergic response to CNS antigens released during injury was causing a production of specifically sensitized lymphocytes or of serum antibodies capable of destroying new axon sprouts either by direct

* Department of Anatomy, Louisiana State University Medical Center, New Orleans, Louisiana 70119 U.S.A.
† Department of Human Anatomy, Texas A&M Medical Center, College Station, Texas 77843 U.S.A.

lysis or through the injury of supportive glial elements. Several immunosuppressives were administered to rats whose spinal cords were transected, and
initial studies indicated that cyclophosphamide treatment resulted in axonal
regeneration. However, no behavioral improvement was reported, and a recent
analysis (Willenborg et al. 1977) of several immunologic mechanisms after
spinal cord injury failed to support the hypothesis put forward by Feringa. It
was considered that any positive effects of cyclophosphamide upon the transected spinal cord were related to its antimitotic capacity, which might inter-
fere with scar formation.

Another approach toward reducing the density of the glio-mesodermal scar
at the site of transection was the application of solutions of trypsin to the
injured spinal cord of dogs and rats (Turbes and Freeman 1953, Freeman et al.
1960). These reports indicated that the density of the collagenous scar could be
reduced by such treatments, but functional changes were not documented.
More recently, Matinian and Andreasian (1976) employed trypsin, hyaluronidase, elastase, and Pyrogenal (a compound with properties comparable to Piromen) percutaneously at the site of transection at T-5 and systematically, either
singly or in combination. They reported that from 30% to 90% of the experimental animals recovered their weight-bearing ability and were able to walk.
However, since many of their morphological and electrophysiological data
were poor and therefore difficult to interpret, it was not possible to assess their
results carefully.

While this study, as well as many previous ones, presented low magnification micrographs of the lesion site in an attempt to document the presence or
absence of axons, there appeared to be a paucity of comprehensive quantitative
studies employing correlated light and electron microscopic techniques undertaken to carefully analyze details of the postoperative events occurring subsequent to a transection. It was also important to determine the nature of any
modification in such pathological sequellae after selected treatments in a single
mammalian animal model.

Objectives

The studies we undertook had several objectives: (1) to describe the types of
cellular elements involved in the formation of the glio-mesodermal scar; (2) to
determine if axons grow into the site of lesion and, if so, to document their
morphological relationship with glial supportive cells as well as cellular elements of the mesodermal matrix; (3) to examine the formation of a glial limiting
membrane in the site of injury and assess its efficacy as a barrier to the passage
of growing axons; (4) to reevaluate, by morphometric methods, the possible
effectiveness of Piromen, cyclophosphamide, and trypsin in reducing scar formation and promoting axon growth; (5) because in lower animal forms ependymal cells actively participate in a well-organized regenerative process resulting
in restitution of neural integrity (Egar and Singer 1972), we decided to examine
the response of the ependymal cells lining the central canal to a transection
injury.

The data to be summarized here have appeared in previous publications (Matthews et al. 1976, 1979,a,b,c, Gelderd et al. 1980).

Techniques

Animals and Surgical Procedures

Mature Long-Evans male rats were used in these experiments. The animals were anesthetized by injection of 7% choral hydrate and subjected to a transection of the spinal cord at the T-5 level. Complete transection was verified by visual inspection using an operating microscope. Subsequent to the surgical procedure, each animal received an injection of Symbio, a wide-spectrum antibiotic, then was allowed to recover from the anesthetic. In order to reduce postoperative morbidity from urinary tract infections, the bladder of each animal was expressed twice daily and 1.5 mg nitrofurantoin was administered orally for a period of 2 weeks.

Treatment Groups

Group A

Piromen, a pyrogenic polysaccharide-nucleic acid complex, prepared in the crude crystalline lyophilized form by Baxter Laboratories, was dissolved in normal saline to a concentration of 1 μg/0.05 ml just prior to application to the lesion site following the transection procedure. Each animal was subsequently given daily intramuscular doses of 1 μg of Piromen throughout the entire postoperative period. Such a regimen of treatment was designed to follow that used in the study by Clemente and Windle (1954).

Group B

Cyclophosphamide was dissolved in normal saline to a concentration of 15 mg/kg and injected intramuscularly on the day of surgery and 24 hours later.

Group C

Crystalline trypsin was dissolved in 0.1 M Sorensen's phosphate buffer adjusted to pH 7.4 and applied to the site of lesion at a dose of 0.35 mg/kg. An equal amount was injected intramuscularly 2 hours later. This procedure was repeated daily for 2 weeks.

Group D

Each animal was subjected to a T-5 transection of the spinal cord. The site of lesion was injected with saline in half the animals in this group, and the remaining half received no further specific treatment.

Fixation and Tissue Processing

Postoperative intervals ranged from 7 to 400 days. Each animal was sacrificed by perfusion following standard procedures (Matthews 1973) and the vertebral column allowed to fix overnight at 4°C. The spinal cord was carefully removed so as not to disturb the area around the lesion site. Cross sections encompassing the lesion site and at fixed distances above and below this zone were taken and kept in separate coded vials. These samples were subsequently postosmicated, dehydrated, and embedded in Epon. Sections cut at a thickness of 1.5 μm and encompassing an entire cross section of the cord were stained with toluidine blue. From this same material thin sections were cut and stained with uranyl acetate and lead citrate and examined with the electron microscope.

For our light microscopic studies, the spinal cord was allowed to remain within the vertebral column and fix for 1–2 weeks, after which a segment approximately 3 cm in length and encompassing the site of transection was removed and processed for embedment in Paraplast. Sections were taken at 10 μm in the longitudinal plane and stained using the Bodian reduced silver method.

Quantitative Analysis

The site of lesion was analyzed in ten animals from each treatment group together with sham-injected controls and the transected animals that had received no further treatment. Transverse sections were cut at 150-μm intervals until 13 evenly spaced groups of sections were accumulated. The cross-sectional area of each section was determined by planimetry and regions of the gliomesodermal matrix classified into one of three subcategories, which included: (1) dense fibrous connective tissue; (2) a loose, areolar matrix containing minimal fibrous elements; and (3) cystic spaces filled with fluid. The cross section of each of these regions was also determined by planimetry and expressed as a percentage of the total area of the cord profile.

Findings

Preliminary Observations

The site of lesion is initially occupied by large numbers of degenerating neural elements and macrophages. During the first week after transection, this zone spreads to include an area of necrosis approximately 2 mm wide within which all recognizable neural elements disappear (Figure 6-1). Following this stage mesenchymal cells invade the wound and begin to produce a collagenous matrix that gradually appears to increase in density throughout the period from 7 to 45 days after injury (Figure 6-2). Reduced silver stains reveal a gradual ingrowth of axons into the scar matrix and surrounding spinal cord paren-

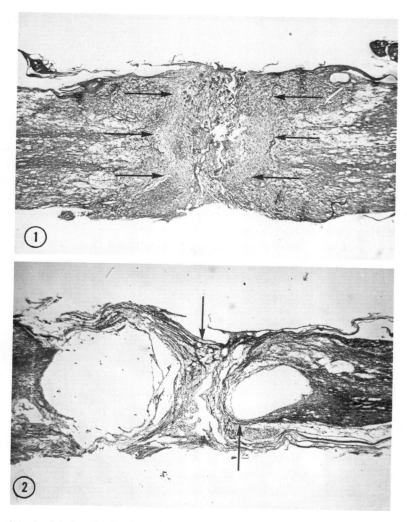

Figure 6-1. In this longitudinal section arrows delineate the zone of necrotic material formed at the injury site. The cranial segment of the spinal cord is located to the left in this figure. Bodian stain; 8 days postoperative (dpo). 22×. From Matthews et al. (1979a).

Figure 6-2. The original site of lesion, into which axons are sprouting (arrows), exhibits a dense, fibrous scar. Two large cysts can be seen both cranial and caudal to this zone. Bodian stain; 45 dpo. 22×. From Matthews et al. (1979a).

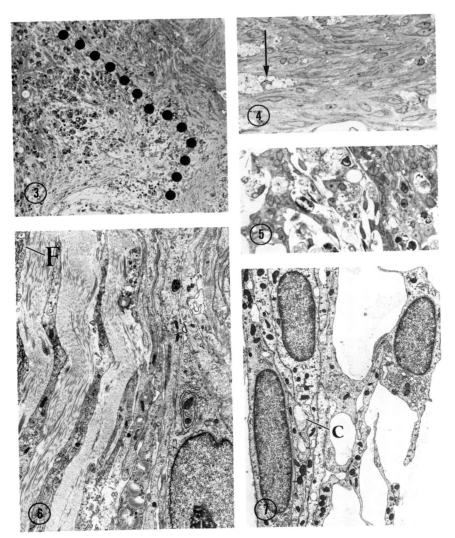

Figure 6-3. This semithin section, cut transversely through the lesion site, illustrates the loose connective tissue component of the scar to the left of the dotted line and the fibrous matrix to the right. Alkaline toluidine blue; 25 dpo. 150×. From Matthews et al. (1979a).

Figure 6-4. Fusiform fibroblasts occur among bundles of collagen fibers. A macrophage, filled with vacuoles and dense bodies, is visible at the lower left (arrow). Alkaline toluidine blue; 25 dpo. 800×. From Matthews et al. (1979a).

Figure 6-5. Cellular aggregates with interposed large areas of extracellular space typify the loose connective tissue portion of the scar. Alkaline toluidine blue; 25 dpo. 800×. From Matthews et al. (1979a).

Figure 6-6. A fibroblast (F) occurs at the upper left. Note alternating collagen fibril bundles and thin cell processes of presumptive fibroblasts; 25 dpo. 10,000×. From Matthews et al. (1979a).

chyma. Most such fibers appear to occur within the dorsal part of the zone of transection and take a tortuous course through the labyrinthine environment of the matrix.

Cystic spaces form within the central gray area of the cord above and below the site of injury. These gradually increase in size, and over a period of several months impinge upon and erode adjacent tissues. Such cysts may represent a major factor hindering the restitution of neural integrity.

Finally, examination of the transected cord revealed a dilation of the central canal in three to four segments rostral to the lesion site. The layer of ependymal cells lining the dilated canal demonstrated a loss of the normal columnar arrangement, reduction in cell height, and the appearance of budlike aggregations of ependymal cells extending for up to 900 μm from the canal.

The following sections will describe in greater detail each of these basic findings and where appropriate relate these to the effects of the different treatment regimens. One of our chief concerns will be to illuminate those alterations interpretable as improving the environment for axonal growth.

Morphological Properties of the Scar Matrix

Two principal patterns of collagen arrangement and density can be found within the scar. The first displays tightly packed bundles of fibers with interposed fusiform fibroblasts and a few scattered macrophages (Figures 6-3 and 6-4). Examination of such areas with the electron microscope reveals closely apposed, parallel collagen fibrils separated periodically by narrow cytoplasmic processes containing granular endoplasmic reticulum, mitochondria, and occasional dense bodies. Many of these processes arise from fibroblasts (Figure 6-6).

The second pattern consists of cords and sheets of cells suspended within a loose matrix with large numbers of blood vessels and extensive areas of extracellular space (Figures 6-3, 6-5, and 6-7). The amount of collagen in such areas appears to be reduced. Upon examination with the electron microscope, cells similar in appearance to fibroblasts are observed, but these display a less dense cytoplasmic matrix. Extensive points of intercellular apposition occur, and many of these are marked by a zonula occludens. Collagen fibrils can also be seen coursing about the abundant extracellular space in small bundles, but most are less dense and poorly organized.

Axonal Infiltration

Axons become evident throughout the scar matrix in relatively large numbers during the period from 45 to 90 days after transection (Figures 6-8, 6-9, and 6-

Figure 6-7. An abundance of extracellular spaces occurs in this micrograph. Collagen fibrils cut transversely in this figure are loosely organized within cavities formed by adjacent cell processes (C); 25 dpo. 10,000×. From Matthews et al. (1979a).

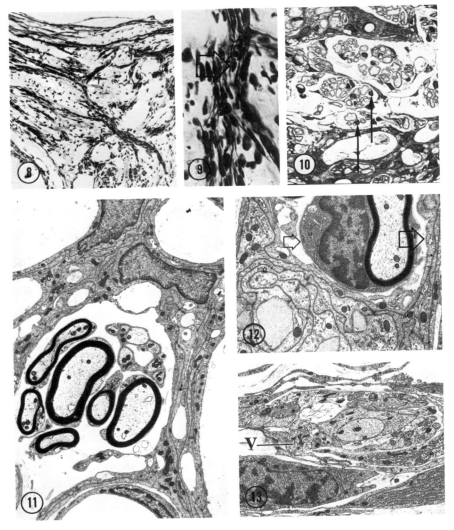

Figures 6-8 and 6-9. Fascicles of axons, darkly stained by silver method, invade the scar matrix. Elongate Schwann cells (arrow) accompany such bundles. Bodian stain; 90 dpo. 84×; 392×. From Matthews et al. (1979a).

Figure 6-10. Cell clusters, characteristic of the loose scar matrix, are associated with numerous axons. Schwann cells are indicated by arrows. Alkaline toluidine blue; 90 dpo. 448×. From Matthews et al. (1979a).

Figures 6-11 and 6-12. Myelinated and unmyelinated axons course through the spaces of the matrix. Schwann cell processes surround such axons and the fascicles are enclosed by groups of mesodermal cellular elements distinct from the Schwann cell-axon complex (small arrow); whereas another basement membrane lines the space through which the axon passes (large arrow); 90 dpo. 4,200×; 5,320×. From Matthews et al. (1979a).

10). They tend to course aimlessly about the matrix, initially appearing as small isolated fibers but with time occurring as fascicles of 5–20 myelinated and unmyelinated fibers associated with Schwann cells. Most are restricted to the loose connective tissue components of the scar (Figures 6-11 and 6-12) and occupy the abundant extracellular spaces in such regions. Often a basement membrane lines these spaces if axons are present, but this membrane is distinct from the basement membrane that encloses axon fascicles (Figure 6-12). Vesicle-filled, axonal swellings associated with groups of unmyelinated axons occur in this matrix at all postoperative periods after 15 days (Figure 6-13).

Examination of segments of the cord at increasing distances from the site of transection revealed that axonal growth extends from the injury zone into these segments. Most occupy the dorsal column area that has been gradually eroding to produce a significant amount of cavitation along this surface for 1–2 mm above and below the original lesion, thereby creating a space facilitating the invasion of axons (Figure 6-14). While these fibers occur as large fascicles adjacent to the lesion site, this well-ordered arrangement is quickly lost and replaced by a more dispersed pattern at distances of 1–3 mm from the lesion site (Figure 6-15). Increasing numbers of fibers appear to grow out into the nearby gray matter of the dorsal horns and may invade the lateral funiculus. Such axons could easily be identified because of their association with a Schwann cell. Bodian-stained longitudinal sections oriented to encompass bundles of such fibers in the dorsal columns together with adjacent gray matter displayed many fibers deviating from the main bundles to course deep into the gray matter as single fibers or small fascicles (Figure 6-16).

An electron microscopic examination of the cavitated dorsal column region as well as the CNS-scar matrix interface revealed a highly irregular and reduplicated surface thrown up into complex folds. Small axons were seen coursing near this surface (Figure 6-17). Some were invested by Schwann cell cytoplasm (Figure 6-18) and, in some instances, a thin myelin sheath, while others seemed to penetrate a short distance into this surface and were enveloped by the pale, filament-filled processes of astrocytes (Figure 6-19). Such cells were found in abundance subjacent to this interface as a new glia limitans formed to seal off the neuropil from components of the periphery. This occurred during the first 2–4 weeks after injury. As increasing numbers of axons grow into these zones and probe deeper into the rifts of the injury surface, examples can be found in which both myelinated and unmyelinated fibers are enclosed by astrocytic processes. This phenomenon is illustrated by the drawing shown in Figure 6-20. An important issue to address was whether some of these axons might have grown so rapidly that they could have entered the CNS. Ultrastructural examination of the dorsal horn and intermediate gray revealed many axons enveloped by Schwann cells at distances of up to 400 μm lateral to the eroded surface.

Figures 6-13. Vescicle-filled axonal profiles (V) occur predominantly in the matrix at earlier survival periods and may possibly represent growth cones; 45 dpo. 5,320×. From Matthews et al. (1979a).

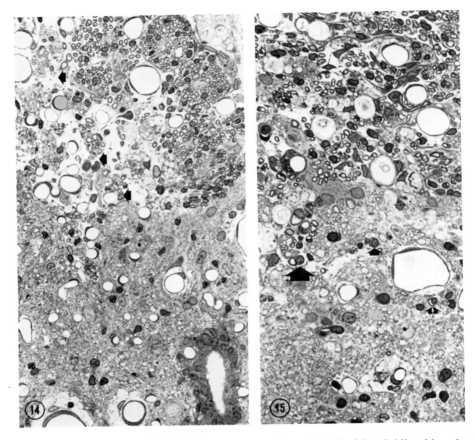

Figure 6-14. An Epon-embedded 2-μm cross section stained with toluidine blue that illustrates the extensive infiltration of the eroded dorsal column region just caudal to the original transection point by fascicles of peripheral axons with associated Schwann cells. The dorsal horn and intermediate gray substance is shown in the lower and upper-left portions of the figure. Arrows delineate the irregular medial borders of the gray substance that has been severely eroded with increasing postoperative periods. The central canal is seen to the lower right; 45 dpo. 250×. From Matthews et al. (1979a).

Figure 6-15. A zone of peripheral axon ingrowth 2 mm rostral to the lesion site is shown at higher magnification. The gray substance of the dorsal horn (lower half of this figure) displays areas of irregularity (large arrow) into which Schwann cell myelinated fibers are insinuated. Some isolated axons are apparently located deep within the neuropil of the gray matter (small arrows); 45 dpo. 575×. From Matthews et al. (1979a).

Some were found within defects in the neuropil lined with a distinct basement membrane and collagen fibers. Examination of 2-μm Epon-embedded serial sections through this region revealed that these spaces were continuous with the extracellular spaces of the matrix. It appeared that the axon–Schwann cell bundles had grown into or perhaps produced deep invaginations into the CNS but never came into direct contact with elements of the neuropil. Instances could, however, be found in which the basement membrane together with astrocytic lamellae deviated away from the ingrowing fibers, thus allowing them to come in contact with CNS tissues. Preterminal peripheral axons leading to a synaptic ending could not be located, although groups of such fibers were found to course into areas displaying concentrations of synapses (Figure 6-21).

Cyst Formation

The dominant feature of the transected spinal cord after 6 months' survival is the appearance and dramatic enlargement of fluid-filled spaces. These cause a gradual atrophy of neural tissue in adjacent cord segments and by 1 year reduce the area of the scar to a narrow septum separating the cysts above and below. Such cysts may in turn extend for several segments and destroy large amounts of adjacent tissue, leaving only a thin shell surrounding the elongated cyst. Those axons that grew into the scar matrix and adjacent neural elements also disappear except for a few that may remain along the cord periphery.

Effects of Treatment Methods

An initial qualitative examination of the lesion site and surrounding tissue at both the light and electron microscopic level in those animals given either Piromen or cyclophosphamide revealed no immediately apparent and distinctive features by which they could be separated from the control series of animals unless a quantitative approach was implemented. This conclusion was based upon observation of individual mesodermal cells within the matrix, the patterns of collagen fibrils, axons and their supportive cells, and the distribution and density of basement membranes.

Administration of trypsin generally followed the methods described by Matinian and Andreasian (1976). This series of animals demonstrated a subtle and somewhat inconsistent change in the arrangement of the fibrous tissue components of the scar matrix characterized by the presence of fibroblasts with large, multilocated cytoplasmic vacuoles associated with areas of collagen loss. Small bundles of unmyelinated axons were infrequently encountered in these areas, but it should be emphasized that this feature as well as the alterations observed in the matrix did not occur in all animals within this treatment group nor was there any apparent dependence upon the length of the postoperative interval.

In order to assess the effects of all the treatments more carefully, a systematic quantitative approach was employed with the purpose of examining the

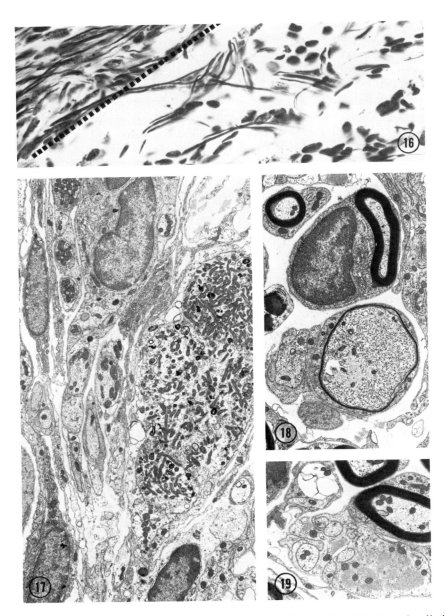

Figure 6-16. A longitudinal section stained by the Bodian method displays the distinctive fascicles of axons appearing in the dorsal columns (upper left) and arrows indicate examples of fibers that course into the adjacent gray substance (lower right). The dotted line indicates the area of demarcation between these two zones; 45 dpo. 495×. From Matthews et al. (1979a).

Figure 6-17. At 15 dpo many unmyelinated axons, encompassed by a Schwann cell and delineated with a basement membrane, are found in the region of the dorsal columns. The large profile, filled with mitochondria and dense bodies in the lower part of this figure, is a terminal club. 5,225×. From Matthews et al. (1979a).

quantity and patterns of distribution of both dense fibrous and loose connective tissue zones within the scar. This was done because of the apparent relationship between these areas and the location of axons infiltrating the scar matrix. The effect of cyst formation and enlargement upon elements of the cord clearly indicated that such areas should be included in the planimetric analysis.

The analysis was performed as follows: At 12 equidistant intervals above and below the lesion site with the original point of transection as the zero point, semithin sections encompassing the entire cross section of the cord were analyzed planimetrically and divided into areas of fibrous connective tissue (FCT), loose connective tissue (LCT), and the fluid-filled cysts. These data were expressed as a percentage of the total cross-sectional area of the cord and plotted in 12 tridimensional graphs as a function of: (1) location of the section in relation to the transection point, denoted as a series of numbers ranging from +6 to −6; and (2) one of five postoperative periods from 15 to 360 days. Three treatment groups were measured against a control group and the results illustrated in Figure 6-22.

Measurement of the cystic spaces confirmed a gradual increase in size to a point at which up to 96% of the cross section becomes occupied by fluid-filled space. No statistically significant differences were found between any of the four treatment groups with respect to cyst size or rate of formation.

Transient reductions in the amount of fibrous connective tissue were detected following administration of Piromen and cyclophosphamide. These occurred during the 45–90-day period and represented moderately significant differences ($P < 0.05$) from controls of the same age. The use of trypsin was associated with a greater reduction of the amount of this tissue that became significant at 45 days postoperatively ($P < 0.01$) and at each interval examined thereafter. It should be reemphasized, however, that some animals showed no effect as a result of treatment with trypsin.

Concomitantly, loose connective tissue areas were somewhat increased in size after treatment with Piromen or cyclophosphamide, although without sufficient consistency to result in a statistically significant difference from control tissue. Trypsin application resulted in significant increases in this component except at the 45-day interval when the amount of LCT was slightly reduced in all animals, possibly owing to the contraction of the scar matrix.

As the loose connective tissue component of the scar became increased in volume following treatment with Piromen, cyclophosphamide, or trypsin, the numbers of axons apparent within the scar matrix also increased, in some cases from two- to fivefold as shown by a separate quantitative study of material

---

Figure 6-18. Three axons in various stages of myelination by Schwann cells are illustrated; 30 dpo. 5,225×. From Matthews et al. (1979a).

Figure 6-19. Several unmyelinated fibers are completely enveloped by an astrocyte. These are usually found near the zone of the glia limitans; 45 dpo. 8,800×. From Matthews et al. (1979a).

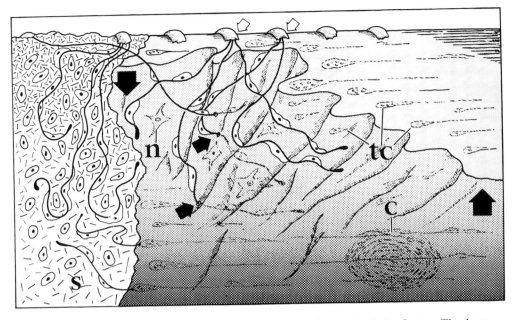

Figure 6-20. The dense scar matrix (S) is shown to the left of the figure. The large eroded zone adjacent to the scar represents schematically the degenerated dorsal white columns. Large, solid arrows delineate this zone from the adjacent scar and from the dorsal surface of the spinal cord shown to the upper right. The surface of the spinal cord is covered by a glia limitans (small dot screen pattern), and this covering becomes reconstituted along the surface of the degenerated and eroded dorsal white columns (large dot screen pattern). Elements of the neuropil including neuronal perikarya (n) and degenerating intrinsic axons are visible beneath this lining. Many of these axons form terminal clubs (tc).

   Injured dorsal roots (small open arrows) are giving rise to new axonal sprouts accompanied by Schwann cells. Some examples have infiltrated the scar matrix while others grow along the irregular surface of the degenerated zone. Occasional axons appear to penetrate the reconstituted glia limitans and enter the spinal cord parenchyma (small solid arrows). Two axons at the lower left of the figure are shown to arise from within the spinal cord and sprout into the scar matrix. The dark, oval profile in the lower right of the figure indicates the location of early stages of cyst formation (c) deep within the grey matter. From Matthews et al. (1979a).

prepared by the Bodian method (Gelderd et al. 1980). This study also included an evaluation of motor function and showed that all animals developed typical signs of spastic paraplegia, including hyper-reflexia, clonus, spontaneous erratic hind-limb movements, and lack of weight-bearing ability, regardless of which treatment was applied. No clearcut behavioral changes were observed that could be associated with any of the treatment groups.

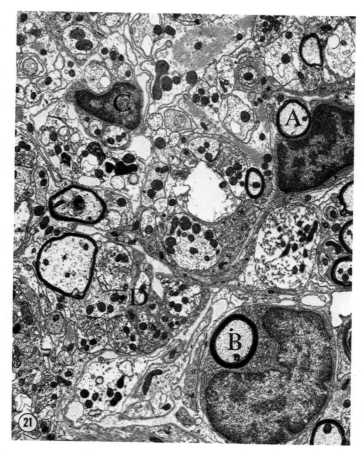

Figure 6-21. This micrograph is a representative cross section of the dorsal horn that illustrates several presumptive peripheral axons associated with Schwann cells which appear to have penetrated this area from the lesion zone. Two myelinated axons (A,B) are seen to the right of the figure. These are completely separated from elements of the neuropil by the intervening astrocyte lining and basement membrane of the glia limitans. A cluster of unmyelinated axons (C) with associated Schwann cells is seen in the upper left. The basement membrane is partially deviated away from these fibers (arrows), allowing them to become directly apposed to the neuropil. Another small cluster of axons (D) is enveloped by supportive cell cytoplasm in a manner typical of Schwann cells. These fibers are in apposition to a cluster of synaptic elements; 45 dpo. 8,750×. From Matthews et al. (1979a).

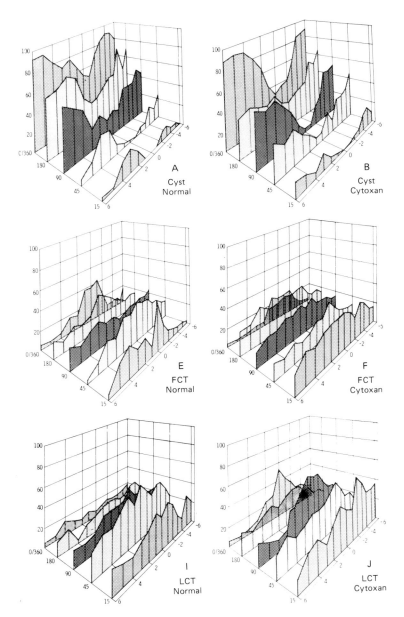

Figure 6-22. A series of tridimensional graphs illustrating the effects of treatment on (1) cysts, (2) fibrous connective tissue (FCT), and (3) loose connective tissue (LCT). Each group depicts three variables. The location of the cross section of the spinal cord in relation to the lesion is plotted along the abscissa at a series of points from +6 through −6 with zero being the transection point. The positive numbers represent the cranial segments and the negative numbers the caudal segments. Postoperative periods in days

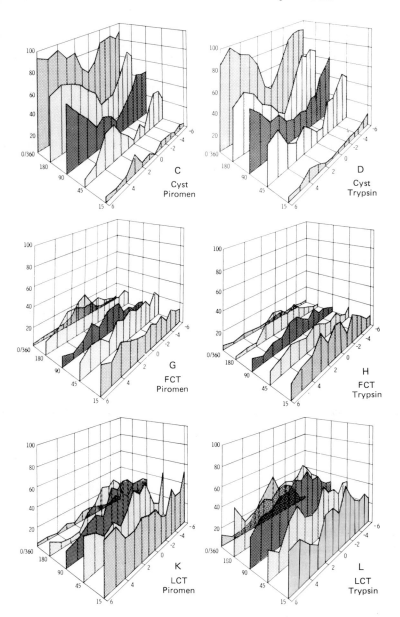

(15–360) are presented along the ordinate. The vertical axis depicts the percentage that each planimetrically determined area constitutes of the total crosssection. Graphs A–D show the effects of three separate treatments and a control series upon cyst formation, graphs E–H give equivalent data for fibrous connective tissue (FCT), and graphs I–L for the loose connective tissue (LCT). From Matthews et al. (1979a).

Ependymal Cell Proliferation

Evidence of ependymal cell proliferation was found in approximately 40% of the animals used in this series of studies. There appeared to be no relationship between the appearance and pattern of distribution of these cells and the type of pharmacologic treatment imposed upon the animal, except that the use of cyclophosphamide was not associated with ependymal cell proliferation, undoubtedly owing to its antimitotic properties.

The portion of the central canal rostral to the lesion site becomes widely dilated during the time when the scar matrix increases in density. With this the height of the ependymal cells is reduced, but buds of such cells begin to form and produce large aggregations that extend for hundreds of microns into adjacent tissues (Figures 6-23 and 6-24). Each cell is characterized by a moderately dense, oval nucleus containing evenly distributed chromatin. The cytoplasm is less dense and displays a few granules. At distances ranging from 300 to 900 μm from the canal and lying either within the scar matrix or adjacent neuropil, clusters of ependymal cells were found arranged into a circular acinar or rosette pattern that displayed a tiny lumen at the center (Figures 6-24 and 6-25). Some clusters of cells encircled a capillary profile.

Electron microscopic examination of the ependymal cells lining the dilated central canal revealed that the internal morphology of individual cells was little altered from normal. In areas near the lesion zone, stacking of cells occurred, together with an increased incidence of zonulae adherentes and gap junctions. However, most retained a typical polarity. Their apices displayed microvilli and cilia, and the base was lined with a basement membrane.

Those ependymal cells located in aggregates at a distance from the central canal also retain their morphological traits and polarity. This latter feature is particularly emphasized by the formation of rosettes (Figure 6-26). Occasionally, other neural or mesodermal elements become incorporated among the cell clusters including synaptic clusters, patches of basement membrane, astrocytic processes, distinguished by their paler cytoplasm and glycogen granules, and collagen fibers.

If the lumen of a rosette is visible within the plane of section, it can be seen to contain profiles of microvilli and cilia, together with basal bodies in the adjacent apices of ependymal cells. Zonulae adherentes were also a prominent feature but these were quite tortuous, consistent with the interdigitation of several ependymal cell processes. The presence of all these components is suggestive of the complete differentiation of the ependymal cells composing the rosettes. However, evidence of abnormality is inferred from the common appearance of intracytoplasmic vacuoles containing whorls of microvilli and cilia, and these resemble similar structures found in the cells composing an ependymoma (Figures 6-27 and 6-28).

The most important finding to arise from this portion of the study was the presence of large numbers of axons coursing in proximity to ependymal cell clusters (Figure 6-29). Some are directly apposed to the ependymal cell surface,

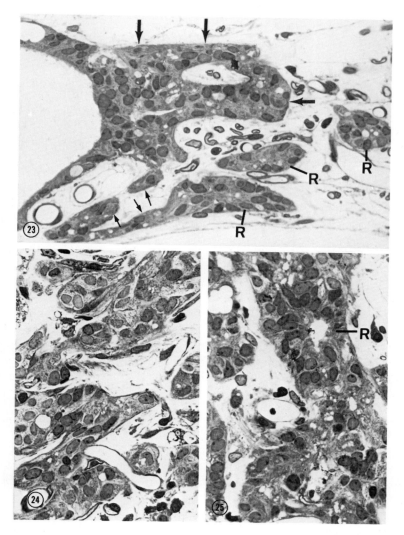

Figure 6-23. A large primary bud (large arrows) of ependymal cell aggregates extends from the dilated central canal in the left of this micrograph. The series of small arrows indicates contiguity of secondary cell clusters with the primary bud. Two rosettes (R) with tiny, centrally located lumina are depicted; 30 dpo. 306×. From Matthews et al. (1979c).

Figures 6-24 and 6-25. Nests of ependymal cells occur both within the degenerating neuropil or white matter. A large rosette (R) with a distinct lumen is shown; 45 dpo. 306×. From Matthews et al. (1979c).

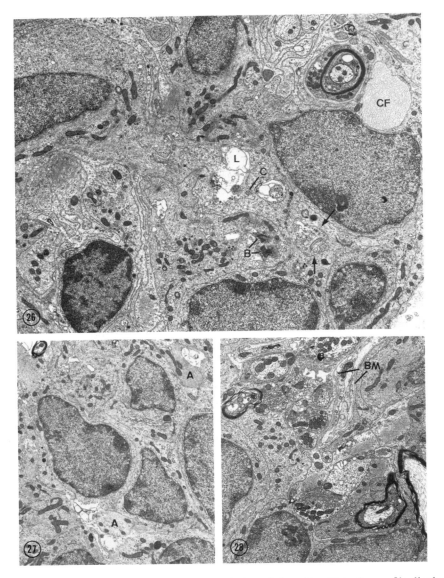

Figure 6-26. A small ependymal rosette consisting of six cells within the profile displays a small central lumen (L) with a single cilium (C). A second tiny lumen (arrows) contains several cilia and microvilli. Two basal bodies (B) are located near this secondary lumen. A bundle of collagen fibrils (CF) is enveloped by an ependymal cell in the upper right of this micrograph; 45 dpo. 6,893×. From Matthews et al. (1979c).

Figure 6-27. This low magnification micrograph illustrates a cluster of ependymal cells. Astrocytic processes (A) are insinuated among the cells but can be distinguished by their paler cytoplasm and thicker filaments; 30 dpo. 3,939×. From Matthews et al. (1979c).

Figure 6-28. Proliferation and clustering of ependymal cells has caused a group of synaptic elements together with portions of the basement membrane (BM) to be incorporated. No structural modifications of appositional membranes of such elements with ependymal cells develop. 60 dpo. 6,565×. From Matthews et al. (1979c).

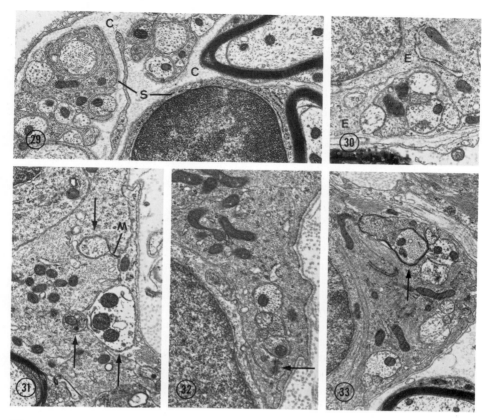

Figure 6-29. A small fascicle of myelinated and unmyelinated axons with Schwann cells (S) is illustrated. This example is found within the scar matrix. Note numerous collagen (C) fibrils; 30 dpo. 18,938×. From Matthews et al. (1979c).

Figure 6-30. A small cluster of five unmyelinated axons indents two adjacent ependymal cell processes (E); 45 dpo. 18,938×. From Matthews et al. (1979c).

Figure 6-31. A small axon (small arrow) is completely enveloped by this ependymal cell and a small mesaxon (M) is formed while two nearby axons (large arrows) merely indent the surface; 45 dpo. 16,665×. From Matthews et al. (1979c).

Figure 6-32. A group of five axons is encompassed and the enveloping processes display a tiny zonula adherens (arrow); 60 dpo. 18,180×. From Matthews et al. (1979c).

Figure 6-33. Several axons are enclosed at various locations within the ependymal cell. A rare myelinated axon (arrow) is included within a fascicle; 60 dpo. 15,908×. From Matthews et al. (1979c).

creating indentations or becoming enveloped by the cell in the manner of a typical Schwann cell mesaxon (Figures 6-30, 6-31, and 6-32). Apposed ependymal cell membranes incorporated into the area of a "mesaxon" sometimes display a tiny zonula adherens. This occurred most frequently if several fibers were enclosed, suggesting an active retention of the fibers. With increasing postoperative periods until 90 days, fascicles of from 3 to 8 axons enclosed within an ependymal cell invagination were a common finding among the cell clusters. Occasionally, a few fibers incorporated in this manner displayed a thin myelin sheath (Figure 6-33).

Discussion

We have used quantitative light and electron microscopic techniques to examine the transected spinal cord in adult rats following administration of Piromen (Clemente and Windle 1954, Puchala and Windle 1977), cyclophosphamide (Feringa et al. 1977), or trypsin (Matinian and Andreasian 1976). These three treatment groups were compared with an equivalent series of animals that received no further treatment following transection.

Our initial thrust was to examine the formation of the glio-mesodermal scar, describe its cellular makeup, and determine if significant numbers of axons can grow into this matrix (Matthews et al. 1979a). We found that two distinctive patterns of distribution and density of connective tissue occur within the scar matrix. One is characterized by concentrations of collagenous fibrils, active fibroblasts, few vascular profiles, and only a modicum of extracellular space. The other pattern found within the matrix was a well-vascularized and much less dense type of tissue with greater numbers of individual cells arranged into sheets and cords, separated by large intercellular lacunae. Axons were able to infiltrate the scar matrix but were largely restricted to those regions containing the loose, areolar, and better vascularized tissue. The application of cyclophosphamide and Piromen was associated with slight reductions in the amount of the dense fibrous connective tissue component of the scar. However, these effects were transient, being found only during the period from 45 to 90 days after spinal cord transection. After this period, the density of the scar increased but was reduced in volume by the gradual encroachment of the adjacent cystic spaces. Cyst formation destroyed large quantities of neural tissue, leaving a mere shell of white matter around the periphery of the spinal cord and eliminating most of the axons that had grown into the matrix of the scar.

Administration of trypsin caused a somewhat more significant reduction in the amount of the dense fibrous component of the scar, which was maintained for a longer period of time than that observed with the previous two treatments. Concomitantly, the number of axons infiltrating the scar was also increased in this treatment group, but evidence of actual bridging of the transection site was lacking. Instead, most axons appeared to enter the scar from the area of the cord dorsum and then course about the matrix in an aimless, serpentine fashion. Regeneration of axons from either the cranial or caudal stump of the severed spinal cord could not be documented despite examination of sets of longitudinally oriented serial sections encompassing the site of lesion and significant expanses of spinal cord above and below this point. This finding, together with the lack of improvement in motor function, fails to provide support for the efficacy of Piromen, cyclophosphamide, or trypsin as therapeutic agents to promote spinal cord regeneration and restitution of function (Puchala and Windle 1977, Feringa et al. 1973, 1974, 1975, 1976, 1977, Matinian and Andreasian 1976). It should be added that we made a special attempt to reproduce the experimental methodology of Matinian and Andreasian as closely as possible in the use of trypsin as an agent to induce cord regeneration. However, their claims of significant spinal cord regeneration could not be substantiated in our study. A more recent study of the possible effectiveness of enzyme therapy in spinal cord injury also showed no significant behavioral, histological, or electrophysiological differences between control animals and those treated with trypsin, hyaluronidase, or elastase (Guth et al. 1980). These investigators concluded that enzyme treatment neither facilitates nerve regeneration nor permits functional restitution in rats with spinal cord transection. The previously reported findings of Matinian and Andreasian were apparently the result of incomplete spinal transection and the retention of a small number of intact axons in the ventral funiculus of the cord. Apparently, this minimal amount of fiber continuity across the partially severed cord is sufficient to allow a dramatic amount of functional return. The underlying mechanism for this remains obscure but is clearly an area requiring further investigation because it may represent a useful model for functional and, possibly, anatomical plasticity in the adult spinal cord.

Our data indicate that the axons infiltrating the scar matrix have no detectable functional significance despite their increased incidence in the three treatment groups. It appears that most of these fibers have sprouted from the central processes of dorsal roots injured during the transection. Large numbers of these axons and their associated Schwann cells not only entered the scar matrix but also grew into the adjacent eroded dorsal white columns and occasionally entered the dorsal horn. However, our electron microscopic studies demonstrated that a newly formed glia limitans almost always intervened between these peripheral fibers and the intrinsic fibers and neurons of the CNS (Matthews et al. 1979b). This barrier effectively seals off the spinal cord from the "peripheral" environment of the lesion zone (Lampert and Cressman 1964, Puchala and Windle, 1977, Windle 1980) and, together with cyst formation and enlargement, may represent one of the most profound barriers to regeneration of the transected spinal cord.

The recent studies of delayed microsurgical nerve autografting following spinal cord transection in dogs (Kao 1980) showed that the presence of the implanted nerve segments was associated with delayed reconstitution of the glia limitans over the injured surface of the cord. This allowed large numbers of new fibers to grow into the autograft using the remaining Schwann elements for support and guidance. His electron micrographs showed axons myelinated by an oligodendrocyte along one internode and by a Schwann cell at an adjacent internode that passed out of the spinal cord tissue and entered the nerve auto-graft. Kao concluded that the principal source of these new fibers in the nerve were sprouts from intrinsic axons of the CNS rather than dorsal roots and stated that 5 of the 40 dogs subjected to this procedure became capable of spontaneous standing or walking. He also performed electrophysiological stud-ies that demonstrated the presence of evoked potentials across the repaired spinal cord. His method of performing the original transection (sub-pial aspira-tion) does not rule out the possibility of an incomplete transection in those five animals displaying an improvement in their motor function, but this study is important in that histological evidence of CNS regeneration into the autograft is provided. The possibility of axons passing through the graft and reentering the opposite segment of the cord is less apparent in this study, but a subsequent investigation by Richardson et al. (1980) of sciatic nerve autografting after removal of a 10-mm segment from the rat spinal cord showed transport of HRP across the autograft. Definitive labeling of neurons was seen in seven of the ten animals receiving an injection of HRP and strongly suggests that a degree of regeneration has occurred. However, as Guth et al. (1980) have pointed out, "Unless complete serial reconstruction is performed in every case of appar-ently successful regeneration, one cannot rule out the possibility of incomplete transection of the spinal cord." Nonetheless, the results of the studies by Kao and Richardson indicate that the biochemical nature of components of the glia limitans should be actively investigated in relationship to axonal growth and repair. The formation of the basal lamina at the site of a spinal cord transection has been examined using an epithelial basal lamina-specific immunohistochemi-cal stain (Feringa et al. 1979). This method demonstrated a gradual formation of the lamina over the out ends of the rat spinal cord between 5 and 20 days after transection and correlated quite closely with the timetable constructed from our ultrastructural data.

Can any examples of regeneration of CNS fibers within the spinal cord be found? The descending monoaminergic pathways of the spinal cord have shown a capacity for regeneration. Thus, if descending noradrenergic axons are selectively lesioned by administration of 6-hydroxy dopamine, significant re-growth of these fibers apparently took place as demonstrated by the use of fluorescence histochemistry and by the measurement of the reestablishment of flexor reflex responses (Nygren and Olson 1976, 1977, Nygren et al. 1971, Björklund and Stenevi 1979). Similarly, descending serotonergic axons can be chemically lesioned by the administration of 5,6- or 5,7-dihydroxytryptamines, and these pathways will also show structural and functional recovery (Björklund and Stenevi 1979, Björklund et al. 1981). These investigators con-cluded that certain long descending fiber systems of the spinal cord can regen-erate lesioned axons if scar formation is absent or minimal. No regeneration of these systems was found if the spinal cord was subjected to a mechanical transection. However, as pointed out by Kalil and Reh (1979, 1982), the actual disintegration of the monoaminergic axons, as a result of the neurochemical method of lesioning the projection system, was not verified at the ultrastruc-tural level but implied by the use of fluorescence histochemical demonstration of the presence or absence of the transmitter. Nonetheless, it seems reasonable to assume that the powerful and specific neurotoxins employed would have severely damaged the susceptible axons and that, as a result, their regrowth must represent a form of regeneration. The lack of mechanical disruption would be expected to allow retention of intrinsic cues to guide the regrowing axons to their proper targets and thereby favor an anatomical and functional restitution. It should be noted that the monoaminergic systems may possess an unusual capacity for regeneration that is not inherent in most tracts of the CNS (Wiklund and Mollgard 1979).

Immature animals seem to have an enhanced ability to recover function after sustaining CNS injury. Much of this recovery has been attributed to the greater potential for functional and anatomical reorganization of uninjured elements of the CNS, rather than an organized regeneration of damaged fibers (Devor 1975, Castro 1978a,b, Hicks and D'Amato 1970, Schneider 1970, Stelzner et al. 1979, Prendergast and Misantone 1980, Cummings et al. 1981). Apparently, those fibers that emit new sprouts rostral to the site of lesion display a random growth and terminate in improper areas (Bernstein and Bernstein 1971, 1973a,b. However, if the surgical lesions are small and are directed to a specific tract, wide expanses of adjacent neural tissue remain to provide a substrate for regrowth of the damaged fibers. Thus, if the pyramidal tract is cut unilaterally in perinatal hamsters, a massive new axonal growth arises from the severed tract rostral to the cut, crosses to the contralateral brainstem, and descends as a compact bundle just medial to the spinal trigeminal nucleus. Despite the abnormal trajectory of the tract, the pattern of termination was normal and synapse formation in appropriate areas was confirmed by electron microscopy following adult cortical lesions (Kalil and Reh 1982). Additionally, restitution of those motor activities specifically mediated by this tract occurred in proportion to the degree of fiber regrowth (Reh and Kalil 1982). Such findings are important and should provide important clues about the mechanisms underlying axonal growth, collateral sprouting, guidance cues, and possible regenerative capacities in specific fiber tracts. However, they further serve to emphasize the fact that the mechanical disruption with subsequent cyst formation following traumatic injury to the spinal cord effectively prevents axonal regeneration, at least in mammalians, and there appear to be no studies to date that have unequivocally overcome this problem.

In addition to the barriers to regeneration created by the glio-mesodermal scar, cysts, etc., most neurons of the mammalian CNS may lack the metabolic machinery to sustain a prolonged period of active synthesis associated with axonal regeneration over long distances. This is in contradistinction to neurons that project to or are located in the periphery (Veraa and Grafstein 1981). Another possibility may be the lack of support for regeneration from glial elements, principally ependymal cells. In nonmammalian animal forms ependymal cells proliferate and actively participate in a well-organized regenerative process. This participation seems essential for the successful regeneration that occurs in these forms after transection of their spinal cord (Simpson 1968, Egar and Singer 1972, Nordlanger and Singer 1978, Michel and Reier 1979). The function of these cells appears to be that of extending out "radial" cytoplasmic processes that envelope and fasciculate regenerating axons. Series of these processes form longitudinal axonal compartments that guide axonal growth. However, Michel and Reier (1979) noted that despite the importance of the ependymal cell surface during axonal outgrowth in the regenerating spinal cord of *Xenopus laevis,* guided neurite elongation did not appear to be dependent upon the prior establishment of a specific type of cytoarchitecture. This suggests that an intrinsic capacity for regeneration exists in the neurons of certain nonmammalian forms and emphasizes the probability that this may not be the case with mammalian CNS neurons.

Our observations of ependymal cell alteration in the rat spinal cord after transection indicated that these cells were undergoing an active proliferation in response to the injury (Matthews et al. 1979c), and this has been confirmed in a study by Gilmore and Leiting (1980) employing [³H]thymidine autoradiography. The trauma of the injury and associated dilation of the central canal represent disruptive factors that alter the cytoarchitecture, spatial arrangement, and appositional relations of the ependymal cells. The normally quiescent ependymal cells may partially revert to a more primitive state and exhibit proliferative patterns similar to those of abnormal neuroepithelium (Shellshear and Emory 1976) or ependymomas (Luse 1961), and subependymomas (Fu et al. 1974, Vick et al. 1977, Azzarelli et al. 1977).

The most intriguing finding in this portion of our studies was the envelopment of axons growing into the lesion site by the abnormally proliferating ependymal cells, a property not usually attributed to the ependyma of mature mammalian neural tissue, although ependymal cell axonal ensheathment occurs on a large scale in human embryonic and fetal spinal cord prior to 6 weeks gestational age (Gamble 1968). Such examples of ependymal proliferation and subsequent envelopment of sprouting axons in the injured adult mammalian spinal cord may represent a minimal attempt to support an abortive regenerative process. In the lizard, *Xantusia vigilis,* implantation of ependymal cells into the stump of an amputated limb initiated regeneration of the limb, suggesting that such cells possess a trophic influence (Bryant and Wozny 1974). However, in our material, the presence of concentrations of ependymal cells was not associated with increased numbers of axon sprouts. Our impression was that those axons that coursed adjacent to the surface of these cells became invaginated into them. No evidence suggestive of a trophic influence could be adduced from our micrographs.

An interesting approach to determine if axons within the mammalian CNS have the capacity for regeneration is that of transplantation of selected areas of the fetal brain to host animals ranging in age from newborn to adult. The concept of such an approach is not new but represents an offshoot of transplantation studies in nonmammalian vertebrates used to analyze problems related to neuronal specificity, plasticity, and mechanisms of axonal guidance (Jacobson 1978). Initial efforts in mammals to transplant spinal ganglia or cerebral cortex to alternative sites in the host were only marginally successful (Saltykow 1905, Ranson 1914, Dunn 1917). The studies by Sugar and Gerard (1940), in which fetal brain tissue or muscle was transplanted to the site of a spinal cord transection, seemed to show that such transplants acted as a bridge for the regenerative growth of CNS axons. These authors reported a return of voluntary hind-limb movement 4–6 weeks following the transplant, but later attempts to confirm their results were unsuccessful (Brown and McCouch 1947, Barnard and Carpenter 1950, Feigin et al. 1951).

The application of improved transplantation techniques have, however, shown that a wide variety of mammalian fetal CNS tissues can be placed in a host brain and that many of these grafts will establish reciprocal connections with the host (Das et al. 1980a,b, Hallas et al. 1980, Stenevi et al. 1976, Björklund et al. 1979, Kormer et al. 1981, Olson and Seiger 1975, Hoffer et al. 1977, Woodward et al. 1977, Perlow et al. 1979, McLoon and Lund 1980a,b, Jaeger and Lund 1979, 1980). Many of these studies, including our own (Matthews et al. 1982, Matthews and West 1982), have shown that the axons originating from the implanted neurons often display a vigorous growth into the host and are directed toward the correct target areas. If the target areas are deafferented by a lesion prior to the transplant, replacement of these axons by implanting the appropriate fetal tissue can be accomplished such that the implanted cells will reestablish the same innervation pattern that was in place prior to the lesion. In many instances, the new connections are physiologically functional and may produce behavioral improvement (Björklund et al. 1979, Björklund and Stenevi 1979).

Recent studies indicate that the use of refined techniques to transplant mammalian spinal cord tissue greatly improve neuronal survival, growth, and axonal elongation into either a co-transplant within the anterior chamber of the eye (Olson et al. 1982) or directly into a host spinal cord (Bregman and Reier 1982, Reier et al. 1983).

The latter studies are particularly interesting in that data was presented to show that appropriate, target-oriented connections extended from the transplant into the host spinal cord for long distances and that cortico-spinal fibers that had not reached the site of transection and were therefore not damaged by the lesion were able to grow through the transplant into the caudal segment of the cord. Such transplants prevented the degeneration of rubrospinal neurons whose axons were injured by the spinal cord lesion (Bregman 1983). These studies are supportive of the work by Sugar and Gerard (1940) and, as the authors concluded, indicate that the implant may serve as a possible relay for supraspinal input or as a bridge for growing fibers.

Many problems remain to be solved in order for such models to become clinically useful (De la Torre 1981), including basic mechanisms of axonal growth, particularly as mediated by axonal transport, specificity and guidance to proper target cells, and synaptogenesis (Veraa and Grafstein 1981). However, these kinds of data allow us to sound a cautious note of optimism about the possibility that the chronic paraplegia or quadriplegia resulting from traumatic spinal cord injury may be overcome by the employment of systematic research approaches to unravel this enigma and bring about a return of function.

Acknowledgments. This study was supported in part by a grant from the Edward G. Schlieder Educational Foundation and by NIH grant NS 14699 from the National Institute of Neurological and Communicative Disorders and Stroke.

References

Azzarelli, B., Rekate, H.L., Roessmann, U. (1977). Subependymona: A case report with ultrastructural study. Acta. Neuropathol. (Berl.) 40, 279–282.

Barnard, J.W., Carpenter W. (1950). Lack of regeneration in the spinal cord of the rat. J. Neurophysiol. 13, 223–228.

Bernstein, J.J., Bernstein, M.E. (1967). Effect of glial-ependymal scar and teflon arrest on the regenerative capacity of goldfish spinal cord. Exp. Neurol. 19, 23–52.

Bernstein, J.J., Bernstein, M.E. (1971). Axonal regeneration and formation of synapes proximal to the site of the lesion following hemisection of the rat spinal cord. Exp. Neurol. 30, 336–351.

Bernstein, J.J., Bernstein, M.E. (1973a). Neuronal alteration and reinnervation following axonal regeneration and sprouting in mammalian spinal cord. Brain Behav. Evol. 8, 135–161.

Bernstein, M.E., Bernstein, J.J. (1973b). Regeneration of axons and synaptic complex formation rostral to the site of hemisection in the spinal cord of the monkey. Int. J. Neurosci. 5, 15–26.

Björklund, A., Kromer, L.F., Stenevi, V. (1979). Cholinergic reinnervation of the rat hippocampus by septal implants is stimulated by perforant path lesion. Brain Res. 173, 57–64.

Björklund, A., Segal, M., Stenevi, U. (1979). Functional reinnervation of rat hippocampus by locus coeruleus implants. Brain Res. 170, 555.

Björklund, A., Stenevi, U. (1979). Regeneration of monoaminergic and cholinergic neurons in the mammalian central nervous system. Physiol. Rev. 59, 62–100.

Björklund, A., Wiklund, N.L., Descarries, L. (1981). Regeneration and plasticity of central serotoninergic neurons: A review. J. Physiol. (Paris) 77, 247–255.

Bregman, B.S. (1983). Neural tissue transplants rescue rubrospinal neurons after neonatal spinal cord lesions. Soc. Neuro. Abs. 13th Annual Meeting.

Bregman, B.S., Reier, P.J. (1982). Transplantation of fetal spinal cord tissue to injured spinal cord in neonatal and adult rats. Soc. Neuro. Abs. 12th Annual Meeting.

Brown, J.O., McCouch, G.P. (1947). Abortive regeneration of the transected spinal cord. J. Comp. Neur. 87, 131–137.

Bryant, S.V., Wozny, K.J. (1974). Stimulation of limb regeneration in the lizard *Xantusia vigilis* by means by ependymal implants. J. Exp. Zool. 189, 399–352.

Campbell, J.B., Windle, W.F. (1960). Relation of millipore to healing and regeneration in transected spinal cords of monkeys. Neurology (Minneapolis) 10, 306–311.

Castro, A.J. (1978a). Projection of the superior cerebellar peduncle in rats and the development of new connections in response to neonatal hemicerebellectomy. J. Comp. Neur. 178, 611–628.

Castro, A.J. (1978b). Analysis of corticospinal and rubrospinal projections after neonatal pyramidotomy in rats. Brain Res. 144, 155–158.

Clemente, D.D., Windle, W.F. (1954). Regeneration of severed nerve fibers in the spinal cord of the adult cat. J. Comp. Neur. 101, 691–731.

Cummings, J.P., Bernstein, D.R., Stelzner, D.J. (1981). Further evidence that sparing of function after spinal cord transection in the neonatal rat is not due to axonal generation or regeneration. Exp. Neurol. 74, 615–620.

Das, G.D., Hallas, B.H., Das, K.G. (1980a). Transplantation of embryonic tissue in the mammalian brain. I. Growth and differentiation of neuroblasts from various regions of the embryonic brain in the cerebellum of neonate rats. TITJ. Life Sci. 4, 93–124.

Das, G.D., Hallas, B.H., Das, K.G. (1980b). Transplantation of brain tissue in the brain of rat. I. Growth characteristics of neocortical transplants from embryos of different ages. Am. J. Anat. 158, 135–145.

De la Torre, J.C. (1981). Spinal cord injury. Review of basic and applied research. Spine 6, 315–335.

Devor, M. (1975). Neuroplasticity in the sparing or deterioration of function after early olfactory tract lesions. Science 190, 998–1000.

Dunn, E. (1917). Primary and secondary findings in a series of attempts to transplant cerebral cortex in the albino rat. J. Comp. Neur. 27, 565–582.

Egar, M., Singer, M. (1972). The role of ependyma in spinal cord regeneration in the urodele, Triturus. Exp. Neurol. 37, 422–430.

Feigin, I., Geller, E.H., Wolfe, A. (1951). Absence of regeneration in the spinal cord of young rats. J. Neuropath. Exp. Neurol. 10, 420–425.

Feringa, E.R., Gurden, G.G., Strodel, W. (1973). Descending spinal motor tract regeneration after spinal cord transection. Neurology (Minneapolis) 23, 599–608.

Feringa, E.R., Johnson, R.D., Wendt, J.S. (1975). Spinal cord regeneration in rats after immunosuppressive treatment. Arch. Neurol (Chicago) 22, 676–683.

Feringa, E.R., Kinning, W.K., Britten, A.G. (1976). Recovery in rats after spinal cord injury. Neurology (Minneapolis) 26, 839–843.

Feringa, E.R., Kowalski, T.F., Vahlsing, H.L. (1980). Basal lamina formation at the site of spinal cord transection. Ann. Neurol. 8, 148–154.

Feringa, E.R., Shuer, L.M., Vahlsing, H.L., Davis, S.W. (1977). Regeneration of corticospinal axons in the rat. Ann. Neurol. 2, 315–321.

Feringa, E.R., Wendt, J.S., Johnson, R.D. (1974). Immunosuppressive treatment to enhance spinal cord regeneration in rats. Neurology (Minneapolis) 24, 287–293.

Freeman, L.W., MacDougall, J., Turbes, C.C. (1960). The treatment of experimental lesions of the spinal cord of dogs with trypsin. J. Neurosurg. 17, 259–265.

Fu, Y., Chen, A.T.L., Kay, S., Young, H.F. (1974). Is subependymoma (subependymal glomerate astrocytoma) an astrocytoma or ependymoma? Cancer 34, 1992–2008.

Gamble, H.J. (1968). Axon ensheathing by ependymal cells in the human embryonic and foetal spinal cord. Nature 218, 182–183.

Gelderd, J.B., Matthews, M.A., St. Onge, M.F., Faciane, C.L. (1980). Qualitative and quantitative effects of ACTH, Piromen, Cytoxan, and isobutyl-2-cyanoacrylate treatments following spinal cord transection in rats. Acta Neurobiol. Exp. 40, 489–500.

Gilmore, S.A., Leiting, J.E. (1980). Changes in the central canal area of immature rats following spinal cord injury. Brain Res. 201, 185–189.

Guth, L., Albuquerque, E.X., Desgpande, S.S., Barrett, C.P., Donati, E.J., Warnicke, J.E. (1980). Ineffectiveness of enzyme therapy on regeneration in the transected spinal cord of the rat. J. Neurosurg. 52, 73–86.

Hallas, B.H., Das, G.D., Das, K.G. (1980). Transplantation of brain tissue in the brain of rat. II. Growth characteristics of neocortical transplants in hosts of different ages. Am. J. Anat. 158, 147–159.

Hicks, S.P., D'Amato, C.J. (1970). Motor-sensory and visual behavior after hemi-sperectomy in newborn and mature rats. Exp. Neurol. 29, 416–438.

Hoffer, B., Seiger, A., Freedman, R., Olson, L., Taylor, D. (1977). Electrophysiology and cytology of hippocampal formation transplants in the anterior chamber of the eye. II. Cholinergic mechanisms. Brain Res. 119, 107–132.

Jacobson, M. (1978). Developmental Neurobiology, Second Edition. New York: Plenum Press.

Jaeger, C.B., Lund, R.D. (1979). Efferent fibers from transplanted cerebral cortex of rats. Brain Res. 165, 338–342.

Jaeger, C.B., Lund, R.D. (1980). Transplantation of embryonic occipital cortex to the tectal region of newborn rats: A light microscopic study of organization and con-nectivity of the transplants. J. Comp. Neur. 194, 571–597.

Kalil, K., Reh, T. (1979). Regrowth of severed axons in the neonatal central nervous system: Establishment of normal connections. Science 205, 1158–1161.

Kalil, K., Reh, T. (1982). A light and electron microscopic study of regrowing pyramidal tract fibers. J. Comp. Neur. 211, 265–275.

Kao, C.C. (1980). Spinal cord reconstruction after traumatic injury. In: The Spinal Cord and Its Reaction to Traumatic Injury. Anatomy, Physiology, Pharmacology Thera-peutics. Modern Pharmacology-Toxicology. Bousquet, W.F., Palmer, R.F. (eds.). New York: Marcel Dekker, Inc.

Kromer, L.F., Björklund, A., Stenevi, V. (1981). Regeneration of the septohippocam-pal pathways in adult rats is promoted by utilizing embryonic hippocampal implants as bridges. Brain Res. 210, 173–200.

Lampert, P., Cressman, M. (1964). Axonal regeneration in the dorsal columns of the spinal cord of adult rats. Lab. Invest. 13, 825–839.

Littrell, J.L. (1955). Apparent functional restitution in Piromen-treated spinal cats. In: Regeneration in the Central Nervous System. Windle, W.F. (ed.). Springfield, IL: C.C. Thomas, pp. 219–228.

Luse, S.A. (1961). Ultrastructural characteristics of normal and neoplastic cells. Prog. Exp. Tumor Res. 2, 1–35.

Matinian, L.A., Andreasian, A.S. (1976). Enzyme therapy in organic lesions of the spinal cord. Tanasescu, E. (transl.). Los Angeles: Brain Information Service, Uni-versity of California.

Matthews, M.A. (1973). Death of the central neuron: An electron microscopic study of thalamic retrograde degeneration following cortical ablation. J. Neurocytol. 2, 265–288.

Matthews, M.A., Gelderd, J.B., St. Onge, M.F. (1976). Electron microscopy of spinal cord injury: Modification of reactive envents with immunosuppressives, pyrogens and antiinflammatory agents. Society for Neuroscience 6th Annual Meeting.

Matthews, M.A.. St. Onge, M.F., Faciane, C.L., Gelderd, J.B. (1979a). Spinal cord transection: A quantitative analysis of elements of the connective tissue matrix formed within the site of lesion following administration of piromen, cytoxan or trypsin. Neuropath. Appl. Neurobiol. 5, 161–180.

Matthews, M.A., St. Onge, M.F., Faciane, C.L., Gelderd, J.B. (1979b). Axon sprouting into segments of rat spinal cord adjacent to the site of a previous transection. Neuropath. Appl. Neurobiol. 5, 181–196.

Matthews, M.A., St. Onge, M.F., Faciane, C.L. (1979c). An electron microscopic analysis of abnormal ependymal cell proliferation and envelopment of sprouting axons following spinal cord transection in the rat. Acta Neuropathol. (Berlin) 45, 27–36.

Matthews, M.A., West, L.C. (1982). Optic fiber development between dual transplants of retina and superior colliculus placed in the occipital cortex. Anat. Embryol. 163, 417–433.

Matthews, M.A., West, L.C., Riccio, R.V. (1982). An ultrastructural analysis of the development of foetal rat retina transplanted to the occipital cortex, a site lacking appropriate target neurons for optic fibers. J. Neurocytol. 11, 533–557.

McLoon, S.C., Lund, R.D. (1980a). Identification of cells in retinal transplants which project to host visual centers: A horseradish peroxidase study in rats. Brain Res. 197, 491–495.

McLoon, S.C., Lund, R.D. (1980b). Specific projections of retina transplanted to rat brain. Exp. Brain Res. 40, 273–282.

McMasters, R.E. (1962). Regeneration of the spinal cord in the rat. Effects of Piromen and ACTH upon the regenerative capacity. J. Comp. Neur. 119, 113–125.

Michel, M.E., Reier, P.J. (1979). Axonal-ependymal associations during early regeneration of the transected spinal cord in *Xenopus laevis* tadpoles. J. Neurocytol. 8, 529–548.

Nordlander, R.H., Singer, M. (1978). The role of ependyma in regeneration of the spinal cord in the urodele amphibian tail. J. Comp. Neurol. 180, 349–374.

Nygren, L.G., Olson, L. (1976). On spinal noradrenaline receptor supersensitivity: Correlation between nerve terminal densities and flexor reflexes various times after intracisternal 6-hydroxydopamine. Brain Res. 116, 455–470.

Nygren, L.G., Olson, L. (1977). A new major projection from locus coeruleus: The main source of noradrenergic nerve terminals in the ventral and dorsal columns of the spinal cord. Brain Res. 132, 85–93.

Nygren, L.G., Olson, L., Seiger, A. (1971). Regeneration of monoamine-containing axons in the developing and adult spinal cord of the rat following intraspinal 6-OH-dopamine injections or transections. Histochemie 28, 1–15.

Olson, I., Björklund, H., Hoffer, B.J., Palmer, M.R., Seiger, A. (1982). Spinal cord grafts: An intraocular approach to enigmas of nerve growth regulation. Brain Res. Bull. 9, 519–537.

Olson, L., Seiger, A. (1975). Brain tissue transplanted to the anterior chamber of the eye. 2. Fluorescence histochemistry of immature catecholamine and 5-hydroxytryptamine neurons innervating the rat vas deferens. Cell Tiss. Res. 158, 141–150.

Perlow, M.J., Freed, W.J., Hoffer, B.J., Seiger, A., Olson, L., Wyatt, R.J. (1979). Brain grafts reduce motor abnormalities produced by destruction of the nigrostriatal dopamine system. Science 204, 643–646.

Pettegrew, R.K. (1976). Trypsin inhibition of scar formation in cordotomized rats (abstract). Anat. Rec. 184, 501.

Prendergast, J., Misantone, L.J. (1980). Sprouting by tracts descending from the midbrain to the spinal cord. The result of thoracic funiculotomy in the newborn, 21-day-old, and adult rat. Exp. Neurol. 69, 458–480.

Puchala, E., Windle, W.F. (1977). The possibility of structural and functional restitution after spinal cord injury. A review. Exp. Neurol. 55, 1–42.

Ramon Cajal, S. (1928). Degeneration and Regeneration of the Nervous System, Vol. II. London: Oxford University Press.

Ranson, S.W. (1914). Transplantation of the spinal ganglion cells. J. Comp. Neur. 24, 547–558.

Reh, T., Kalil, K. (1982). Functional role of regrowing pyramidal tract fibers. J. Comp. Neur. 211, 276–283.

Reier, P.J., Perlow, M.J., Guth, L. (1983). Development of embryonic spinal cord transplants in the rat. Dev. Brain Res. In press.

Richardson, P.M., McGuinness, U.M., Aguayo, A.J. (1980). Axons from CNS neurons regenerate into PNS grafts. Nature 284, 264–265.

Saltykow, S. (1905). Versuche über gehirnplantation Zugleich einbeitrag zür Kenntniss der Borgange an den zelligen gehirnelementen. Arch. Psych. 40, 320.

Schneider, G.E. (1970). Mechanisms of functional recovery following lesions of visual cortex or superior colliculus in neonate and adult hamsters. Brain Behav. Evol. 3, 295–323.

Shellshear, I., Emory, J.L. (1976). Gliosis and aqueductule formation in the aqueduct of Silvius. Dev. Med. Child. Neurol. Suppl. 37, 22–28.

Simpson, S.B. (1968). Morphology of the regenerated spinal cord in the lizard, *Anolis carolinensis*. J. Comp. Neurol. 134, 193–210.

Stelzner, D.J., Weber, E.D., Prendergast, J. (1979). A comparison of the effect of mid-thoracic spinal hemisection in the neonatal or weanling rat on the distribution and density of dorsal root axons in the lumbosacral spinal cord of the adult. Brain Res. 172, 407–426.

Stenevi, V., Björklund, A., Svendgaard, N. (1976). Transplantation of central and peripheral monoamine neurons to the adult brain. Techniques and conditions for survival. Brain Res. 114, 1–20.

Sugar, O., Gerard, R.W. (1940). Spinal cord regeneration in the rat. J. Neurophysiol. 3, 1–19.

Turbes, C.C., Freeman, L.W. (1953). Apparent spinal cord regeneration following intramuscular trypsin. Anat. Rec. 117, 288.

Veraa, R.P., Grafstein, B. (1981). Cellular mechanisms for recovery from nervous system injury: A conference report. Exp. Neurol. 71, 6–75.

Vick, N.A., Lin, M., Bigner, D.D. (1977). The role of the subependymal plate in tumorigenesis. Acta Neuropathol. (Berlin) 40, 63–71.

Wiklund, L., Mollgard, K. (1979). Neurotoxic destruction of the serotonergic synaptic innervation of the rat subcommissural organ if followed by reinnervation through collateral sprouting of non-monaminergic neurons. J. Neurocytol. 8, 469–480.

Willenborg, D.O., Staten, E.A., Eidelberg, E. (1977). Studies on cell-mediated hypersensitivity to neural antigens after experimental spinal cord injury. Exp. Neurol. 54, 383–392.

Windle, W.F. (1980). Concussion, contusion and severence of the spinal cord. In: The Spinal Cord and Its Reaction to Traumatic Injury. Anatomy, Physiology, Pharmacology, Therapeutics. Modern Pharmacology-Toxicology. Bousquet, W.F., Palmer, R.F. (eds.). New York: Marcel Dekker, Inc.

Woodward, D.J. Seiger, A., Olson, L., Hoffer, B.J. (1977). Intrinsic and extrinsic determinants of dendritic development as revealed by Golgi studies of cerebellar and hippocampal transplants in oculo. Exp. Neurol. 57, 984–998.

Chapter 7

Regenerative Growth of Retinofugal Axons into and through Neocortical Transplants Following Transection of the Optic Tract in Adult Rats

Douglas T. Ross* and Gopal D. Das†

Historical Background

Injury to the CNS of adult mammals usually results in functional deficits that are incompletely recovered. Complete functional recovery from brain or spinal cord injury is impeded by (1) the inability of the adult mammalian CNS to produce new neurons to replace those lost, and (2) the apparent inability of most intrinsic CNS neurons to regenerate their axons following damage. The successful elongative axonal regeneration and functional reinnervation that typically follows crush or transection of teleostean and amphibian optic nerves (Sperry 1945, Jacobsen and Gaze 1965, Murray 1976) does not normally occur following transection of the optic nerve or other long myelinated fiber tracts in the adult mammalian CNS. The regenerative failure of intrinsic CNS neurons has been well documented in the last 80 years (Ramon y Cajal 1928, Windle 1955, Clemente 1964, Guth and Windle 1970, Kiernan 1979), but the cause or causes of this failure remain almost as obscure as they were in Ramon y Cajal's time.

It is now clear that some CNS neurons, most notably noradrenergic locus coruleus neurons and cholinergic "septohippocampal" neurons, do express a significant capacity for axonal regeneration following damage (Björklund and Stenevi 1979). Cholinergic and catecholaminergic neurons in the adult mammalian CNS have also been found to express a high degree of "neuroplasticity," manifest as "reactive synaptogenesis" in response to local deafferentation (Lynch and Cotman 1975) or "compensatory collateral hypertrophy" of one axonal branch following damage to another part of its arbor (Gage et al. 1983). The *regenerative capacity* of these neurons, whose axons branch diffusely within the CNS, has been attributed to their high degree of *neuroplasticity* (Björklund and Stenevi 1979). In contrast, neurons that give rise to most spe-

* Center for Neural Science, Brown University, Providence, Rhode Island 02912 U.S.A.

† Department of Biological Sciences, Purdue University, West Lafayeete, Indiana 47907 U.S.A.

cific projection systems within the adult mammalian CNS, including those that may use excitatory amino acids as their neurotransmitters (McGeer et al 1978), do not appear to retain a high degree of neuroplasticity into adulthood (Schneider 1979). The issue of regenerability in the majority of intrinsic CNS neuronal systems, however, remains largely unresolved. Do the neurons in these specific projection systems possess an intrinsic capacity for axonal regeneration? Is it possible that some adult mammalian CNS neurons that do not manifest a high degree of neuroplasticity may express a capacity for sustained axonal regeneration?

The response of adult mammalian retinal ganglion cells to optic nerve injury is often cited as a representative example of the apparent irregenerability of intrinsic CNS neurons. Damaged retinal ganglion cell axons exhibit a transient phase of terminal and collateral sprouting following optic nerve injury (Ramon y Cajal 1928, Richardson et al. 1982). These sprouts are soon resorbed and the axotomized retinal ganglion cells degenerate (Leinfelder 1933, Mantz and Klein 1951, Eayrs 1952, Grafstein and Ingoglia 1982, Richardson et al. 1982, Misantone et al. 1984). In contrast to the regenerative failure that occurs in response to optic nerve injury, axonal sprouts that persist for up to 1 year have been reported following focal lesions in the ganglion cell fiber layer in the retina of adult mice and rats (Goldberg and Frank 1980, McConnel and Berry 1983). In silver-impregnated preparations it appears that axonal sprouts arise from the axotomized retinal ganglion cells and ramify proximal to the lesion site. Although these regenerated axons did not course through or around the lesion site to reenter the ganglion cell fiber layer, they do represent a form of *sustained* axonal regeneration that is not resorbed following a *transient* phase of abortive sprouting.

Our studies (Ross and Das 1981, 1982a,b, 1983, Ross 1983) have established that adult rat retinal ganglion cells do possess an intrinsic capacity for sustained axonal regeneration and demonstrate that this capacity may be expressed in several forms. The regenerative metamorphosis of retinofugal axons damaged by transection of the optic tract or stratum opticum progresses through three phases (Ross 1983). The first phase, the acute response to axotomy, is characterized by the hypertrophy of proximal axonal segments and the formation of swollen terminal clubs within the proximal stump of the transected retinofugal projection (Figure 7-1a). These hypertrophied segments extend retinopetally from 400 to 1,600 microns and define the *Zone of Traumatic Reaction (ZTR)*. The second phase appears to represent the sprouting of numerous fine processes from damaged axons within the zone of traumatic reaction (Figure 7-1b). A third phase in the metamorphosis of damaged retinofugal axons, sustained axonal regeneration, follows the phase of abortive sprouting. The phase of sustained regenerative growth is characterized by the formation of dense fascicles and neuroma-like tangled masses of retinofugal axons within the zone of traumatic reaction (Figure 7-1c). Because the zone of traumatic reaction is evident at all times from 1 hour to 1 year after transection of the optic tract or stratum opticum, it is possible to reliably differentiate between regions of spared and damaged axons in the retinofugal projection.

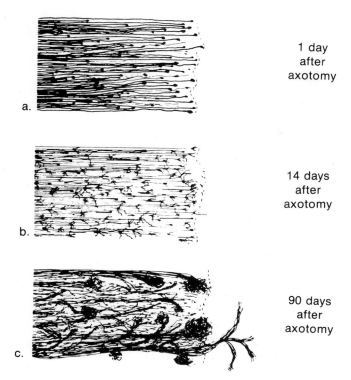

1 day
after
axotomy

a.

14 days
after
axotomy

b.

90 days
after
axotomy

c.

Figure 7-1. Stages in the metamorphosis of damaged retinofugal axons within the zone of traumatic reaction. (a) Acute phase of traumatic reaction, characterized by the formation of hypertrophied segments capped by swollen terminal clubs. (b) Phase of "abortive" sprouting of fine terminal and collateral processes within the zone of traumatic reaction. (c) Phase of sustained axonal regeneration, characterized by the formation of dense fascicle and neuroma-like neoformations within the zone of traumatic reaction and the elongative growth of regenerating axons across the wound margin of the zone.

Both the dense fascicle and tangled mass neuroma-like neoformations are evident within the ZTR 1 month after transection of the optic tract, brachium, or stratum opticum and become more pronounced following longer survival intervals. In cases where the lesion surfaces of the brain had fused together, dense fascicle and neuroma-like tangled mass neoformations of retinofugal axons within the zone of traumatic reaction extend up to but never across or around the thin scar of fusion marking the lesion site (Figure 7-2). In cases where cavitation had occurred at the lesion site, fascicles of retinofugal axons were found to cross the margin of the lesion cavity and course upon connective tissue elements in the lumen (Figure 7-3). These fascicles extend in all directions from the zone of traumatic reaction and course up to 2.5 mm through the non-neuronal matrix present in the diencephalon. Fascicles of regenerated retinofugal axons were never found to either reenter the host brain parenchyma

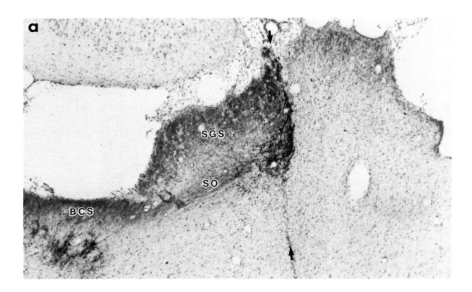

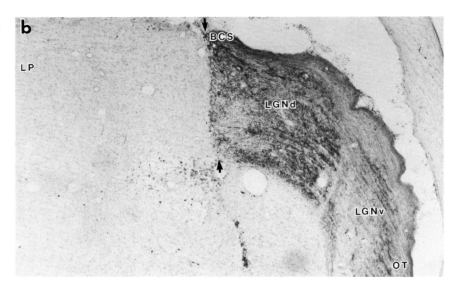

Figure 7-2. Failure of regenerating retinofugal axons to cross a scar of fusion. (a) Sagittal section through the optic layers of the superior colliculus, 90 days after transverse transection of the stratum opticum. Retinofugal axons anterogradely labeled following intravitreal injection of HRP into the contralateral eye extend up to but not across the scar of fusion marking the lesion site (arrows). Note the dense axonal neoformations proximal to the scar. (b) Coronal section through the lateral geniculate, 30 days after sagittal transection of the brachium of the superior colliculus. HRP-labeled axons from the contralateral retina extend up to but not across the scar of fusion in the diencephalic parenchyma. Abbreviations: BCS, brachium of the superior colliculus; SO, stratum opticum; SGS, stratum griseum superficiale; LGNd, lateral geniculate nucleus pars dorsalis; LGNv, lateral geniculate nucleus pars ventralis; OT, optic tract; LP, lateroposterior thalamic nucleus.

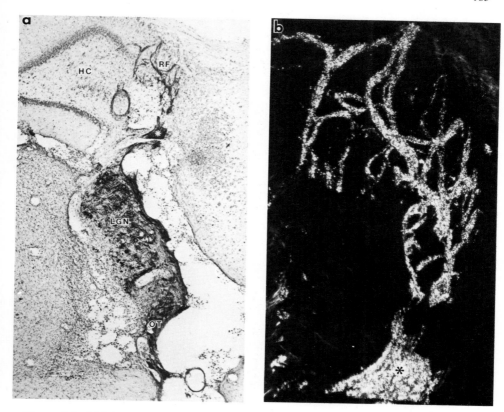

Figure 7-3. Thick fascicles of regenerated retinofugal axons extending dorsally into the lesion cavity. (a) Coronal section through the LGN, 9 months after sagittal transection of the brachium. Fascicles of HRP-labeled retinofugal axons cross the wound margin of the zone of traumatic reaction and course up to 2.5 mm upon connective tissue elements in the lumen of the lesion cavity in the hippocampal formation. (b) Detail of regenerated fascicles of retinofugal axons in the lesion cavity, polarized light optics. Abbreviations: HC, hippocampal formation; LGN, lateral geniculate nucleus; OT, optic tract; RF, regenerated fascicles of retinofugal fibers.

from the lesion cavity or course around the lesion cavity within the undamaged regions.

When embryonic neural tissue is transplanted at the lesion site immediately following transection of the retinofugal projection, the retinal ganglion cells' capacity for sustained regenerative growth may be expressed as retinal afferent ingrowth to the transplant. Two forms of retinal afferent ingrowth have been documented (Ross and Das 1981, 1982a,b, Ross 1983). Ingrowth of retinal afferents across transplant interface positions with *terminal* areas in the retinofugal projection (lateral geniculate nuclei, pretectal nuclei, optic layers of the superior colliculus) was restricted to relatively dense, bushy patches of apparent terminal labeling within 150 μm of the transplant interface (Figure 7-4a). In

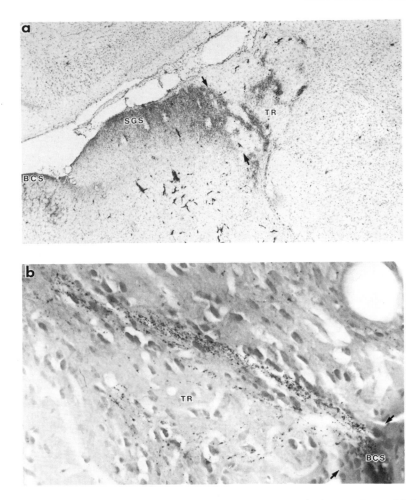

Figure 7-4. Two types of retinal afferent ingrowth to neocortical transplants. (a) Sagittal section through the superior colliculus of a case that had received a transplant of 17-day embryonic neocortical tissue following transverse transection of the stratum opticum. HRP-labeled axons from the contralateral eye cross the transplant interface, penetrate into the transplant parenchyma, and arborize in regions of dense termination. Ninety days after transverse transection/transplantation surgery. (b) A fascicle of retinofugal axons enters the transplant across the lateral interface with the brachium of the superior colliculus and penetrates deeply into the transplant parenchyma. Fink Heimer silver impregnation of degenerating axons, 5 days after enucleation of the contralateral eye, 90 days after transplantation of 17-day embryonic neocortical tissue into the caudal diencephalon. Abbreviations: BCS, brachium of the superior colliculus; SGS, stratum griseum superficiale; TR, transplant.

contrast, retinal afferent ingrowth across transplant interface positions with *main trunk* regions of the retinofugal projection (optic tract, brachium of the superior colliculus) was characterized by fascicles of axons that penetrated deep, 250 μm or more, into the transplant parenchyma before arborizing diffusely (Figure 7-4b).

Retinal afferent ingrowth to transplants was found to be highly dependent upon the position of the transplant relative to the host's retinofugal projection and the type of interface the transplant shared with structures within the host's retinofugal projection (Ross and Das 1981). Only those transplants that were well integrated with the parenchyma of structures in the host's retinofugal projection were found to receive retinal afferents (Figure 7-5). Transplants that were apposed to intact surfaces of structures in the host's retinofugal projection were devoid of retinal afferents (Figure 7-5a). Similarly, transplants that were well integrated with the host brain parenchyma but did not share interface regions with the host's retinofugal projection were also devoid of retinal afferents (Figure 7-5b). Retinal afferent ingrowth clearly required several conditions: *(1) that the retinofugal projection be damaged at the transplantation site, (2) that the embryonic tissue be transplanted at positions where it became adherent to the damaged parenchymal surfaces of the host brain, and (3) that the transplants developed well-integrated interface positions with structures in the host's retinofugal projection.* In cases where *any* of these necessary conditions were not met, the transplants were devoid of retinal afferents.

The ingrowth of retinal afferents was clearly not dependent upon the type of embryonic tissue transplanted. Heterotopic transplants of embryonic neocortical tissue (which were used in most cases) were found to receive retinal afferents across well-integrated interface regions in 35 of 62 cases examined (Ross, 1983). Those transplants that failed to receive a retinal afferent projection failed to meet at least one of the necessary conditions. Similarly, transplants of embryonic hippocampal, olfactory bulb, cerebellar, hypothalamic, mesencepha-

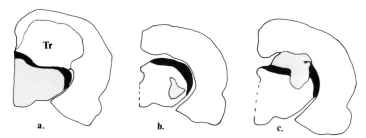

Figure 7-5. Transplant position and retinal afferent ingrowth. (a) Transplants apposed to intact regions of the host's retinofugal projection were devoid of retinal afferents. (b) Transplants that were well integrated with the diencephalic or tectal parenchyma but did not share interface positions with structures in the host's retinofugal projection were devoid of retinal afferents. (c) Transplants that were well integrated with structures in the host's retinofugal projection received retinal afferents across these interface positions.

lic, tectal, and diencephalic tissues were found to receive retinal afferents *only* when they met the above three conditions (Ross and Das, unpublished observations). There was no indication that homotopic tectal or diencephalic transplants were hyper-innervated by retinal afferents relative to the heterotopic transplants.

The ingrowth of retinal afferents to neocortical and other embryonic neural transplants is consistent with the "principle of nonspecific ingrowth" that has been repeatedly illustrated in studies of afferent ingrowth to heterotopic transplants of embryonic neural tissue. This principle holds that the afferents of a neural transplant are determined by the site to which it is transplanted and are not specified by the region of the embryonic neuraxis from which the tissue was obtained. Hine (1977) found that transplants of embryonic cerebellar tissue received afferents characteristic of the basal ganglia following transplantation into the caudate-putamen of neonatal rats. Oblinger (1981, Oblinger et al 1980, Oblinger and Das 1982) found that embryonic neocortical tissue transplanted into the cerebellar cortex of neonatal and adult rats received afferents from the pontocerebellar, olivocerebellar, and spinocerebellar projections. Both tectal and diencephalic transplants in the cerebellar cortex of neonatal rats were also found to receive precerebellar afferents (Hallas et al 1980). Similarly, Graziadei and Kaplan (1980) found that olfactory sensory axons innervated transplants of embryonic neocortical tissues placed in lesion cavities in the olfactory bulbs of adult mice.

The afferent ingrowth of axons from host brain fiber systems may represent either the normal developmental growth of neonatal host fiber systems, the sprouting of new processes from undamaged axons proximal to the transplant interface, or the regeneration of axons damaged during the transplantation procedure. Several lines of evidence strongly suggest that *retinal afferent ingrowth to transplants in adult host rats is due to the regenerative growth of damaged axons*. First, retinal afferents entered the transplants only across well-integrated interface regions where damaged axons were present, the interface with the *zone of traumatic reaction* (Ross, 1983). In cases where ingrowth was observed retinal afferents crossed the transplant interface from the zone of traumatic reaction with their *normal trajectory*. Second, retinal afferents were never found to enter the transplants across interface positions with spared, undamaged regions of the retinofugal projection. Despite the fact that up to 97% of the transplant's interface with the retinofugal projection was with spared portions of the projection, *no ingrowth was ever found to arise from regions outside the zone of traumatic reaction and course with aberrant trajectory into the transplants* (Ross and Das 1983, Ross, 1983). Third, for transplants of embryonic neocortical tissue in the superior colliculus of adult rats a highly significant correlation was seen between the area of a transplant's interface with the zone of traumatic reaction in the optic layers and the volume of the transplant innervated by the retinofugal projection (Ross and Das 1983, Ross 1983). *These results suggest that the magnitude of retinal afferent ingrowth to the transplants is dependant upon the number of damaged axons within the zone of traumatic reaction*. Unlike the ingrowth of precerebellar afferents to neocortical transplants in the cerebellum (Oblinger 1981, Oblinger and Das 1983), there was no correlation seen between the total transplant interface area with the host fiber projection and the volume of afferent ingrowth from the projection. This difference may reflect the ability of intact precerebellar axons to sprout (Oblinger 1981, Oblinger and Das 1983), a capacity that undamaged adult retinal ganglion cells may not possess.

Kromer et al. (1981a) reported the ingrowth of presumptive cholinergic axons from the septohippocampal projection into transplants of embryonic hippocampal tissue. This ingrowth was apparently due to the regeneration of axons damaged by fimbrial transection at the transplantation site. The regenerative ingrowth of retinal afferents to neocortical and other transplants of embryonic tissues (Ross and Das 1981, 1982a,b, 1983 Ross 1983) together with the cholinergic ingrowth to transplants in the fimbria (Kromer et al. 1981a) and the innervation of implants of iris muscle by cholinergic and catecholaminergic axons (Björklund and Stenevi 1971, Svendgaard et al. 1975, 1976, Emson et al. 1977) may all represent the ''proximal'' regenerative growth of damaged axons. The term ''proximal axonal regeneration'' was introduced by Kiernan (1970) to describe a form of regenerative growth manifest by hypothalamic neurosecretory axons following transection of the median eminence. These axons sprouted locally, terminated upon blood vessels proximal to the site of transection, and did not cross the lesion site to reinnervate their normal target, the neurohypophysis (Kiernan 1970). All types of sustained regeneration that fall short of reinnervating the deafferented normal target structure may be considered as examples of *proximal* regenerative growth. This may include axonal ingrowth to transplants of peripheral nerve, muscle, and embryonic neural tissue in the CNS of adult mammals, local synapse formation proximal to sites of injury in the CNS (Bernstein and Bernstein, 1971), and the formation of neuromatous tangled masses of regenerated axons near long-standing lesions in the CNS (Sung 1981, Ross 1983).

Proximo-distal regenerative growth, characterized by the regeneration of axons across the plane of transection and reinnervation of their normal target areas, was described by Kiernan (1970) in some cases following transection of the median eminence. Such proximo-distal regenerative growth is well documented to occur following transection or crush of telostean and amphibian optic nerves (Sperry 1945, Jacobsen and Gaze 1965, Murray 1976) and mammalian peripheral nerves (Ramon y Cajal 1928, Guth 1956, Sunderland 1968, Morris et al. 1972). Though there have been many claims of apparent proximo-distal regenerative growth following injuries to the adult mammalian CNS, few of the claims have proven to be valid. Kromer et al. (1981b) reported that homotopic transplants of embryonic hippocampal tissues may support the proximo-distal regenerative growth of damaged septohippocampal axons back to their normal target regions. They observed that presumed cholinergic axons, visualized using acetylcholinesterase histochemistry, in some cases appeared to grow out of the transected fimbria, ''bridge'' transplants of embryonic hippocampal tissue, and reinnervate areas in the hippocampus deafferented by the fimbrial transection. The source of guidance cues for this type of growth was suggested to reside in a specific affinity of the cholinergic axons for substrate pathways normally encountered in development and/or a specific trophic attraction to their normal target (Kromer et al. 1981b).

In light of our findings on the regenerability of adult rat retinofugal axons, the following experiment was designed, in part, to determine whether heterotopic neocortical transplants could support the proximo-distal regenerative growth of retinofugal axons. The optic tract or brachium of the superior colliculus was transected in adult rats, and embryonic neocortical tissue, a tissue not normally encountered by retinofugal axons, was transplanted at the site of transection. Since retinofugal axons do regenerate following optic tract transection, and the magnitude of retinal afferent ingrowth to transplants appears to be a function of the number of damaged axons within the zone of traumatic reaction, it was reasoned that transplants placed at the site of optic tract or brachium transection might receive a profuse ingrowth of retinofugal axons that penetrate deep into the transplant parenchyma. The regenerative growth of retinofugal axons was visualized using HRP that was anterogradely transported following intravitreal injection at various times after transplantation. This specific anatomical tract tracing method was chosen because of the discrete pattern of retinofugal labeling produced by intravitreal HRP injection. Both the positive and negative findings from this study are presented here, and the entire process of proximo-distal axonal regeneration is considered in the discussion.

Methods

Lesion-Transplantation Surgeries

Adult female Long-Evans rats (4 months old, 280–320g) were anesthetized with an intramuscular injection of a ketamine (87 mg/kg) xylazine (13 mg/kg) mixture and prepared for stereotaxic surgery. A modified # 11 scalpel blade was stereotactically lowered into the brain and moved in either the sagittal plane, partially transecting the brachium of the superior colliculus, or the transverse plane, partially transecting the optic tract. Immediately following the partial transection, 2.5–3.5 mm³ of 17-day embryonic neocortical tissue was stereotactically transplanted at the lesion site. The stereotaxic coordinates used for the lesion/transplantation surgeries are given in Table 7-1. A detailed description of the stereotaxic transplantation apparatus, instructions on its assembly, and technical comments on its use have been published elsewhere (Das and Ross 1982).

Connectivity Studies and HRP Histochemistry

Approximately 80% of the experimental animals survived the operative procedures. Of the 53 transection/transplantation cases used for histological analysis

Table 7-1. Coordinates for Partial Transection of the Optic Tract or Brachium of the Superior Colliculus and Transplantation of Embryonic Neural Tissues

	Lesion type	A.P. (mm posterior to the Bregma)[1]	M.L. (mm lateral to midline)[2]	S.D. (mm below dura)
Partial transections of the brachium of the superior colliculus	Complete caudal (SCC)	3.0–5.0 (4.0)	3.0	6.0
	Complete rostral (SCR)	2.0–4.0 (3.0)	3.0	6.0
	Incomplete rostral and caudal (SI)	3.0–4.0 (3.5)	3.0	6.0
Partial transections of the optic tract	Complete ventral (TCV)	2.5	2.0–4.0 (3.0)	7.5
	Incomplete ventral (TIV)	2.5	2.0–4.0 (3.0)	6.5
	Superficial (TS)	2.5	3.0–4.0 (3.5)	6.0

[1] Antero-posterior transplantation coordinates following sagittal brachium transection given in parentheses.
[2] Medio-lateral transplantation coordinates following transverse optic tract transection given in parentheses.

in this study, 13 had received unilateral transections and transplants and 40 had received transections and transplants bilaterally. Between 3 days and 18 months after the transplantation surgery most of the animals were reanesthetized with the ketamine–xylazine mixture and given an intravitreal injection of HRP (4 μl of 25% Sigma type VI in lactated Ringer's solution) in each eye contralateral to a transplant. Twenty-four hours following the HRP injection the experimental animals were etherized, exsanguinated by transcardial perfusion with a 0.1 M phosphate buffer (pH 7.4), fixed by transcardial perfusion with a solution of 0.5% paraformaldehyde and 2.0% glutaraldehyde in phosphate buffer, and post fixed by perfusion with a 10% sucrose-phosphate buffer solution (4° C). The brains were removed and stored in the cold sucrose-phosphate solution for 1 hour - 3 days. Frozen sections were cut at 40 μm in the coronal plane and alternate sections were collected in cold phosphate buffer for HRP histochemistry. Sections were reacted free-floating for HRP histochemistry using Adams' (1980) modification of Mesulam's (1978) tetramethylbenzadine (TMB) chromagen procedure. The sections were stored in cold (4° C) 0.1 M acetate buffer for 20 minutes - 3 days, serially mounted onto gelatin subbed slides from a 0.3% gelatin solution, then allowed to air dry overnight at room temperature. The TMB–HRP reaction product was stabilized by immersing the mounted sections in methyl salicylate for 3 minutes as per Adams (1980). The slides were then quickly hydrated through a decreasing series of alcohols and rinsed well in distilled water before counterstaining for 1.25 minutes in 0.025% Thionin (aq). Differentiation and dehydration were accomplished quickly owing to the high alcohol lability of the TMB–HRP reaction product (Mesulam 1978, 1982, Adams 1980). The slides were then cleared in methyl salicylate, transferred to xylene, and cover-slipped with permount. The HRP reaction product in sections stabilized with methyl salicylate did not fade and has remained very clearly detectable for as long as 3 years. The second set of alternate 40-μm sections was mounted, dried, and stained with either cresyl violet, hematoxalin and eosin, or a modified Bodian's silver impregnation technique (Loots et al. 1979).

Analysis of HRP Labeling Patterns and Retinal Afferent Ingrowth

Both brightfield and polarized light optics were used for qualitative analysis of the patterns of HRP labeling of retinofugal axons in the zone of traumatic reaction (ZTR), retinal afferent projections to the transplants, and retinal innervation patterns in the optic layers of the superior colliculus (Figure 7-6). The type and extent of the partial transection was verified for each lesion-transplantation case using several criteria determined from a study of partial transection alone (Ross 1983). Complete ventral transverse transections of the optic tract (T.C.V., n = 22) were identified by: (1) the absence of spared fascicles of intact retinofugal axons in the optic tract ventral to the lesion-transplantation site and caudal to the zone of traumatic reaction, and (2) the absence of HRP terminal labeling in the LGN caudal to the lesion-transplantation site (see Figure 7-13). TCV lesions produced complete retinal deafferentation in the lateral ¼ to ½ of the optic layers, depending upon their medial extent. Incomplete ventral transverse transections of the optic tract (T.I.V., n = 20) were identified by: (1) the presence of spared fascicles in the optic tract ventral to the lesion-transplanta-

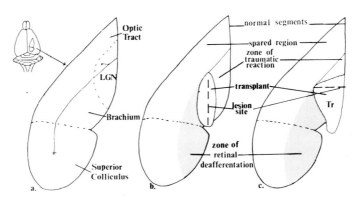

Figure 7-6. Regions of the retinofugal projection in transection/transplantation cases. (a) Schematic dorsal view of the normal rat retinofugal projection. (b) Regions examined in cases where transplantation had followed sagittal transection of the brachium of the superior colliculus. (c) Regions examined in cases where transplantation followed transverse transection of the optic tract.

tion site, and (2) the presence of HRP terminal labeling in the LGNd caudal to the transplantation site (see Figure 7-16). TIV lesions produced complete retinal deafferentation in the middle $1/4$ to $1/3$ of the optic layers depending upon the ventral and medial extent of the lesion. Superficial focal transverse lesions (T.S., n = 7) were identified by sparing of the LGNd and optic tract lateral to transplants in the caudal diencephalon or sparing of the optic tract and retinofugal terminal labeling pattern in the LGNd medial to transplants located in the subarachnoid space lateral to the optic tract. Complete caudal transections of the brachium of the superior colliculus (S.C.C., N = 15) were identified by: (1) the absence of spared fascicles of HRP-labeled axons in the brachium of the superior colliculus caudal to the transplant, and (2) the presence of a zone of traumatic reaction in the optic tract, brachium, and LGN lateral to the transplant that extended to the caudal limit of the brachium (see Figure 7-9). SCC lesions produced complete retinal deafferentation in the lateral $1/2$ to $1/3$ of the optic layers depending upon the rostral extent of the lesion. Complete rostral sagittal transections of the brachium (S.C.R., n = 14) were identified by: (1) the absence of spared fascicles of HRP-labeled axons in the brachium that coursed mediolaterally across the plane of transection rostral to the transplant, and (2) the presence of a zone of traumatic reaction lateral to the transplants that extended up to the rostral-most limit of the brachium. Sagittal transections of the brachium that were incomplete both rostrally and caudally (S.I.) were identified by: (1) fascicles of axons in the brachium that coursed medio-laterally across the plane of transection both rostral and caudal to the transplant, and (2) zones of traumatic reaction in the brachium, optic tract, and LGN that did not extend to either the rostral or caudal limits of the brachium.

The identification of HRP-labeled axons as retinal afferents to transplants was made using criteria from a previous study (Ross and Das 1981, Ross 1983). These criteria were: (*1*) *penetration of HRP-labeled axons or fascicles of axons at least 50 μm across a clearly defined transplant interface in at least two consecutive sections, (2) the presence of positively identified neocortical neurons both at the position of the suspected ingrowth and at corresponding positions in immediately adjacent serial sections, and (3) the absence of spared fascicles of intact retinofugal axons in adjacent sections at positions that corresponded to the position of the suspected ingrowth.* Using these criteria it was possible to insure with a high degree of certainty that labeled axons interpreted as retinal afferents to the transplants were not parts of the spared host retinofugal projection that only appeared to enter the transplants due to the plane of sectioning.

The patterns of sparing and deafferentation in the optic layers of the superior colliculus were determined for each experimental case using brightfield and polarized light optics. These patterns were compared to those seen in lesion control cases that had received similar partial transections (Ross 1983). Only those cases in which HRP-labeled retinofugal axons were found to course through the transplant parenchyma and HRP terminal labeling was seen in regions of the optic layers deafferented by the partial transection were classified as examples of proximo-distal regeneration.

Results

Was the Presence of a Transplant at the Site of Partial Transection in the Optic Tract/Brachium Sufficient to Ensure Retinal Afferent Ingrowth to the Transplants?

Amputation neuroma-like structures within the zone of traumatic reaction (ZTR) and in the connective tissue matrix of the lesion cavity adjacent to the zone were the only evidence of regenerative growth from damaged retinofugal axons in 40% (25 of 62) of the lesion-transplantation cases that survived for 30 days or more. Those transplants that were otherwise well integrated with the diencephalic parenchyma but had not established well integrated interface regions with the ZTR in the retinofugal projection (n = 20) were devoid of retinal afferents. Although many of these transplants were well integrated with spared portions of the brachium of the superior colliculus medially and the distal stump of the optic tract/brachium caudally, no retinal afferent ingrowth was seen from these positions. In all of these cases dense fascicles of retinofugal axons appeared to terminate in neuroma-like tangled masses proximal to the ZTR's lesion margin or transplant interface region (Figure 7-7a). In many cases the retinofugal terminal zones in the LGN regions of the ZTR were characterized by a denser than normal HRP labeling pattern. This pattern of dense labeling tapered off markedly toward the retinopetal end of the ZTR. In some cases where the transection had extended into the hippocampal formation dorsal or lateral to the diencephalon, the wound margin of the zone of traumatic reaction in the retinofugal projection had fused with the hippocampal parenchyma. Retinofugal axons did not regenerate across the scar of fusion at these positions into either the transplants or the hippocampal parenchyma. In other cases (n = 5) the transplants were celarly necrotic or extraparenchymal and had not developed well integrated interface regions with the host brain at all. In some cases fascicles of retinofugal axons coursed from the ZTR onto the connective tissue matrix in the lesion cavity. Although fascicles of HRP-labeled axons appeared to course upon the outer surface of some extraparenchymal transplants, axons from these fascicles neither penetrated into the transplant parenchyma nor reentered the host's brain parenchyma (Figure 7-7b).

Although dense fascicles and neuroma-like tangled masses of retinofugal axons were never found rostral to the ZTR in any of the 93 cases examined between 3 days and 18 months after the lesion-transplantation surgery, there was evidence suggestive of a dying back of some damaged retinofugal axons from the ZTR. In all cases that survived for 30 days or longer a few axons characterized by swollen or varicose segments capped by swollen terminal clubs could be found among the normal segments rostral to the ZTR in the optic tract. This type of reaction was very isolated and did not appear to represent a regression *en masse* of damaged retinofugal axons from the ZTR.

The presence of an embryonic neural transplant at the site of a partial tran-

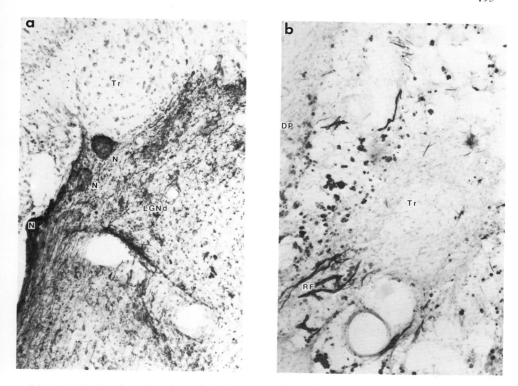

Figure 7-7. Neoformations of regenerated retinofugal axons that failed to grow into neocortical transplants. (a) Neuroma-like tangled mass neoformations of HRP-labeled retinofugal axons (N) at the interface between the transplant and the zone of traumatic reaction in the host's LGNd, 140 days after transection/transplantation. HRP injected into the eye contralateral to the transplant. (b) Thick fascicles of regenerated retinofugal axons that course through the connective tissue in the lesion cavity and onto the surface of an extraparenchymal neocortical transplant, 140 days after transection/transplantation. HRP injected into the eye contralateral to the transplant. Abbreviations: N, neuroma-like tangled mass neoformations of retinofugal axons; RF, regenerated fascicles of retinofugal axons; Tr, transplant; DP, diencephalic parenchyma; LGNd, lateral geniculate nucleus pars dorsalis.

section in the optic tract/brachium was clearly not sufficient to ensure retinal afferent ingrowth to the transplants. For retinal afferent ingrowth to occur it was necessary for the transplant to become anatomically integrated with the host brain parenchyma through interface positions with the zone of traumatic reaction in the retinofugal projection. The lack of ingrowth across some apparently well-integrated transplant interface regions with the ZTR suggests that the development of a confluent extracellular space between the ZTR and the transplant may also be necessary for ensuring that the retinofugal axons' regenerative capacity is expressed as retinal afferent ingrowth.

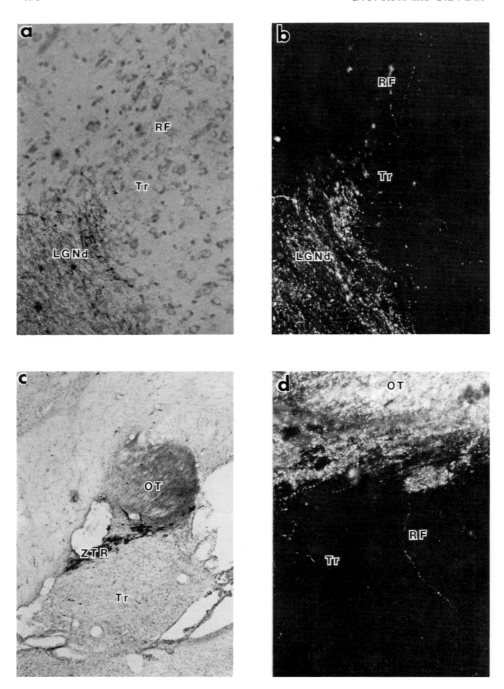

Figure 7-8. Retinal afferent ingrowth to neocortical transplants arising from different positions in the zone of traumatic reaction. (a) Retinal afferent ingrowth into a neocortical transplant across an interface with the *lesion margin* of the zone of traumatic

Did Partial Transection of the Optic Tract/Brachium at the Transplantation Site Result in a Profuse Ingrowth of Retinal Axons to the Transplants?

Although some transplants received relatively profuse retinal afferent projections, others received projections that were quite meager and qualitatively no different from the amount of ingrowth seen when only very focal lesions were made in the LGN and optic tract (Ross and Das 1981, Ross 1983). As noted earlier, a few transplants received no retinal afferents at all.

Retinal afferent ingrowth was seen in 60% (37 of 62) of the transplants that had survived 30 days or longer after lesion-transplantation surgery. The most frequent form of retinal afferent ingrowth (n = 20) was a profusion of HRP-labeled axons and fascicles of axons that penetrated 150–500 μm into the transplant parenchyma and arborized in regions where they appeared to terminate. In 13 of these 20 cases the transplants had developed interface regions with the damaged surface of the retinofugal projection at the wound margin of the zone of traumatic reaction. Retinal afferents most often appeared to arise from the optic tract and brachium regions of the ZTR (Figure 7-8a,b). However, in a few cases there was also evidence of retinal afferent ingrowth that penetrated less that 150 μm across transplant interface regions with retinofugal terminal zones in the LGN and pretectal nuclei.

In a few cases retinal afferents were found to enter the transplants across interface positions with the more retinopetal regions of the ZTR. These transplants had not become well integrated with the zone of traumatic reaction at the wound margin but had become well integrated with the ZTR at more retinopetal positions (Figure 7-8c). Across these retinopetal ZTR interface positions HRP-labeled retinofugal axons penetrated up to 500 μm into the transplant parenchyma (Figure 7-8d).

The most profuse ingrowth of retinofugal axons was found in those cases (n = 17) where the retinofugal axons coursed through the transplant parenchyma. In these cases several fascicles of retinofugal axons were found to arise from the zone of traumatic reaction in the optic tract or brachium, cross well-integrated transplant interface regions, and course through the transplant parenchyma from 500 μm to 4 mm. In these cases some axons were found that split off from the main fascicles and arborized within the transplant parenchyma. This type of ingrowth appears to represent a more profuse form of the deeply penetrating fascicles that arise from main trunk regions of the retinofugal projections (Ross and Das 1981, 1982b).

The variability in the patterns of retinal afferent ingrowth to transplants

---

reaction in the LGN, 120 days after transection/transplantation surgery. (b) Same field as A seen using polarized light optics. (c) A neocortical transplant anatomically integrated with the retinopetal end of the zone of traumatic reaction (ZTR) in the optic tract, 545 days after transection/transplantation surgery. (d) Detail of retinal afferent ingrowth from the *retinopetal end* of the zone of traumatic reaction in the optic tract OT. Abbreviations: RF, regenerated fibers; Tr, transplant; LGNd, lateral geniculate nucleus pars dorsalis; OT, optic tract.

placed at sites of transection in the optic tract and brachium of the superior colliculus may be due, in part, to the severity of vascular damage at the transplantation site. Extensive vascular damage at the transection/transplantation site may have induced pathological reactions within the host brain, particularly in the zone of traumatic reaction, which prevented complete anatomical integration in some cases or severely restricted the access of the regenerating retinofugal axons to the transplant interface in others.

Can Heterotopic Transplants of Embryonic Neocortical Tissue Support the Proximo-Distal Regenerative Growth of Axons from the Transected Optic Tract or Brachium through the Transplants?

In 17 cases retinofugal axons were found to arise from the zone of traumatic reaction in the optic tract/brachium, penetrate across the transplant interface, course through the transplant parenchyma, reenter the distal stump of the transected retinofugal projection, and reinnervate regions in the optic layers that had been deafferented by the partial transection. Proximo-distal regenerative growth through the transplants took three general forms. The first form was seen in four cases that had survived for 30–360 days after the lesiontransplantation surgery. In these cases HRP-labeled axons and fascicles of retinofugal axons penetrated into the transplants across the lateral interface from the zone of traumatic reaction in the optic tract or brachium, coursed deeply (1–2 mm) through the transplant parenchyma, reentered the host brain at the distal stump of the transected optic tract/brachium across the medial transplant interface, and reinnervated zones of complete deafferentation in the lateral half of the superior colliculus. A case showing this form of retinofugal projection is illustrated in Figures 7-10 and 7-11. In this representative case the experimental animal received a transplant of embryonic neocortical tissue immediately following a sagittal transection of its brachium that was complete caudally (S.C.C.). The characteristic pattern of sparing and deafferentation in the retinofugal projection associated with lesions of this type (S.C.C.) is illustrated for a lesion control case in Figure 7-9. In all four of the cases exhibiting this type of retinofugal projection, the axons entered the transplant parenchyma only across well-integrated interface regions with the zone of traumatic reaction in the optic tract or brachium. No axons were ever found to course from fascicles of spared retinofugal axons into the transplants. Within the transplant parenchyma retinofugal axons coursed through both neuron-dense and relatively neuron-free zones. Axons and fascicles of axons were found to reeenter the host brain only across portions of the medial transplant interface with the distal stump of the transected brachium of the superior colliculus (Figure 7-12). There were no zones of complete retinal deafferentation remaining in the optic layers in these four cases. It appeared that axons which had coursed through the transplants and grown down the distal stump reinnervated the deafferented regions in the optic layers. It was unclear whether the pattern of HRP labeling in these regions actually represented the formation of synaptic contacts since none of these cases were examined ultrastructurally. However, the pattern of anterograde HRP labeling in these reinnervated zones appeared similar to regions of terminal labeling seen in the normal retinofugal projection.

That these cases actually represented the proximo-distal regenerative growth of damaged axons and not the misinterpretation of spared fascicles of axons was supported by several observations on the response of retinofugal axons to trauma and the development of the retinal afferent projections to the transplants. In lesion control cases there was no evidence of teased fascicles of retinofugal axons that appeared to course through the lesion cavity. Similarly, axons that coursed through transplants were never seen in lesion-transplantation cases sacrificed less than 30 days after the surgery. The first retinal afferents were detected 14 days after lesion-transplantation surgery, and fascicles of axons that coursed through the transplants and reentered the distal stump of the transected retinofugal projection were only seen 30 days or more following transplantation. In all cases interpreted as representing proximo-distal regeneration, it was clear that the host's retinofugal projection had been transected rostral, caudal, dorsal, and ventral to the fascicles of axons that coursed through the transplants. We conclude that the labeled retinofugal axons that coursed through the transplants' parenchyma represent the proximo-distal regenerative growth of damaged retinofugal axons.

A second form of retinofugal axonal projection through the transplants was seen in 6 cases that had survived for 60 days to 1 year after lesion-transplantation surgery. In all of these cases the host's optic tract had been partially transected in the transverse plane immediately prior to transplantation. In each of these six cases a profusion of HRP-labeled fascicles of retinofugal axons had crossed the rostral transplant interface from the zone of traumatic reaction in the optic tract, coursed through the transplant parenchyma traversing along the contour of the transplants' lateral border with the hippocampal formation, reentered the host brain across the caudo-medial transplant interface with the distal stump of the transected brachium, and reinnervated regions of the optic layers that had been deafferented by the partial transection. Figures 7-14 and 7-15 illustrate this type of retinofugal projection through a transplant in an experimental case that received a complete ventral transverse transection of the optic tract (T.C.V.) immediately prior to transplantation. The patterns of sparing and deafferentation in the retinofugal projection associated with this type of partial transection are illustrated for a (T.C.V.) lesion control case in Figure 7-13. Retinofugal axons were found to arise from the zone of traumatic reaction in the host's optic tract and penetrate across the rostral transplant interface. No retinofugal axons were ever found to enter the transplants from positions outside the zone of traumatic reaction. Within the transplant parenchyma retinofugal axons and fascicles of axons traversed through relatively neuron-free regions along the contour of the transplants' lateral border with the hippocampal formation (Figure 7-15a). At these positions the transplants were apposed to, but not anatomically integrated with, the host's hippocampal parenchyma. Pia mater could be seen at this border region along its entire length in most cases. The HRP-labeled fascicles of retinofugal axons within the transplants translocated dorso-medially as they coursed caudally through the transplant parenchyma. HRP-labeled retinofugal axons reentered the host brain in all six of these cases across the transplants' caudo-medial interface with the distal stump of the transected brachium of the superior colliculus. Retinofugal axons were never found to penetrate into the host brain at aberrant positions. Many of the fascicles of axons that reentered the distal stump of the transected optic tract/brachium took extremely tortuous courses in doing so. Some of these fascicles coursed through the transplant parenchyma at positions dorsal or ventral to their normal position in the brachium of the superior colliculus while other fascicles coursed completely around the caudal-most lobes of the transplants and reentered the distal stump of the brachium coursing rostrally and ventrally (Figure 7-15b,c). A sparse pattern of HRP terminal labeling had replaced the zones of complete retinal deafferentation in the optic layers (Figure 7-15d). Although the labeling in these zones was not as dense as that

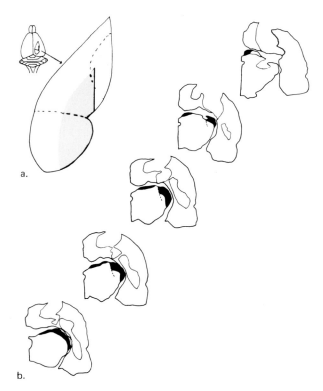

Figure 7-9. Schematics and drawings of regions associated with complete caudal transections of the brachium (S.C.C.). (a) Schematic dorsal view of the retinofugal projection illustrating patterns of sparing (white) and deafferentiation (shaded) associated with a S.C.C. lesion. (b) Drawings of representative serial sections through the various regions of the retinofugal projection.

normally seen in the optic layers, no zones of complete retinal deafferentation remained.

Several observations suggest that this form of retinofugal axon penetration through the transplants actually represents the proximo-distal regenerative growth of damaged retinofugal axons. No fascicles of axons that appeared to have been distended around growing transplants were found in any of the 31

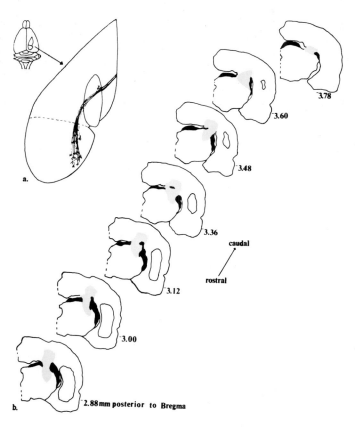

Figure 7-10. Schematic drawing and representative serial sections of a case in which retinofugal axons had regenerated (1.25 mm) through a neocortical transplant placed at the site of a complete caudal sagittal transection of the brachium (S.C.C.). (a) Schematic dorsal view of the retinofugal projection, the caudal diencephalon, and superior colliculus showing the relative position of the transplant, the extent of the brachium transection, and the course of retinofugal axons through the transplant. (b) Representative serial sections from various regions of the retinofugal projection depicting retinofugal axons that penetrate across the transplant interface with the zone of traumatic reaction in the optic tract, course deeply through the transplant parenchyma, reenter the distal stump of the transected brachium, and reinnervate regions of the optic layers that had been deafferented by the complete caudal transection of the brachium.

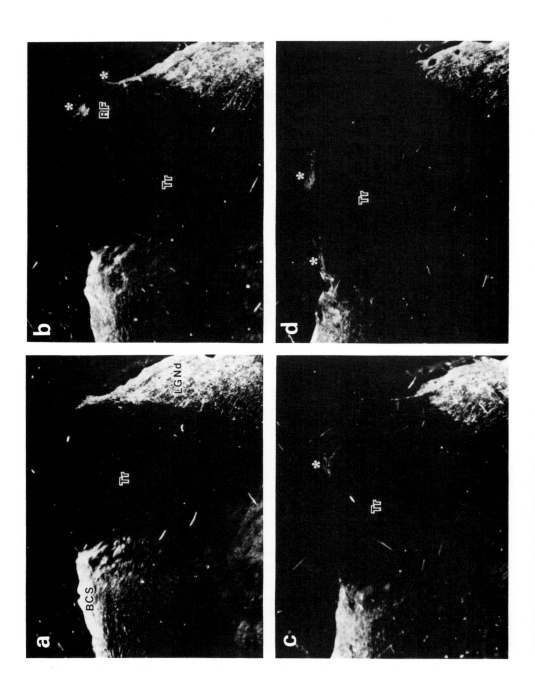

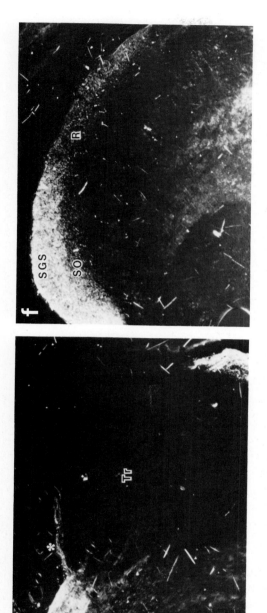

Figure 7-11. A fascicle of HRP-labeled retinofugal axons that crosses the transplant interface from the zone of traumatic reaction, courses through the transplant parenchyma 1.25 mm, reenters the distal stump of the brachium, and reinnervates the lateral half of the optic layers. (a) Axons from the optic tract region of the zone of traumatic reaction enter the transplant. (b–d) Axons course caudomedially through the transplant parenchyma, across the plane of distal transection. (e) Regenerated axons entering the distal stump of the brachium across the medial transplant interface. (f) Moderately dense pattern of HRP terminal labeling in the lateral half of the optic layers. HRP injected into the contralateral eye 30 days following transection/transplantation surgery, polarized light optics. Abbreviations: Tr, transplant; BCS, brachium of the superior colliculus; LGNd, lateral geniculate nucleus pars dorsalis; RF, regenerated fasciles of retinofugal axons; SGS, stratum griseum superficiale; SO, stratum opticum; R, reinnervated.

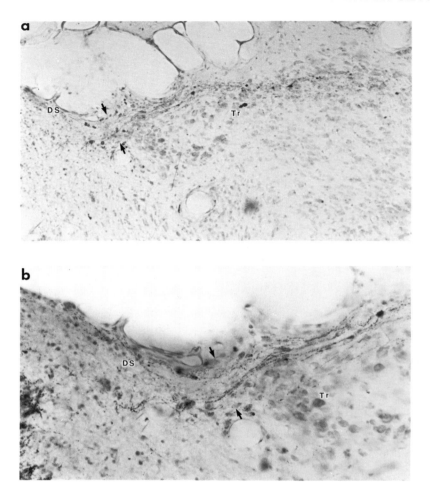

Figure 7-12. Reentry of regenerated retinofugal axons across the medial transplant interface into the distal stump. (a) HRP-labeled axons coursing through a neuron-dense region of the transplant parenchyma (Tr). (b) Detail of the medial transplant interface from a. HRP-labeled axons cross the medial transplant interface (arrows) and reenter the distal stump of the brachium (DS).

cases examined between 3 and 21 days after transplantation. In other cases where transplant growth had clearly distended the optic tract, the zone of traumatic reaction rostral to the transplants was exaggerated retinopetally and axons capped by terminal balls and neuromalike neoformations were evident throughout the region of distention (Ross 1983). In the six cases that made up the present group the fascicles of axons that coursed through the transplants were not characterized by either terminal clubs on indivivdual axons, dense fascicles, or neuroma-like tangled masses of axons within the transplant parenchyma. Similarly, at the point of reentry into the distal stump of the transected optic tract/brachium no aggregations of swollen terminal clubs or neuroma-like neoformations were ever found. Axons that arborized within the transplant parenchyma were found to branch off of the regenerated optic tract fascicles in all six of these cases. These cases represent retinofugal axonal regeneration through the molecular zone at the apposed, unintegrated margins of the neocortical transplants.

The third form of retinofugal projection through the transplants was seen in seven cases that had survived 30–240 days after surgery. In these cases numerous HRP-labeled axons crossed into the transplants from interface positions with the zone of traumatic reaction in the optic tract or brachium, coursed between 500 μm and 1.5 mm through neuron-dense regions of the transplant parenchyma with a trajectory generally parallel to spared fascicles of retinofugal axons outside the transplants, and reentered the distal stump of the brachium across the transplant's caudo-medial interface. The case presented in Figure 7-17 is characteristic of this form of growth. In this case the pretransplantation lesion was an incomplete ventral transverse transection of the optic tract. In Figure 7-16 a lesion control case with a similar T.I.V. lesion is shown for comparison. In this case and three others in this group, zones of sparse labeling in the optic layers were attributed to reinnervation of the denervated zones by the axons that had coursed through the transplant's parenchyma. In three other cases the pretransplantation stab wounds had only superficially damaged the host retinofugal projection, and the zones of partial deafferentation found in the optic layers in these cases could not confidently be attributed to reinnervation by axons that coursed through the transplant parenchyma. In none of the 31 cases examined between 3 and 21 days following transplantation surgery was there any indication that transplant neuroblasts had migrated into the white matter of the optic tract or brachium or into the parenchyma of the LGN. Because the volumetric growth of embryonic neocortical transplants is expansive and not infiltrative, a clearly discernible border is present between the transplant and the host brain parenchyma at all times following transplantation. The fascicles of retinofugal axons that course through the transplant parenchyma parallel to spared fascicles of host optic tract axons represent the proximo-distal regeneration of damaged retinofugal axons.

Discussion

Regenerative Growth of Retinofugal Axons through Neocortical Transplants

The results of these experiments indicate that embryonic neocortical tissue provides a physical matrix sufficient to support the proximo-distal regenerative growth of retinofugal axons through the transplants. Given the history of claimed proximo-distal regeneration in the adult mammalian CNS, a considerable amount of skepticism is warranted when any new claims are made. Our

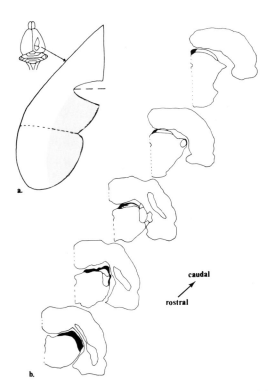

Figure 7-13. Schematics and drawings of regions associated with complete ventral transverse transection of the optic tract (TCV). (a) Schematic dorsal view of the retinofugal projection illustrating patterns of sparing (white) and deafferentation (shaded) associated with a TCV lesion. (b) Drawings of representative serial sections through the various regions of the retinofugal projection.

conclusion that the HRP-labeled retinofugal axons which coursed through the transplants actually represent proximo-distal regenerative growth of damaged axons is based upon several very strong lines of evidence. First, adult rat retinal ganglion cells posses an intrinsic capacity for axonal regeneration following transection of the retinofugal projection (Ross 1983). This capacity is expressed as the growth of thick fascicle and tangled mass neuroma-like neoformations following transection of the retinofugal projection at the level of the optic tract and is expressed as retinal afferent ingrowth to transplants of embryonic neural tissue that develop well-integrated interface regions with the zone of traumatic reaction in the damaged retinofugal projection (Ross and Das 1982a,b, 1983, Ross 1983). The proximo-distal regeneration of retinofugal axons appears to represent another form of expression of the retinal ganglion cells' intrinsic regenerative capacity. Second, it was clear that the fascicles of retinofugal axons which coursed through the transplant parenchyma were not spared fascicles of axons that had been passively displaced or enwrapped by

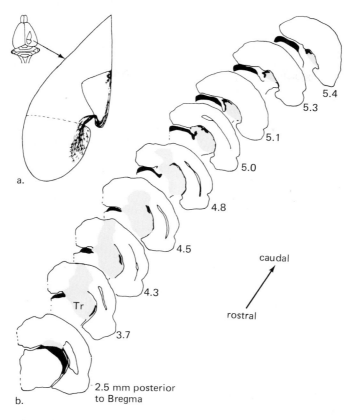

Figure 7-14. Schematic drawing and representative serial sections of a case in which retinofugal axons had regenerated through a neocortical transplant placed at the site of a complete ventral transverse transection of the optic tract (TCV). (a) Schematic dorsal view of the caudal diencephalon and superior colliculus showing the relative position of the transplant, the extent of the optic tract transection, and the course of retinofugal axons through the transplant. (b) Representative serial sections from various regions of the retinofugal projection depicting retinofugal axons that penetrate across the transplant interface with the zone of traumatic reaction in the optic tract, traverse the transplant parenchyma along the contour of the lateral surface of apposition with the hippocampal formation, course around the caudal-most lobe of the transplant, reenter the distal stump of the transected brachium coursing rostrally and ventrally, and reinnervate the lateral regions of the optic layers that had been deafferented by the TCV lesion.

the volumetric expansion of the developing transplants. In the 47 lesion control cases examined between 3 days and 18 months following transection of the optic tract or brachium, there were no cases where teased fascicles were found to bridge the lumen of the lesion cavity (Ross 1983). In the 31 cases that had survived from 3 to 21 days following lesion-transplantation surgery no fascicles of axons were found to course through any of the transplants and there was no

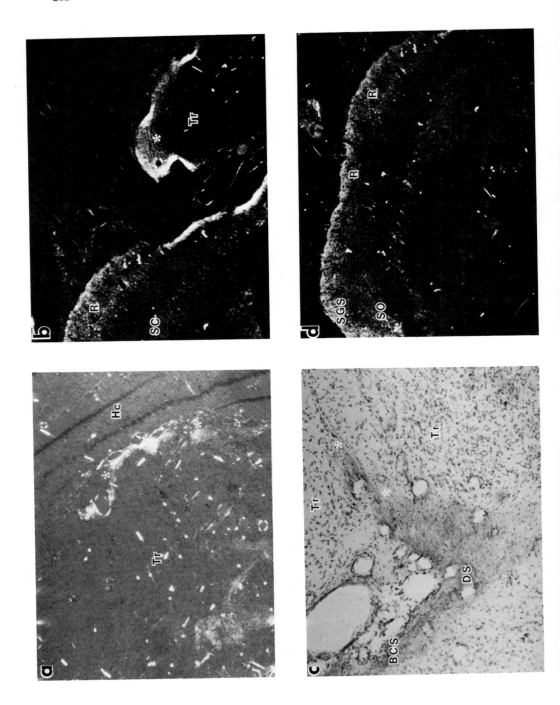

indication that neurons from the developing transplants had either migrated into the optic tract or enwrapped fascicles of spared retinofugal axons at the edge of the lesion cavity. Axons that coursed through the transplant parenchyma were always found to arise from the zone of traumatic reaction and never from spared regions of the retinofugal projection. In each case where fascicles of retinofugal axons had coursed through the transplant parenchyma it appeared that some axons branched off the main fascicle and terminated within neuron-dense regions of the transplant parenchyma. Finally, it was possible to be certain that HRP retinofugal terminal labeling in zones of the optic layers of the superior colliculus deafferented by optic tract transection was due to reinnervation by regenerated retinofugal axons. Due to the topographic ordering of axons in the caudal retinofugal projection (Yamadori 1981, Ross 1983) it was possible to accurately predict patterns of deafferentation in the optic layers based upon the location and extent of the transection. The patterns of sparing and deafferentation in the optic layers associated with different types of partial transections were determined from the analysis of 47 control cases that received partial transections alone and 76 lesion-transplantation cases in which retinofugal axons had not regenerated through the transplants (Ross 1983). In these cases there was no evidence that spared retinofugal axons had massively sprouted into the deafferented zones. The large zones of complete deafferentation persisted from 4 days to 1 year after transection. The reinnervation of the optic layers observed in the cases where retinofugal axons had regenerated through the transplant parenchyma was clearly not due to the sprouting of spared retinofugal axons. In every case interpreted as representing proximo-distal regeneration the HRP-labeled retinofugal axons were found to arise from the zone of traumatic reaction, cross the transplant interface, course through neuron-dense regions of the transplant parenchyma, reenter the distal stump of the transected optic tract, and reinnervate regions of the optic layers deafferented by the transection.

Although retinal ganglion cells may express their regenerative capacity as proximo-distal regenerative growth through neocortical transplants, this form of sustained regenerative growth was found in only about 25% of all cases

Figure 7-15. A large fascicle of regenerated retinofugal axons that traversed the transplant parenchyma along the contour of the apposed lateral surface, around the caudal lobe of the transplant, reentered the distal stump of the brachium, and reinnervated the lateral regions of the optic layers. HRP injected into the eye contralateral to the transplant 90 days after transection/transplantation surgery. (a) HRP-labeled axons coursing within the transplant parenchyma along the contour of the apposed surface with the hippocampal formation (Hc). (b) Facsicle of HRP-labeled axons coursing around the caudal lobe of the transplant. (c) Regenerated retinofugal axons crossing the caudomedial transplant interface into the distal stump of the brachium (DS). (d) Reinnervation of the lateral regions of the optic layers by regenerated retinofugal axons. a,b,d polarized light optics. Abbreviations: TR, transplant; SC, superior colliculus; R, reinnervated; BCS, brachium of the superior colliculus; SGS, stratum griseum superficiale; SO, stratum opticum.

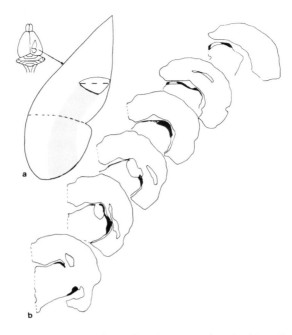

Figure 7-16. Schematics and drawings of regions associated with an incomplete ventral transverse transection of the optic tract (TIV). (a) Schematic dorsal view of the retinofugal projection illustrating patterns of sparing (white) and deafferentation (shaded) associated with a TIV lesion. (b) Drawings of representative serial sections through the various regions of the retinofugal projection.

examined in this study. Clearly, the transplantation of embryonic neural tissue at the site of transection in the adult rat's retinofugal projection did not guarantee the proximo-distal regenerative growth of retinofugal axons through the transplants.

Spatial and Temporal Stages in the Proximo-Distal Regeneration of Damaged CNS Tracts

The process of proximo-distal regeneration of retinofugal axons may break down at a number of intermediate points. The number and frequency of these forms of "arrested" or proximal regenerative growth suggest that resolution of the enigma of regeneration in the mammalian CNS may necessitate a systematic identification of all conditions that constrain the process. Rather than ascribing the regenerative failure of retinofugal axons to any one cause, the conditions that may constrain the process of axonal regeneration in the adult mammalian CNS may best be considered in a sequence of spatial and temporal stages. Sunderland (1968) described a sequence of stages in the regeneration of peripheral nerves after injury that provides an excellent conceptual model for

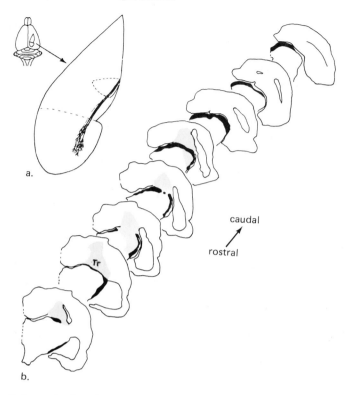

a.

caudal

rostral

Tr

b.

Figure 7-17. Schematic drawing and representative serial sections of a case in which retinofugal axons had regenerated through a neocortical transplant placed at the site of an incomplete ventral transverse transection of the optic tract (TIV). (a) Schematic dorsal view of the caudal diencephalon and superior colliculus showing the relative position of the transplant, the extent of the optic tract transection, and the course of retinofugal axons through the transplant. (b) Representative serial sections from various regions of the retinofugal projection depicting retinofugal axons that penetrate across the transplant interface with the zone of traumatic reaction in the optic tract, course through the transplant parenchyma parallel to fascicles of spared retinofugal axons in the optic tract, reenter the distal stump of the optic tract, and reinnervate regions in the medial ⅓ of the optic layers that had been deafferented by the TIV lesion.

considering regeneration in any system. In the following sections observations of successful and failed regeneration of retinal ganglion cells will be considered throughout this sequence of stages:

1. recovery of neurons from the retrograde effects of axotomy,
2. sprouting and regeneration within the zone of traumatic reaction,
3. regeneration of axons between the proximal and distal stumps of the transected tract,
4. regenerative growth down the distal stump of the transected tract,
5. reinnervation of the normal target area,

6. formation of functional synaptic contacts, and
7. functional recovery from behavioral deficits produced by the transection of the CNS tract.

Observations of both successful and failed regeneration of retinofugal axons will be considered together with observations of successful and failed axonal regeneration in other systems at each stage.

Stage 1: Recovery of Neurons from the Retrograde Effects of Axotomy

Barron (1983) suggested that many intrinsic CNS neurons may not regenerate their axons due to the severity of their perikaryal response to axotomy. It is clear, however, that all intrinsic CNS neurons do not exhibit the same retrograde response to axotomy (Lieberman 1971, Beresford 1965). The perikaryal response of CNS neurons to axotomy can be separated into three general classes; (1) those neurons, such as the thalamic relay neurons, that undergo rapid retrograde degeneration following axotomy (Wong-Riley 1972, Matthews 1973, Barron et al. 1973); (2) those neurons, such as neocortical pyramidal neurons, that gradually atrophy following axotomy (Kalil and Schneider 1975); and (3) those neurons, such as the noradrenergic locus coruleus neurons, whose perikarya display little if any obvious morphological response to axotomy (Reis et al. 1981). These three classes of perikaryal response to axotomy may correspond to the three types of retrograde reaction of axons to injury: "indirect Wallerian degeneration," gradual retrograde atrophy, and axonal regeneration, respectively (Beresford 1965).

Although some neurons recover from the retrograde effects of axotomy, many do not. The basis for the observed differences in sensitivity of intrinsic CNS neurons to axotomy is unclear. It has been suggested that the presence of "sustaining" collaterals proximal to the cell body or the distance of the axotomizing injury from the perikarya may account for the variability of perikaryal responses observed (Rose and Woolsey 1949, Cragg 1970, Lieberman 1971). It is also possible that differences in the metabolic patterns of neurons may bias their sensitivity to axotomizing trauma. Neurons that regenerate their axons may shift their metabolic priorities from a synaptic mode, in which a large amount of their metabolic energy is devoted to the production of neurotransmitters, molecules related to synaptic transmission, and the maintenance of excitable membrane properties, to a synthetic or regenerative mode, characterized by a down regulation of transmitter-related metabolism and an increase in the synthesis of structural elements, such as cytoskeletal components (Lasek and Hoffman 1976) needed for axonal regeneration (Grafstein 1975). Pathological alterations consequent upon traumatic injury to the CNS may prevent certain types of neurons from making this shift in metabolic priorities. These pathological processes may underlie the failure of many intrinsic CNS neurons to regenerate their axons and result in their subsequent degeneration.

The response of retinal ganglion cells to axotomy is highly dependent upon the position at which the retinofugal axons are cut. It is well established that most, if not all, retinal ganglion cells degenerate following transection or crush of the optic nerve in adult mammals (Leinfelder 1933, Mantz and Klein 1951, Eayrs 1952, Grafstein and Ingoglia 1982, Misantone et al. 1984). In contrast, neither the transection of the optic tract in adult cats (Chow and Dewson 1966) nor the ablation of the superior colliculus in adult rats (Perry and Cowey 1979) results in any detectable retinal ganglion cell death within 3 months after the axotomizing injuries. Our observations of sustained axonal regeneration following transection of the optic tract, brachium, or stratum opticum of the superior colliculus are consistent with the suggestion that damage farther out on the axonal arbor may result in a less severe retrograde response. However, the regenerative failure and neuronal degeneration that follows transection of the mammalian optic nerve may not be entirely due to the proximity of the injury to the perikarya. Observations of sustained axonal regeneration following focal injury of the ganglion cell fiber layer in the retina (Goldberg and Frank 1980, McConnell and Berry 1983) suggest that injuries even more proximal to the retinal ganglion cell perikarya may not result in marked retrograde neuronal degeneration. It is possible that transection or crush of the optic nerve creates a pathological condition in the retina that does not occur following focal retinal lesions or extensive transection of the caudal retinofugal projection. Vascular insufficiency resulting from severance of the central retinal vein in the core of the optic nerve may produce ischemia within the retina, precipitating a metabolic crisis that results in the degeneration of the axotomized retinal ganglion cells. Retinal ganglion cells in the poikilothermic teleostean fishes and amphibians may be less sensitive to the metabolic alterations induced by optic nerve transection due to the ability of these cold-blooded animals to efficiently alter their metabolic activity over a wide range.

Stage 2: Sprouting and Regeneration within the Zone of Traumatic Reaction

Ramon y Cajal (1928) described three phases in the metamorphosis of axons in the proximal stumps of damaged peripheral nerves: (1) an acute phase of traumatic reaction characterized by the formation of hypertrophied segments capped by swollen terminal clubs, (2) a phase characterized by the sprouting of fine processes from the terminal club (terminal sprouts) and from positions on the hypertrophied segment at a distance from the terminal club (collateral sprouts), and (3) sustained regenerative growth of axons from the proximal stump into the lesion site that may reenter the distal stump and reinnervate deafferented target areas. The regenerative metamorphosis of retinal ganglion cells, like that of peripherally projecting neurons, central cholinergic, and catecholaminergic neurons (Björklund et al. 1971, Katzman et al. 1971), appears to proceed beyond the phase of terminal and collateral sprouting into a phase of sustained axonal regeneration (Ross 1983). The phase of "abortive" terminal and collateral sprouting appears to begin within 2 days following transection of the optic tract, brachium, or stratum opticum of the superior colliculus. This phase is characterized by an increased density of fine processes near the wound margin of the zone. The density of HRP labeling within the zone of traumatic reaction appears to reach a peak between 7 and 10 days but then undergoes a marked decrease such that between 18 and 21 days after the injury the density of HRP labeling within the zone appears to return to normal. This phase may represent the transient sprouting of fine terminal and collateral processes described by Ramon y Cajal (1928). As with the abortive sprouting Ramon y Cajal observed in the "metamorphic" zone of traumatic reaction, it appears that most of the processes within the retinofugal zone of traumatic reaction are resorbed within 3 weeks after the injury. A few scattered processes within the zone of traumatic reaction and at the wound margin that have clearly aberrant orientation are the only evidence of this phase that persists 21 days after transection. It is unclear exactly when the onset of the phase of sustained axonal regeneration occurs. This phase may temporally overlap the end of the abortive sprouting phase.

Following the phase of abortive sprouting some neurons may express a capacity for sustained axonal regeneration that is manifest in the development of axonal neoformations and/or new synaptic contacts. Some regenerated axons may find their way out of the zone of traumatic reaction, but it appears that many do not. Neoformations found within the zone of traumatic reaction may include dense fascicles and neuroma-like tangled masses of regenerated axons and the formation of local synaptic contacts. The existence of these forms of sustained regenerative growth suggests that conditions within the zone of traumatic reaction may place serious constraints upon proximo-distal regeneration. Since dense fascicle, neuroma-like tangled mass and local synaptic contact formation may reflect different local conditions encountered by the regenerating axons, each will be considered separately.

Formation of Dense Fascicles of Regenerated Axons. Within the zone of traumatic reaction the phase of sustained axonal regeneration progresses very slowly. By one month after transection of the retinofugal projection dense fascicles of retinofugal axons are found within the zone of traumatic reaction. The formation of dense fascicles appears to be analogous to the "compartmentalization" of regenerating peripheral nerve axons within the proximal stump of transected peripheral nerves (Morris et al. 1972). The normal fascicular organization of axons in the proximal stump of the transected sciatic nerve is replaced by numerous small funiculi, each of which is enwrapped by a distinct perineurial sheath. Morris et al. (1972) suggested that the compartmentalization process reflects an alteration in the glial and connective tissue matrix within the proximal stump of the damaged peripheral nerve which ensures the survival of the regenerating axons but impairs the progress of their regenerative elongation. Alterations in the axon-glial relationships within the zone of traumatic reaction may underlie the formation of dense fascicles of regenerating retinofugal axons and restrict their growth through the zone.

Disruption of epineurial and perineurial elements within damaged peripheral nerves results in a proliferation of glial and connective tissue elements both at the lesion site and within the proximal stump (Morris et al. 1972). The severity of disruption in the normal three-dimensional matrix of supporting tissues within a nerve strongly influences the accuracy and completeness of regeneration. Whereas nerves that receive mild crush injuries that do not severely disrupt either the perineuriun, epineurium, or endoneurium regenerate with a high degree of accuracy, nerves that suffer more severe injuries which disrupt their supporting tissues are characterized by axonal regeneration accompanied by the formation of neuromas both within the connective tissue matrix of the scar and within the proximal stump itself (Sunderland 1968). Within the zone of traumatic reaction in the proximal stump of the transected optic tract or brachium the normal matrix of non-neuronal elements may reorganize into a reactive tangle of astrocytic, oligodendroglial, and vascular processes. Although this altered glial environment does not prevent the sustained regeneration of damaged retinofugal axons, it clearly does not provide an oriented matrix to guide their growth. In studies of retinofugal axon regenerability, the dense fascicle and tangled mass neuroma-like neoformations within the zone of traumatic reaction are the most frequently encountered form of sustained axonal regeneration. The predominance of the neuroma-like and dense fascicle neoformations appears to reflect the severity of the trauma induced by transection of the optic tract, brachium, or stratum opticum of the superior colliculus. Since the regeneration of damaged retinofugal axons may be initiated from points deep within the zone of traumatic reaction, it appears that the access of the regenerating axons to the wound margin is extremely restricted. This does not suggest that the "glial barrier" at the margin of the lesion cavity is impenetrable, only that the regenerating axons encounter an environment within the zone of traumatic reaction that does not contain a highly oriented physical matrix for the contact guidance (Harrison 1910) of the regenerating retinofugal axons.

Neuroma formation represents the expression of a capacity for sustained regenerative growth that is severely restricted to a proximal axonal growth and may not result in the formation of synaptic contacts on dendritic or perikaryal elements. Bernstein et al. (1978) observed similar neuroma-like structures (neuromata) following transection of the spinal cord of adults rats. Ultrastructurally these neuromata contained axons that appeared to form presynaptic contacts upon other axons within the neuromata. Neuromata in the transected spinal cord are apparently resorbed because they become less evident at periods longer than 30 days and appear to disappear completely by 90 days after transection. Unlike the neuromata in the spinal cord, the dense fascicle and neuroma-like neoformations in the zone of traumatic reaction of the retinofugal projection become more pronounced at times longer than 1 month after optic tract or brachium transection. Neuroma-like tangled mass neoformations have also been described in association with lesions of long standing in the human brainstem and spinal cord (Sung 1981).

The growth of regenerating retinofugal axons to the wound margin of the zone of traumatic reaction may be constrained by the availability of physically uninterrupted extracellular space. The formation of dense fascicle and neuromalike neoformations by regenerating axons that never reach the wound margin may represent growth within *cul-de sac* regions that are physically enclosed by a dense meshwork of reactive non-neuronal elements. These neoformations would appear to be highly analogous to peripheral nerve neuromas (Sunderland 1968) and Probst bundles that form in congenitally or experimentally acallosal animals during development (Silver et al. 1982). All of these phenomena represent sustained axonal growth within abnormal physical environments.

Local Synapse Formation. Bernstein and Bernstein (1971) observed increases in synaptic density proximal to sites of spinal cord transection in the adult rat. They suggested that the increased synaptic density may represent the local termination of damaged axons that normally terminate distal to the site of spinal cord transection and that the formation of these connections may prevent the axons from regenerating any farther. In our experiments an increase in the HRP-labeling density of retinofugal terminal zones within the zone of traumatic reaction was evident, particularly in cases that had survived for periods longer than 90 days following transection of the retinofugal projection. These increases in HRP-labeling density in the lateral geniculate and stratum griseum regions of the retinofugal projection following transection of the optic tract and stratum opticum, respectively, may represent an increased density of termination by damaged retinofugal axons proximal to the lesion site. If this occurs, a point that can only be resolved by quantitative electron microscopic analysis, the local termination of regenerating retinofugal axons within the zone of traumatic reaction may limit the number of retinofugal axons that gain access to the wound margin in the zone of traumatic reaction.

Stage 3: Regeneration of Axons between the Proximal and Distal Stumps of the Transected Tract

The successful regenerative growth of axons between the proximal and distal stumps of a transected tract requires (1) the regeneration of axons across the lesion margin of the zone of traumatic reaction, (2) axonal regeneration through the lesion cavity or tissue tranplanted into the lesion cavity, and (3) the reentry of regenerated axons into the brain parenchyma at the position of the distal stump of the transected tract. Since regenerative failure may occur at any of these three points, each will be considered separately.

Regenerative Growth of Axons across the Wound Margin of the Zone of Traumatic Reaction. Under some conditions regenerating axons cross the wound margin and either penetrate into peripheral nerve (Tello 1911, Sugar and Gerard 1950, Kao 1974, Kao et al. 1977, Richardson et al. 1980, David and Aguayo 1981), muscle (Glees 1955, Nathaniel and Clemente 1959, Horvat 1967, Björklund and Stenevi 1971, Svendgaard et al. 1975, 1976, Emson et al. 1977, Heinicke 1978, Schoenfeld and Katzman 1980), or embryonic neural tissue (Kromer et al. 1981a,b, Ross and Das 1982b, 1983, Ross 1983) transplanted at the site of transection in adult mammalian CNS tracts, or enter the lumen of lesion cavities. These findings indicate that the glial scarring which may occur around lesion sites within the adult mammalian CNS is not absolutely refractory to axonal regeneration.

Fascicles of regenerated retinofugal axons were found which crossed the wound margin and extended into the lumen of the lesion cavity in all cases examined 2 months or more after transection of the optic tract or brachium where cavitation had occured at the lesion site. Similarly, transplants of embryonic neocortical and other neural tissues were found to receive retinal afferents across well-integrated interface regions with the zone of traumatic reaction in the host's retinofugal projection. Although it appeared that the anatomical integration of embryonic neocortical tissues may have supplanted cicatrization at the wound margin of the zone of traumatic reaction, the anatomical integration of a transplant was not always sufficient to ensure retinal afferent ingrowth at these positions. In some cases tangled mass neuroma-like neoformations were found at transplant interface positions that appeared to be well integrated with the zone of traumatic reaction in the retinofugal projection. The development of a confluent extracellular space between the zone of traumatic reaction and the transplant parenchyma may be necessary for the regeneration of retinofugal axons into the transplants. In cases where the margins of lesion cavities created by optic tract, brachium, or stratum opticum transection were found to have fused together, regenerated retinofugal axons never crossed the thin glial scars that marked these lesion sites. It would appear that fusion of the wound margins may prevent the development of a confluent extracellular space between the proximal and distal stumps of the transected retinofugal projection.

Regenerative Growth of Axons through the Lumen of a Lesion Cavity or through Tissue Transplanted at the Lesion Site. Retinofugal axons that regenerate into the lumen of lesion cavities at the sites of optic tract or brachium transection appear to course with random orientation upon the connective tissue elements present there (Ross 1983). This type of unoriented regenerative growth is similar to that seen following transection of the optic nerve and removal of a large length of the distal stump in adult goldfish (Bohn et al. 1982). The failure of these axons to reenter the distal stump of the transected retinofugal projection appears to be due to the lack of an oriented physical matrix for contact guidance (Harrison 1910) or odogenesis (Dustin 1910) of the regenerating axons. Although the milieu may contain "substrate pathways" (Weiss 1934, Letourneau 1975, Katz et al. 1980) or cell adhesion molecules (Edelman 1983) that the regenerating axons may recognize, they do not appear to orient the regenerating axons toward the distal stump of the transected optic tract.

Heterotopic transplants of embryonic neocortical tissue appear to be similar to grafts of predegenerated peripheral nerves (Sugar and Gerard 1950, Kao 1974, Kao et al. 1977, David and Aguayo 1981) and homotopic transplants of embryonic hippocampal tissue (Kromer et al. 1981b) in that they may provide an oriented physical matrix that is sufficient to support the regenerative growth of axons between the proximal and distal stumps of transected tracts in the adult mammalian CNS. In the present study only half of the cases in which retinofugal axons had entered the transplants were characterized by regeneration that extended between the proximal and distal stumps of the transected retinofugal projection. In the other half of the cases the retinofugal axons ramified and appeared to terminate within the transplants. In all cases where retinofugal axons had coursed between the proximal and distal stump it also appeared that some axons ramified and terminated within the transplant parenchyma. It is possible that the regenerative growth of axons through transplants of embryonic neural tissue may be diminished by the formation of local synaptic contacts upon elements in the transplants. Regenerating retinofugal axons appear to exhibit a relative affinity for some elements in neocortical tissue. This may involve the recognition by the regenerating retinofugal axons of postsynaptic receptor sites on neocortical neurons. The nature of the affinity of regenerating retinofugal axons for elements in heterotopic transplants remains to be established. However, it is clear that retinofugal axons do not express an absolute disaffinity for neocortical tissue as suggested by Lund et al. (1983).

The regenerative growth of axons through the parenchyma of embryonic neural transplants may be dependent upon the contact of the regenerating axons with ''substrate pathways'' (Katz et al. 1980) within the transplanted tissue that are oriented toward the distal stump. No attempt was made to control the orientation of the transplanted embryonic neural tissue. The lack of alignment between the zone of traumatic reaction and appropriate substrate pathways may, in part, account for the fact that regenerative growth of retinofugal axons through the transplants occurred in less than half of the transplants that received retinal afferents. The existence of several forms of axonal regeneration through the transplants suggests that the regenerating axons may have employed several different substrate pathways. One type of regenerative growth through the transplants, the form characterized by axons that traversed the transplant parenchyma along the contour of the transplant's apposed lateral surface with the hippocampus, appears to represent growth through the relatively neuron-free glial matrix in the transplants' molecular zone. Growth of neurons through deep regions of the transplant parenchyma may be made possible by the fasciculation of regenerating retinofugal axons along bundles of intrinsic transplant projections. It is likely that regenerating retinofugal axons may be able to follow multiple guidance cues as they course through the parenchyma of embryonic neural transplants.

It appears unlikely that the proximo-distal regenerative growth of retinofugal axons through the transplants represents a strong neurotropic attraction to their normal target or growth along a gradient of diffusable factors made by elements in the distal stump or the optic layers of the superior colliculus. If proximo-distal regenerative growth of axons was guided predominantly by neurotropic attraction then (1) successful proximo-distal regenerative growth through transplants should have occurred with greater frequency, and (2) should have been manifest in the orientation of regenerated fascicles within the lumen of lesion cavities toward the distal stump of the transected retinofugal projection. The limited number of cases where proximo-distal regeneration did occur suggests that if neurotropic influences are operating in this system their expression is constrained by the physical nature of the milieu encountered by the regenerating axons.

Reentry of Regenerating Axons into the Distal Stump of the Transected Tract. Reentry of regenerating retinofugal axons into the host brain parenchyma occurred only across transplant interface regions with the distal stump of the transected optic tract or brachium. The anatomical integration of embryonic neocortical transplants placed at the site of transection in the optic tract or brachium includes the formation of interface regions between the transplant and the distal stump of the transected retinofugal projection. The mechanisms that provide guidance of regenerating axons across this interface are unknown. Efferent projections from neocortical transplants in the caudal diencephalon have been found to enter the brachium and course toward the superior colliculus (Ross and Das, unpublished observations). It is possible that regenerating retinofugal axons fasciculated along transplant efferent pathways, following axons that had previously grown into the distal stump. The absence of retinofugal axon reentry across transplant interface regions with the host brain outside the distal stump suggests that the outgrowth of axons from transplants may be constrained by the availability of physical space in the host brain parenchyma. The density of the neuropil in the host brain, particularly in regions surrounding lesions, has often been suggested as a possible cause of regenerative failure in the mammalian CNS (Clemente 1964, Guth et al. 1983) and a barrier to the ingrowth of axons from transplanted neural tissues into the adult mammalian CNS (LeGros Clark, 1943). It is possible that a greater amount of extracellular space may be available at interface regions with the distal stump of transected CNS tracts. The outgrowth of transplant efferents and regenerating axons that coursed through the transplant parenchyma may preferentially occur at these interface positions.

The reentry of septohippocampal axons into the adult host's hippocampal formation from transplants of embryonic hippocampal tissue apparently does not occur at the distal stump of the transected septohippocampal projection in the fimbria (Kromer et al. 1981b). Since the fimbria, unlike the optic tract, is a two-way tract (Raisman et al. 1965) the distal stump of the transected septohippocampal projection in the fimbria is also the proximal stump of the transected hippocampal efferent projection. It is possible that within the zone of traumatic reaction in the proximal stump of the hippocampal efferent projection there is not sufficient extracellular space to permit the entry of regenerating septohippocampal axons. These axons may meet less physical resistance to outgrowth at well-integrated transplant interface positions with the Ammon's horn or dentate gyrus regions of the adult host's hippocampal formation. Both the reentry of regenerating septohippocampal axons from transplants of embryonic hippocampal tissue (Kromer et al. 1981b) and the efferent outgrowth of axons from transplants of embryonic septal (Björklund and Stenevi 1977, Björklund et al. 1979, Lewis and Cotman 1980) and mesencephalic (Björklund et al. 1976) tissues have been found to penetrate across interface regions where the transplants had "fused" with the gray matter of the hippocampal formation. However, in order for the transplant to become anatomically integrated with the hippocampal parenchyma, the embryonic tissue had to be transplanted at positions apposed to damaged surfaces of Ammon's horn and or the dentate gyrus (Björklund et al. 1976). Damage to the host hippocampal formation would be expected to produce degeneration of axons in the hilus of the dentate gyrus and the perforant path. The axons that enter the host's hippocampal formation from the transplants may penetrate across interface positions that correspond to the distal stump of damaged tracts within the hippocampal formation. It appears that the nature and position of a transplant's interface with the host brain parenchyma has a great influence upon the pattern of axonal outgrowth from the transplants (Raisman and Ebner 1983).

Fragments of predegenerated peripheral nerves have been grafted between the proximal and distal stumps of transected spinal cord in several species of adult mammals (Sugar and Gerard 1950, Kao 1974, Kao et al. 1977, Richardson et al. 1980) and between the spinal cord and medulla of adult rats (David and Aguayo 1981). Although axons are found to penetrate into the transplants and grow between the proximal and distal stumps of the cord, few axons are found to reenter the parenchyma of the distal stump (Kao et al. 1977). These nerve grafts do not appear to become well integrated with the damaged surfaces of the CNS (Kao et al. 1977). David and Aguayo (1981) reported that axons may penetrate several hundred microns into the spinal cord and medulla following their elongative growth through a sciatic nerve graft. However, since the antero-grade labeling of the ingrowing fibers was accomplished by transecting the graft and applying HRP to the ends, it is possible that the labeled fibers repre-sent the ingrowth of peripheral sympathetic axons that possess a demonstrated capacity for penetrating into the CNS as the sites of injury (Loy and Moore 1977).

Stage 4: Regenerative Growth down the Distal Stump of the Transected Tract

Within the distal stump of the transected retinofugal projection there appears to be sufficient extracellular space for regenerating axons to grow in. Cook and Wisnewski (1973) found that there was significant extracellular space surround-ing the myelin sheaths of degenerating retinofugal axons in the cat and monkey optic nerve both during the early period (0–35 days) and later times (196–413 days) after enucleation of an eye. The growth of axons down the distal stump of the transected retinofugal projection appears to be very similar to the growth of peripheral nerve axons down the distal stump. Since we analyzed cases of proximo-distal regenerative growth of retinofugal axons only at the light micro-scopic level it is unclear whether the regenerating axons coursed within or outside of the old myelin sheaths in the distal stump. It appears that the distal stump provided a highly oriented pathway for the guidance of the regenerating retinofugal axons back to their "appropriate" terminal regions in the optic layers of the superior colliculus. In some cases a moderate amount of HRP terminal labeling was found in the deeper layers of the superior colliculus, ventral to regions that had been reinnervated by the regenerated axons (Ross 1983). Since partial transections of the optic tract also partially transect the corticotectal projections, the presence of aberrant projections to deeper layers suggests that the regenerating axons may have grown along pathways made available by degenerating corticotectal axons. Regenerating retinofugal axons in adult goldfish have also been found to grow along degenerating tectal efferent pathways following transection of the optic tract (Lo and Levine 1981). This form of mechanical guidance along degenerating host brain pathways may also account for the aberrant projections that are found among the basically appropriate innervation patterns of host brain sites by axons from transplanted tissues (Björklund et al. 1976).

Stage 5: Reinnervation of the Normal Target Area

The formation of new synaptic contacts upon deafferented postsynaptic elements due to the sprouting of intact axons has been well documented to occur in some systems in the adult mammalian CNS (Raisman 1969, Raisman and Field 1973, Matthews et al. 1976, Tsukahara 1981). However, it has yet to be demonstrated that axons which have *regenerated* back into the brain parenchyma actually make synaptic contacts with neuronal elements in their appropriate target regions.

The patterns of HRP labeling in regions of the optic layers that had been deafferented by the transection of the optic tract or brachium were clearly similar to HRP terminal labeling in the superior colliculus of normal adult rats. These reinnervated zones generally appeared to be only slightly less densely labeled with the anterogradely transported HRP. The nature of the termination patterns of retinofugal axons that had regenerated through the transplants and reinnervated the optic layers remains to be established ultrastructurally. It is unclear whether the reinnervation of the optic layers represents a specific affinity of retinofugal axons for their appropriate targets (Sperry 1963). The apparent termination of regenerated retinofugal axons within heterotopic transplants of embryonic tissues and in the deeper layers of the superior colliculus below the reinnervated optic layers suggests that the regenerating axons at least have a relative affinity for other targets, similar to developing retinofugal axons (Frost, 1981).

As yet there is no evidence that the proximo-distal regeneration of retinofugal axons in adult rats proceeds through the final two stages, the formation of synaptic contacts and the recovery of lost visual function. If the regenerated retinofugal axons do form synaptic terminals in the optic layers the functionality of these contacts can only be established in an unequivocal manner by electrophysiological recording from the reinnervated areas during photic or optic nerve stimulation. Only after ultrastructural and electrophysiological studies have established the synaptic patterns and possible functionality of these projections can behavioral studies establish whether the anatomically identified patterns of proximo-distal regeneration may actually underly "true" functional regeneration or recovery of function. As yet these criteria have not been met for the regenerated retinofugal projection or any other adult mammalian CNS system in which proximo-distal regeneration has been studied.

The ultrastructural identification of the synaptic terminations of regenerated axons and the electrophysiological characterization of their efficacy are clearly important in establishing whether the proximo-distal regeneration of retinofugal axons is accompanied by functional reinnervation of the optic layers. However, the importance of demonstrating these properties is overshadowed by the fact that the regenerative growth of most damaged retinofugal axons was arrested at intermediate stages in this process. Clearly, no claims of complete "reconstruction" of damaged tracts or "functional" transplantation are warranted by the meager positive findings of proximo-distal axonal regeneration in this study. Further research needs to be directed at identifying the optimal conditions for surmounting the obstacles to successful proximo-distal axonal regeneration at each stage of this process.

References

Adams, J.C. (1980). Stabilizing and rapid thionin staining of TMB based reaction product. Neurosci. Lett. 17, 7–9.

Barron, K.D. (1983). Comparative observations on the cytologic reactions of central and peripheral nerve cells to axotomy. In: Spinal Cord Reconstruction. Kao, C.C., Bunge, R.P., Reier, P.J. (eds.). New York: Raven Press, pp. 1–14.

Barron, K.D., Means, E.D., Larsen, E. (1973). Ultrastructural evidence of retrograde degeneration in thalamus of rat. I. Neuronal soma and dendrites. J. Neuropath. Exp. Neurol. 32, 218–244.

Beresford, W.A.A. (1965). A discussion on retrograde changes in nerve fibers. In: Mechanisms of Neural Regeneration. Singer, M., Schade, J.P. (eds.). Prog. Brain Res. 14, 33–56.

Bernstein, J.J., Bernstein, M.E. (1971). Axonal regeneration and formation of synapses proximal to the site of lesion following hemisection of the rat spinal cord. Exp. Neurol. 30, 336–351.

Bernstein, J.J., Wells, M.R., Bernstein, M.E. (1978). Effect of puromycin treatment on the regeneration of hemisected and transected rat spinal cord. J. Neurocytol. 7, 215–228.

Björklund, A., Katzman, R., Stenevi, U., West, K.A. (1971). Development and growth of axonal sprouts from noradrenaline and 5-hydroxytryptamine neurons in the rat spinal cord. Brain Res. 31, 21–33.

Björklund, A., Kromer, L.F., Stenevi, U. (1979). Cholinergic reinnervation of the rat hippocampus by septal implants is stimulated by perforant path lesions. Brain Res. 173, 57–64.

Björklund, A. Stenevi, U. (1971). Growth of central catecholamine neurons into smooth muscle grafts in the rat mesencephalon. Brain Res. 31, 1–20.

Björklund, A., Stenevi, U. (1977). Reformation of the severed septohippocampal cholinergic pathway in the adult rat by transplanted septal neurons. Cell Tiss. Res. 185, 289–302.

Björklund, A., Stenevi, U. (1979). Regeneration of monoaminergic and cholinergic neurons in the mammalian central nervous system. Physiol. Rev. 59, 62–100.

Björklund, A., Stenevi, U., Svendgaard, N.A. (1976). Growth of transplanted monoaminergic neurons into the adult hippocampus along the perforant path. Nature (London) 262, 787–790.

Bohn, R.C., Reier, P.J., Sourbeer, E.B. (1982). Axonal interactions with connective tissue and glial substrata during optic nerve regeneration in Xenopus larvae and adults. Am. J. Anat. 165, 397–419.

Chow, K.L., Dewson, J.H. (1966). Numerical estimates of neurons and glia in the lateral geniculate body during retrograde degeneration. J. Comp. Neurol. 128, 63–74.

Clemente, C.D. (1964). Regeneration in the vertebrate central nervous system. Int. Rev. Neurobiol. 6, 257–301.

Cook, R.D., Wisnewski, H.M. (1973). The role of oligodendroglia and astroglia in Wallerian degeneration of the optic nerve. Brain Res. 61, 191–206.

Cragg, B.G. (1970). What is the signal for chromatolysis? Brain Res. 23, 1–21.

Das, G.D., Ross, D.T. (1982). Stereotaxic technique for transplantation of neural tissues in the brain of adult rats. Experientia 38, 848–850.

David, S., Aguayo, A.J. (1981). Axonal elongation into peripheral nervous system "bridges" after central nervous system injury. Science 214, 931–933.

Dustin, A.P. (1910). Le role des tropismes et de l'odogenese dans la regeneracion du systeme nerveux. Arch. Biol. (Liege) 25, 269–388.

Eayrs, J.T. (1952). Relationships between the ganglion cell layer of the retina and the optic nerve in the rat. Brit. J. Ophthalmol. 36, 453–459.

Edelman, G.M. (1983). Cell adhesion molecules. Science 217, 450–457.

Emson, P.C., Björklund, A., Stenevi, U. (1977). Evaluation of the regenerative capacity of central dopaminergic, noradrenergic and cholinergic neurons using iris implants as targets. Brain Res. 135, 87–105.

Frost, D. (1981). Orderly anomalous retinal projections to the medial geniculate, ventrobasal and lateral posterior nuclei of the hamster. J. Comp. Neurol. 203, 227–256.

Gage, F.H., Björklund, A., Stenevi, U. (1983). Re-innervation of the partially deafferented hippocampus by compensatory collateral sprouting from spared cholinergic and noradrenergic afferents. Brain Res. 268, 27–37.

Glees, P. (1955). Studies on cortical regeneration with special reference to cerebral implants. In: Regeneration in the Central Nervous System. Windle, W.F. (ed.). Springfield, IL: C.C. Thomas, pp. 809–822.

Goldberg, S., Frank. B. (1980). Will central nervous systems in the adult mammal regenerate after bypassing a lesion? A study in the mouse and chick visual system. Exp. Neurol. 70, 675–689.

Grafstein, B. (1975). The nerve cell body response to axotomy. Exp. Neurol. 48, 32–51.

Grafstein, B., Ingoglia, N.A. (1982). Intracranial transection of the optic nerve in adult mice: Preliminary observations. Exp. Neurol. 76, 318–330.

Graziadei, P.P.C., Kaplan, M.S. (1980). Regrowth of olfactory sensory axons into transplanted neural tissue. I. Development of connections with occipital cortex. Brain Res. 201, 39–44.

Guth, L. (1956). Regeneration in the mammalian peripheral nervous system. Physiol. Rev. 36, 441–478.

Guth, L., Reier, P.J. Barrett, C.P., Donatti, E.J. (1983). Repair of the mammalian spinal cord. Trends Neurosci. 6, 20–24.

Guth, L., Windle, W.F. (1970). The enigma of central nervous system regeneration. Exp. Neurol. Supp. 5, 1–43.

Hallas, B.H., Oblinger, M.M., Das, G.D. (1980). Heterotopic neural transplants in the cerebellum of the rat: Their afferents. Brain Res. 196, 242–246.

Harrison, R.G. (1910). The outgrowth of the nerve fiber as a form of protoplasmic movement. J. Exp. Zool. 9, 787–846.

Heinicke, E.A. (1978). Vascular permeability and axonal regeneration into tissue auto-transplanted into the brain. Proc. Canad. Fed. Biol. Sci. 21, 40.

Hine, R. (1977). Transplanted cerebellar tissue in rats: Its growth and afferents. Anat. Rec. 187, 605.

Horvat, J.C. (1967). Réactiones régénératives provoquées au niveau de la moelle épinière thoracique de la souris par la greffe de nerfs et de quelques tissus non nerveux. Comp. Rend. Assoc. Anat. 52, 659–669.

Jacobsen, M., Gaze, R.M. (1965). Selection of appropriate tectal connections by regenerating optic nerve fibers in adult goldfish. Exp. Neurol. 13, 418–430.

Kalil, K., Schneider, G.E. (1975). Retrograde cortical and axonal changes following lesions of the pyramidal tract. Brain Res. 89, 15–27.

Kao, C.C. (1974). Comparison of healing processes in transected spinal cords grafted with autologous brain tissue, sciatic nerve, and nodose ganglia. Exp. Neurol. 44, 424–437.

Kao, C.C., Chang, L.W., Bloodworth, J.M.B. (1977). The mechanism of spinal cord cavitation following spinal cord transection. Part 3. Delayed grafting with and without spinal cord re-transection. J. Neurosurg. 46, 757–766.

Katz, M.J., Lasek, R.J., Nauta, H.J.W. (1980). Ontogeny of substrate pathways and the origin of the neural circuit pattern. Neuroscience 5, 821–833.

Katzman, R., Björklund, A., Owman, C., Stenevi, U., West, K.A. (1971). Evidence for regenerative axon sprouting of central catecholamine neurons in the rat mesencephalon following electrolytic lesions. Brain Res. 25, 579–596.

Kiernan, J.A. (1970). Two types of axonal regeneration in the neurohypophysis of the rat. J. Anat. 107, 187.

Kiernan, J.A. (1979). Hypotheses concerned with axonal regeneration in the mammalian central nervous system. Biol. Rev. 54, 155–197.

Kromer, L.F., Björklund, A., Stenevi, U. (1981a). Innervation of embryonic hippocampal implants by regenerating axons of cholinergic septal neurons in the adult rat. Brain Res. 210, 153–171.

Kromer, L.F. Björklund, A., Stenevi, U. (1981b). Regeneration of the septohippocampal pathways in adult rats is promoted by utilizing embryonic hippocampal implants as bridges. Brain Res. 210, 173–200.

Lasek, R.J., Hoffman, P.N. (1976). The neuronal cytoskeleton, axonal transport and axonal growth. In: Cell Motility. Goldman, R., Pollard, T., Rosenbaum, J. (eds.). Cold Spring Harbor Laboratory, pp. 1021–1051.

LeGros Clark, W.E. (1943). The problem of neuronal regeneration in the central nervous system. II. The insertion of peripheral nerve stumps into the brain. J. Anat. 77, 251–259.

Leinfelder, P.S. (1933). Retrograde degeneration in the optic nerves and retinal ganglion cells. Trans. Am. Ophthalmol. Soc. 36, 307–315.

Letourneau, P.C. (1975). Cell-to-substratum adhesion and guidance of axonal elongation. Dev. Biol. 44, 92–101.

Lewis, E.R., Cotman, C.W. (1980). Mechanisms of septal lamination in the developing hippocampus revealed by outgrowth of fibers from septal implants. I. Positional and temporal factors. Brain Res. 196, 307–330.

Lieberman, A.R. (1971). The axon reaction: A review of the principal features of perikaryal response to axonal injury. Int. Rev. Neurobiol. 14, 49–124.

Lo, R.Y.S., Levine, R.L. (1981). Anatomical evidence for the influence of degenerating pathways on regenerating optic fibers following surgical manipulations in the visual system of the goldfish. Brain Res. 210, 61–68.

Loots, G.P., Loots, J.M., Brown, M., Schoeman, J.L. (1979). A rapid silver impregnation method for nervous tissue: A modified protargol-peroxide technique. Stain Tech. 54, 97–100.

Loy, R., Moore, R.Y. (1977). Anomalous innervation of the hippocampal formation by peripheral sympathetic axons following mechanical injury. Exp. Neurol. 57, 645–650.

Lund, R.D. Harvey, A.R., Jaeger, C.B., McLoon, S.C. (1983). Transplantation of embryonic neural tissues to the tectal region of the rat. In: Changing Concepts of the Nervous System. Morrison, A.P., Strick, F.L. (eds.). New York: Academic Press, pp. 361–375.

Lynch, G.S., Cotman, C.W. (1975). The hippocampus as a model for studying anatomical plasticity in the adult brain. In: The hippocampus, Vol. 1. Isaacson, R., Pribram, K. (eds.). New York: Plenum Press, pp. 123–155.

Mantz, J., Klein, M. (1951). Recherches experimentales sur la section et la ligature du nerf optique chez le rat. Comp. Rend. Soc. Biol. Paris 145, 920–924.

Matthews, D.A., Cotman, C.W., Lynch, G.S. (1976). An electron microscopic study of lesion induced synaptogenesis in the dentate gyrus of the adult rat. I. Magnitude and time course of degeneration. Brain Res. 115, 1–21.

Matthews, M.A. (1973). Death of a central neuron: An electron microscopic study of thalamic retrograde degeneration following cortical ablation. J. Neurocytol. 2, 265–288.

McConnell, P., Berry, M. (1983). Regeneration of ganglion cells in the adult mouse retina. Brain Res. 241, 362–365.

McGeer, P.L., Eccles, J.C., McGeer, E.G. (1981). Molecular Biology of the Mammalian Brain. New York: Plenum Press, pp. 183–197.

Mesulam, M.M. (1978). Tetramethyl benzadine for horseradish peroxidase neurohistochemistry: A non-carcinogenic blue reaction product with superior sensitivity for visualizing neural afferents and efferents. J. Histochem. Cytochem. 26, 106–117.

Mesulam, M.M. (1982). Principles of horseradish peroxidase neurohistochemistry and their applications for tracing neural pathways; axonal transport, enzyme histochemistry and light microscopic analysis. In: Tracing Neural Connections with Horseradish Peroxidase. Mesulam, M.M. (ed.). New York: Wiley, pp. 1–152.

Misantone, L.J., Gerschbaum, M., Murray, M. (1984). Viability of retinal ganglion cells after optic nerve crush in adult rats. J. Neurocyt. 13, 449–465.

Morris, J.H., Hudson, A.R., Wedell, G. (1972). A study of degeneration and regeneration in the divided rat sciatic nerve based on electron microscopy. IV. Changes in fascicular microtopography, perineurism and endoneurial fibroblasts. Z. Zellforsch. 124, 165–203.

Murray, M. (1976). Regeneration of retinal axons into the goldfish optic tectum. J. Comp. Neurol. 168, 175–196.

Nathaniel, E.J.H., Clemente, C.D. (1959). Growth of nerve fibers into skin and muscle grafts in rat brains. Exp. Neurol. 1, 65–81.

Oblinger, M.M. (1981). Afferent and efferent connectivity of neocortical transplants in the cerebellar hemisphere. Ph.D. Thesis, Purdue Univ., West Lafayette, IN.

Oblinger, M.M., Das, G.D. (1982). Connectivity of neural transplants in adult rats: Analysis of afferents and efferents of neocortical transplants in the cerebellar hemisphere. Brain Res. 249, 31–49.

Oblinger, M.M., Das, G.D. (1983). Connectivity of transplants in the cerebellum: A model of developmental differences in neuroplasticity. In: Neural Tissue Transplantation Research. Wallace, R.B., Das, G.D. (eds.). New York: Springer-Verlag, pp. 105–133.

Oblinger, M.M., Hallas, B.H., Das, G.D. (1980). Neocortical transplants in the cerebellum of the rat: Their afferents and efferents. Brain Res. 189, 228–232.

Perry, V.H., Cowey, A. (1979). Changes in the retinofugal pathways following cortical and tectal lesions in neonatal and adult rats. Exp. Brain Res. 35, 97–108.

Raisman, G. (1969). Neuronal plasticity in the septal nuclei of the adult rat. Brain Res. 14, 25–48.

Raisman, G., Cowan, W.M., Powell, T.P.S. (1965). The extrinsic afferent, commisural and associational fibers of the hippocampus. Brain 88, 963–996.

Raisman, G., Ebner, F.F. (1983). Mossy fiber projections into and out of hippocampal transplants. Neuroscience 9, 783–901.

Raisman, G., Field, P.M. (1973). A quantitative investigation of the development of collateral innervation after partial deafferentation of the septal nuclei. Brain Res. 50, 241–264.

Ramon y Cajal, S. (1928). Degeneration and Regeneration in the Nervous System, Vols. I and II. May, R. (trans.). New York: Hafner.

Reis, D.J., Ross, R.A., Iacovitti, C., Gilad, G., Joh, T.H. (1981). Changes in neurotransmitter synthesizing enzymes during regeneration, compensatory and collateral sprouting of central catecholaminergic neurons in adult and developing rats. In: Lesion Induced Plasticity in Sensorimotor Systems. Flohr, H., Precht, W. (eds.). New York: Springer-Verlag, pp. 87–102.

Richardson, P.M., Issa, V.M.K., Shemie, S. (1982). Regeneration and retrograde degeneration of axons in the rat optic nerve. J. Neurocytol. 11, 949–966.

Richardson, P.M., McGuiness, V.M., Aguayo, A.J. (1980). Axons from CNS neurons regenerate into PNS grafts. Nature 284, 264–265.

Rose, J.E., Woolsey, C.N. (1949). Organization of the mammalian thalamus and its relationship to the cerebral cortex. Electroenceph. Clin. Neurophysiol. 1, 391–401.

Ross, D.T. (1983). Regenerative growth of adult rat retinofugal axons: Traumatic reaction, neuroma formation, and the regeneration of axons into and through transplants of embryonic neocortical tissue. Ph.D. Thesis, Purdue Univ., West Lafayette, IN.

Ross, D.T., Das, G.D. (1981). Adult rat optic tract axons sprout into neocortical transplants. Anat. Rec. 199, 217A.

Ross, D.T., Das, G.D. (1982a). Lesion size and position influence the magnitude of retinal afferent ingrowth to neocortical transplants. Anat. Rec. 202, 161A.

Ross, D.T., Das, G.D. (1982b). Regeneration of axons from the transected optic tract of adult rats into and through neocortical transplants. Soc. Neurosci. Abstr. 8, 758.

Ross, D.T., Das, G.D. (1983). Retinal afferent ingrowth to neocortical transplants in the adult rat superior colliculus is due to the regeneration of damaged axons rather than sprouting from intact axons. Anat. Rec. 205, 167A.

Schoenfeld, A.R., Katzman, R. (1980). Autoradiographic demonstration of the central origin of regenerating fibers into iris tissue implants in the rat mesencephalon. Brain Res. 197, 355–363.

Schneider, G.E. (1979). Is it really better to have your brain lesion early? A revision of the "Kennard principle." Neuropsychologia 17, 557–583.

Silver, J., Lorenz, S.E., Whalston, D., Couglin, J. (1982). Axonal guidance during the development of the great cerebral commisures: Descriptive and experimental studies in vivo on the role of preformed pathways. J. Comp. Neurol. 210, 10–29.

Sperry, R.W. (1945). Optic nerve regeneration with return of vision in anurans. J. Neurophysiol. 7, 57–70.

Sperry, R.W. (1963). Chemoaffinity in the orderly growth of nerve fiber patterns and connections. Proc. Nat. Acad. Sci. 50, 703–710.

Sugar, O., Gerard, R.W. (1950). Spinal cord regeneration in the rat. J. Neurophysiol. 3, 1–19.

Sunderland, S. (1968). Nerves and Nerve Injuries. Baltimore: Williams and Wilkins.

Sung, J.H. (1981). Tangled masses of regenerated central nerve fibers (non myelinated central neuromas) in the central nervous system. J. Neuropath. Exp. Neurol. 40, 645–657.

Svendgaard, N.A., Björklund, A., Stenevi, U. (1975). Regenerative properties of central monoamine neurons. Ergebn. Anat. Entwick. Gesch. 51, 1–77.

Svendgaard, N.A., Björklund, A., Stenevi, U. (1976). Regeneration of central cholinergic neurons in the adult rat brain. Brain Res. 102, 1–22.

Tello, F. (1911). La influencia del neurotropismo en la regeneracion de los centros nerviosos. Trab. Inst. Cajal. Invest. Biol. 5, 123–159.

Tsukahara, N. (1981). Synaptic plasticity in the mammalian central nervous system. Ann. Rev. Neurosci. 4, 351–379.

Weiss, P. (1934). *In vitro* experiments on the factors determining the course of the outgrowing nerve fiber. J. Exp. Zool. 68, 393–448.

Windle, W.F. (1955). Regeneration in the Central Nervous System. Springfield, IL: C.C. Thomas.

Wong-Riley, M. (1972). Changes in the dorsal lateral geniculate nucleus of the squirrel monkey after unilateral ablation of the visual cortex. J. Comp. Neurol. 146, 519–548.

Yamadori, T. (1981). An experimental anatomical study on the topographic termination of the optic nerve fibers in the rat. J. Hirnsforsch. 22, 313–326.

Chapter 8

The Role of Neuroglia in Axonal Growth and Regeneration

Amico Bignami, Nguyen H. Chi, and Doris Dahl*

Introduction

Compared to other organs, cicatrization and tissue repair in the brain and spinal cord are unique processes because of the participation of a CNS-specific cell, the astrocyte. A remarkable feature of the astrocytic response to injury is the intracytoplasmic accumulation of intermediate (10 nm) filaments resulting in dense glial scars (fibrous gliosis). Since the classical observations of Cajal, Penfield, and Windle it has been proposed that fibrous gliosis is relevant to the problem of CNS regeneration and that astrocytes exert an inhibitory influence on axonal growth (reviewed by Reier et al. 1983).

In this review we will discuss some experiments aimed at elucidating the role of neuroglia in CNS regeneration. Only a few of the manifold aspects of this problem will be considered, the selection being guided by personal experience and interest in specific questions, i.e., the reason why axons are able to grow in immature brains and readily regenerate in peripheral nerve but fail to do so in adult CNS.

Immunohistological Markers

In the experiments to be discussed in the following pages, immunohistological markers allowed the identification of the main structures relevant to the problem:

1. GFA protein, the subunit of astrocyte-specific intermediate filaments (reviewed by Dahl and Bignami 1983);

---

* Department of Neuropathology, Harvard Medical School and Spinal Cord Injury Research Laboratory, Veterans Administration Medical Center, Boston, Massachusetts 02132 U.S.A.

2. neurofilament proteins, the subunits of neuron-specific intermediate filaments (reviewed by Dahl and Bignami 1985); and
3. laminin, a basal membrane glycoprotein (Timpl et al. 1980). Laminin allows the identification of reactive Schwann cells, i.e., Schwann cells reacting to Wallerian degeneration of peripheral nerve (Bignami et al. 1984a) and of the basal lamina delineating the PNS–CNS boundary (Bignami et al. 1984b).

Transplantation of Peripheral Nerve into Brain and Spinal Cord

Since the beginning of the century, a large number of anatomoclinical observations have repeatedly demonstrated that regeneration in the spinal cord is abortive at best and never functional. However, as pathologists have known for many years, lesions in this location are never "clean," that is, they always produce extensive tissue necrosis resulting in cavitation and/or extensive scarring, both glial scarring and connective tissue scarring mainly proceeding from the leptomeninges. As emphasized by Kao and his collaborators (1977), even the most carefully conducted surgical procedure often results in extensive tissue necrosis separating the stumps of the transected spinal cord. The possibility could thus be considered that the absence of regeneration in long fiber tracts was not a matter of principle but mainly operational. After all, one would not expect regeneration in peripheral nerve nor in the skin under these conditions, that is, extensive tissue necrosis and scarring. With this in mind, many investigators, starting with Tello in 1911, have tried to devise procedures to bridge the gap and thus promote regeneration. For obvious reasons, in view of the vigorous regeneration occurring in PNS, the most popular approach was the introduction of peripheral nerve grafts in the brain and the spinal cord. It was repeatedly demonstrated that some of these grafts become well innervated and the origin of nerve fibers from CNS neurons has been convincingly demonstrated by the use of tracing methods more recently introduced in neuroanatomy (reviewed by Richardson et al. 1983).

In our laboratory we have studied some of the glial and axonal reactions occurring in these grafts, with particular regard to the brain–graft interface, i.e., the zone of entry of regenerating axons.

Peripheral nerve grafts were first implanted in the rat spinal cord (Chi et al. 1980). Some grafts became extremely well innervated. However, regenerated axons were strictly confined to the site of surgery, i.e., they never extended into nontraumatized tissues above and below the lesion. As a specific example the posterior columns undergoing ascending Wallerian degeneration in the proximal stump remained invariably devoid of axons.

Since it is difficult to avoid posterior root damage during spinal cord surgery in the rat, the experiments were repeated in the brain under conditions that did not allow invasion of peripheral nerve fibers (Chi and Dahl 1983). The results were identical to those previously reported in the spinal cord as to the innervation of the graft. Moreover, the brain–graft interface was more amenable to histological analysis allowing some observation as to glio-axonal interactions in this region. It appeared that the mesh of GFA-positive astrocytic fibers forming at the brain–graft interface did not constitute an insuperable barrier as to the penetration of axons inside the graft. However, axonal growth in this location was highly disorganized, with bundles of fibers criss-crossing in all directions, in marked contrast with the rectilinear and orderly course taken by the axons once they had reached the graft (Figure 8-1). It was only when the surgical

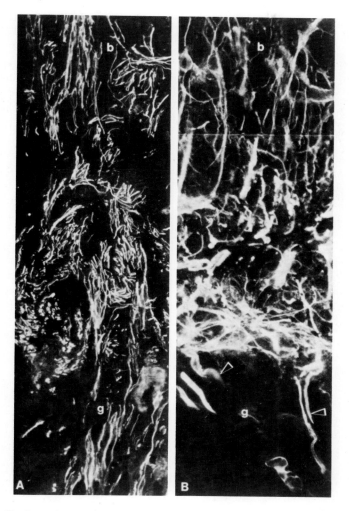

Figure 8-1. Brain graft with severe brain damage. (A) Immunofluorescence with neurofil-ament antisera. (B) Immunofluorescence with GFA protein antisera. (A) Axonal sprouts at the brain–graft interface took a tangled course so that direct continuity between brain (b) and graft (g) was difficult to demonstrate. (B) Astrocytes formed a thick mesh of randomly oriented fibers at the brain–graft interface. From this glial "capsule" longitu-dinally oriented astrocytic fibers extended into the graft (arrowheads). A, 240×; B, 480×. From Chi and Dahl (1983).

damage to the brain facing the graft was reduced to a minimum that a direct penetration from the brain into the graft could be observed and continuity thus easily demonstrated (Figure 8-2). Under these conditions the orientation of the glial fibers at the brain–graft interface was essentially the same as that of the axons (isomorphic gliosis).

In conclusion, the findings suggest that gliosis does not prevent axonal growth and that extensive elongation is the rule rather than the exception when regenerating fibers are able to penetrate into a peripheral nerve graft. However,

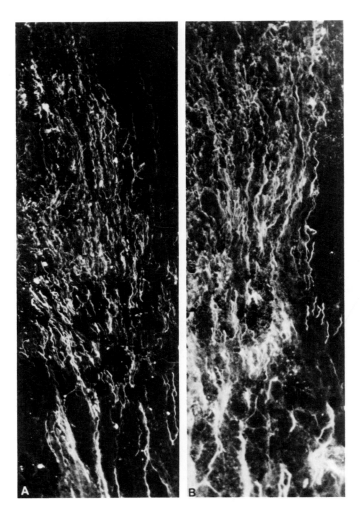

Figure 8-2. Brain–graft interface with minimal brain damage (Same orientation as in Figure 8-1). (A) Immunofluorescence with neurofilament antisera. (B) Immunofluorescence with GFA antisera. Axonal sprouts and glial fibers at the brain–graft interface followed a rectilinear course. Note absence of a glial "capsule" at the brain–graft interface. 240×. From Chi and Dahl (1983).

the growth ceases abruptly when the axons reach CNS tissue that is not traumatized by the surgical procedure. This is why peripheral nerve transplants
have not found clinical application. The axons growing in the graft are unable to
reach their target and thus reestablish functional connections.

Regenerating Dorsal Roots and the Nerve Entry Zone

Experiments conducted by Stensaas et al. (1979) and more extensively reported in a recent review (Reier et al. 1983) also point in the same direction,
i.e., regenerating axons are unable to grow in normal CNS. In these experiments the posterior roots of adult cats were injured and particular care was
taken to avoid damage to the spinal cord. Posterior roots, like peripheral
nerves, regenerate vigorously. However, in these experiments, they stopped
growing precisely at the root entry zone, that is, at the boundary between PNS
and CNS. It was thus suggested that "regenerating dorsal root axons are
blocked by spinal cord astrocytes" forming the glia limitans (Stensaas et al.
1979).

We recently confirmed these electron microscopic observations by immuno-
histology at the light microscopic level (Bignami et al. (1984b). As previously
shown in sciatic nerve undergoing Wallerian degeneration (Bignami et al.
1984a), reactive Schwann cells forming the bands of Büngner in crushed dorsal
roots stained intensely with laminin antisera (Figure 8-3). Within these bands
bundles of regenerating axons were present, as indicated by double labeling
with neurofilament antisera (Figure 8-4). With very few exceptions, regenerating axons were not observed in the laminin-negative intramedullary division of
the root (Figures 8-3 and 8-4).

In the following sections we will discuss experimental approaches that may
help to understand these apparently contradictory observations, i.e., (1) reinnervation of peripheral nerve grafts through reactive gliosis forming at the
brain–graft interface, and (2) the "blocking" effect of nonreactive astrocytes.

Laminin and Nerve Regeneration

Adhesive interactions play a key role in the initiation, elongation, and guidance
of axons. Among the several components of the extracellular matrix, particular
attention has been paid recently to laminin, a basal lamina glycoprotein (Timpl
et al. 1980). Laminin is a potent stimulator of neurite growth *in vitro* (Baron-
Van Evercooren et al. 1982, Manthorpe et al. 1983). Moreover, regenerating
axons in peripheral nerves grow on a substratum of intensely laminin-positive
Schwann cells (Figures 8-5 and 8-6). In normal nerve, laminin immunoreactivity is confined to endoneural basal laminae (Figure 8-7). It is thus conceivable
that astrocytes responding to trauma may provide an adhesive factor required
for axonal growth. Some recent observations by Liesi et al. (1983) are interest-

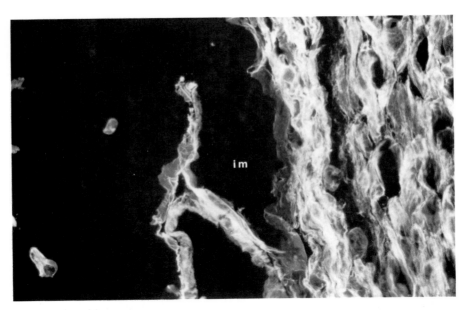

Figure 8-3. Longitudinal section of rat spinal cord 5 weeks after crushing of dorsal roots stained by immunofluorescence with laminin antisera. The laminin-negative domelike protrusion of spinal cord identifies the intramedullary division of the dorsal root (im). Note the intense laminin immunoreactivity of crushed dorsal roots (on the right of the figure). Within the spinal cord laminin immunoreactivity is confined to blood vessels. 272×.

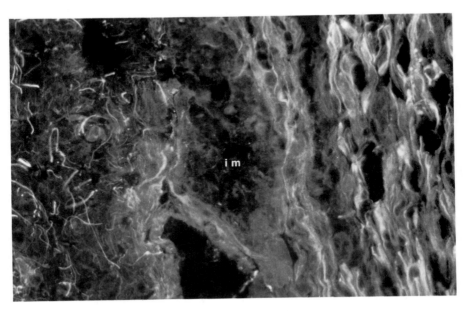

Figure 8-4. Same section as in Figure 8-3 double labeled with neurofilament antisera. The intramedullary division of the dorsal root (im) is empty of axons although bundles of regenerated fibers within laminin-positive cell bands of Büngner (Figure 8-3) are in close proximity (on the right of the figure). 272×.

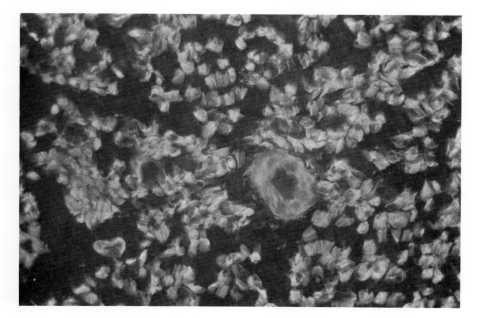

Figure 8-5. Distal stump of crushed rat sciatic nerve stained with laminin antisera 11 days after operation (transverse section). Note the intense laminin immunoreactivity of the cell bands of Büngner. To facilitate orientation in Figure 8-6, a field including a large blood vessel was chosen. 292×. From Bignami et al. J. Neuropathol. Exp. Neurol. 1984a.

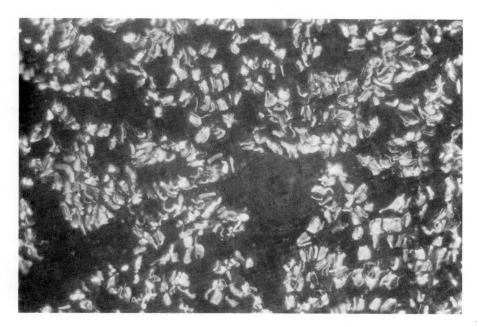

Figure 8-6. Same section as in Figure 8-5 double-labeled with neurofilament antisera. Compare with Figure 8-5 and note the close correspondence between laminin-positive cell bands of Büngner and bundles of regenerated axons. 292×. From Bignami et al. J. Neuropathol Exp. Neurol. 1984a.

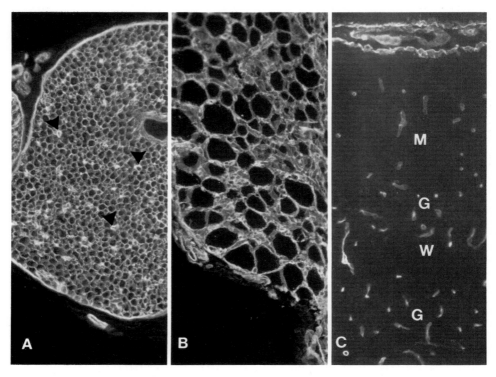

Figure 8-7. Normal pattern of laminin immunoreactivity in the peripheral nerve (A), posterior root ganglion (B), and brain (C) of the rat. (A) Transverse section of sciatic nerve. Laminin immunoreactivity is confined to perineurium, endoneurium, and small blood vessels (arrowheads). The connective tissue of the epineurium is not decorated (staining in this location is confined to blood vessels). (B) Posterior root ganglion. Sensory neurons are surrounded by a basal lamina. (C) Gyrus of cerebellum. Laminin immunoreactivity is confined to meninges and blood vessels. Note the different patterns of vascularization in the molecular layer (M), granular layer (G), and white matter (W). From Bignami et al. (1984c).

ing in this respect. It was found that newborn murine astrocytes in primary culture express laminin but lose this property as they mature *in vitro*. However, reactive astrocytes at the brain–graft interface were laminin-negative and the same was also true for reactive astrocytes in stabbed rat cerebral cortex (Bignami and Chi, unpublished observation).

The possibility still exists that other components of the extracellular matrix may serve as an adhesive substratum for axonal growth *in vivo*. Immature glia are laminin-negative in the rat embryo. Peripheral nerves identified with neuro-filament antisera were laminin-negative until late in development (Figures 8-8 and 8-9).

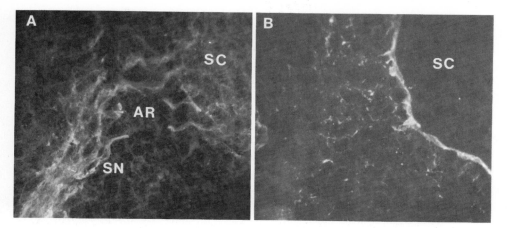

Figure 8-8. Double staining with neurofilament and laminin antisera in a 13-day rat embryo. (A) The antero-lateral region of the spinal cord (SC), the anterior roots (AR), and the spinal nerve (SN) are stained with neurofilament antisera (fluorescein optics). (B) The basal lamina surrounding the spinal cord (SC) is stained while anterior roots and spinal nerve are laminin-negative (rhodamine optics). The fine immunofluorescent dots in the region of the anterior roots were not within the nerve bundles when examined directly under the microscope. 260×. From Bignami et al. (1984c).

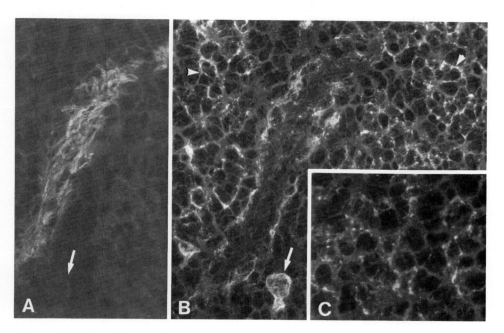

Figure 8-9. A small neurofilament positive intramuscular nerve trunk (A, fluorescein optic) is still laminin-negative in a 17-day embryo perineurium excepted (B, rhodamine optics). Arrows in A and B indicate the position of the same laminin-positive blood vessel. On day 17 several myotubes are surrounded by a basal lamina (arrowheads in B) while on day 16 laminin immunoreactivity in this location is in the form of dots (C). A and B, 292×; C, 467×. From Bignami et al. (1984c).

Hyaluronectin and the Vimentin-GFA Transition

The protein subunits forming intermediate filaments can be viewed as taxo-
nomic characters identifying the principal cells of the body, i.e., epithelia (kera-
tins), mesenchyma (vimentin), muscle (desmin), astroglia (GFA protein), and
neurons (neurofilament triplet proteins). There are, however, exceptions to this
general rule, such as the expression of vimentin by immature non-mesenchy-
mal cells, specifically CNS neuroglia and skeletal muscle, before the appearance of the specific intermediate filament proteins (Bennett et al. 1979, Bignami
et al. 1982, Schnitzer et al. 1981, Tapscott et al. 1981). Figure 8-10 illustrates
the remarkable vimentin-GFA transition occurring during glial differentiation
(Dahl 1981, Dahl et al. 1981, 1982, Yokoyama et al. 1981). The possibility was
thus considered that immature vimentin-positive neuroglia would display mesenchymal properties important for morphogenesis, such as the production of
an extracellular matrix playing a role in cell migration and neurite formation.

Hyaluronectin is the name given by B. Delpech to a glycoprotein that specifically binds hyaluronate, a mucopolysaccharide of the extracellular matrix
(Delpech 1982, Delpech and Halavent 1981). In normal adults, hyaluronectin is
essentially localized in the nervous system. Before the discovery of its hyaluronic acid-binding properties it was referred to as "nervous system-associ-
ated antigen 3" (Delpech et al. 1976). In adult rats, hyaluronectin was immuno-
histologically localized at the nodes of Ranvier of central and peripheral
myelinated fibers and around approximately 10% of rat cerebral neurons
(Delpech et al. 1982).

We recently studied the distribution of hyaluronectin immunoreactivity in
the rat embryo (Bignami and Delpech 1985). Our findings suggest that hyaluronectin is first distributed along radial glia and then accumulates in regions
of axonal growth and neuropil formation. On day 11–12 of gestation, when the

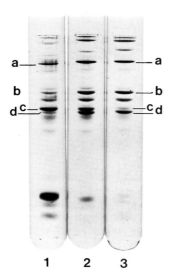

Figure 8-10. Progressive decrease of vimentin and
progressive increase of GFA protein during postnatal
development in cytoskeletal preparations of rat brain
resolved on SDS-PAGE. Identified bands: a, 150K
neurofilament polypeptide; b, 70K neurofilament polypeptide; c, vimentin; d, GFA protein. Gel 1, day 5; gel
2, day 12; gel 3, 3 weeks. From Dahl (1981).

wall of the telencephalic vesicle is formed by perpendicularly oriented bipolar cells, delicate immunofluorescent profiles spanning the entire thickness of the wall were observed with hyaluronectin antisera (Figure 8-11). The distribution of the immunoreactive material was similar to that observed with vimentin antisera. On day 13, concomitant with the formation of a primordial plexiform layer resulting from ingrowth of axonal bundles and from the development of neuronal processes, a marked accumulation of hyaluronectin immunoreactivity was observed in the external layer (Figure 8-12).

Fibrinolytic System

Another possibility to be considered is that the lack of CNS regeneration is the price we have to pay for a tight blood–brain barrier only temporarily and locally disrupted by trauma. This hypothesis would account for the abortive attempts at regeneration occurring at the site of injury and for the absence of regenera-

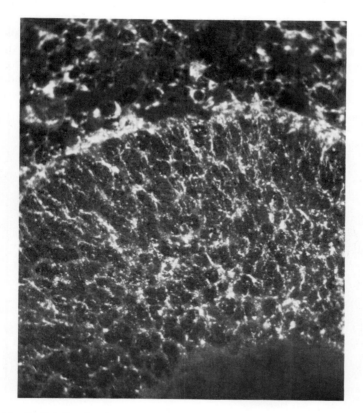

Figure 8-11. Radial distribution of hyaluronectin immunoreactivity in the neural tube of a 12-day rat embryo. Also note the presence of hyaluronectin in the surrounding mesenchyma. 480×

tion beyond the site of injury. Moreover, it would account for the only well-documented example of regeneration of a fiber tract within the mature CNS, i.e., the regeneration of hypothalamic-hypophysial tract, since the tuber cinereum and the neurohypophysis are two of the brain regions lacking a blood–brain barrier. If the problem is in the blood–brain barrier, the question may be asked as to which macromolecules in the blood circulation are required for axonal growth. Recently, we have been interested in the fibrinolytic system (Bignami et al. 1982), because apparently it plays an important role in cellular events involving cell migration and tissue remodeling in embryogenesis. Plasminogen is a 90K dalton plasma protein produced in the liver that is catalyzed to plasmin, the active fibronolytic enzyme, by tissue plasminogen activators (PA's). In accordance with other investigators (Krystosek and Seeds 1981, Moonen et al. 1982, Soreq and Miskin 1981), we found that compared to adult cerebellum, PA activity was markedly increased in neonatal murine cerebellum both at the time of granule cell division (first postnatal week) and at the time of granule cell migration (second postnatal week). Moreover, we found that PA activity was markedly increased in peripheral nerve undergoing Wallerian degeneration and this both in crushed nerves and in transected nerves that had been tightly ligated to prevent regeneration, thus suggesting that proliferating Schwann cells rather than growing axons were the sources of tissue PA's. Conversely, we could not demonstrate an increase of PA activity in a central tract (optic nerve) undergoing Wallerian degeneration, although admittedly

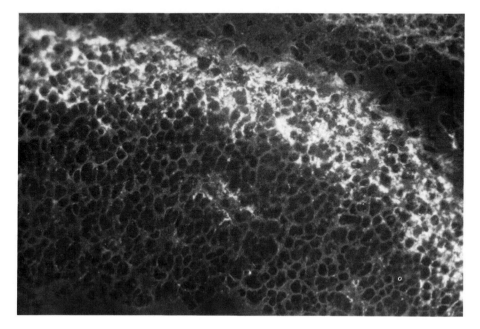

Figure 8-12. Accumulation of hyaluronectin immunoreactive material in the primordial plexiform layer of the cerebral cortex in a 14-day rat embryo. 268×.

with a rather insensitive method (Todd's fibrin slide technique). It would thus appear that if the fibrinolytic system is an essential requirement not only for embryonic development but also for adult tissue regeneration, at least two factors may be taken into account to explain the lack of regeneration in CNS tracts: (1) a blood–brain barrier to plasminogen, and (2) a deficient production of PA's by central glia in tracts undergoing Wallerian degeneration. Another finding pointing in the same direction is the sluggish proliferation of neuroglia in central tracts undergoing Wallerian degeneration (Bignami and Ralston 1969) as compared to the striking proliferation of Schwann cells in peripheral nerve under the same conditions. It was recently proposed that plasmin serves as a proliferation factor in developing spinal cords in culture (Kalderon 1982).

Acknowledgments. This research was supported by NIH Grant NS 13034 and by the Veterans Administration.

References

Baron-Van Evercooren, A., Kleinman, H.D. Ohno, S., Marangos, P., Schwartz, J.P., Dubois-Dalcq, M.E. (1982). Nerve growth factor, laminin and fibronectin in human fetal sensory ganglia cultures. J. Neurosci. Res. 8, 179–193.

Bennett, G.S., Fellini, S.A., Toyama, Y., Holtzer, H. (1979). Redistribution of intermediate filament subunits during skeletal myogenesis and maturation *in vitro*. J. Cell Biol. 82, 577–584.

Bignami, A., Cella, G., Chi, N.H. (1982). Plasminogen activators in rat neural tissues during development and in Wallerian degeneration. Acta Neuropathol. (Berlin) 58, 224–228.

Bignami, A., Chi, N.H. Dahl, D. (1984a). Laminin in rat sciatic nerve undergoing Wallerian degeneration. Immunofluorescence study with laminin and neurofilament antisera. J. Neuropath. Exp. Neurol. 43, 94–103.

Bignami, A., Chi, N.H., Dahl, D. (1984b). Regenerating dorsal roots and the nerve entry zone. Immunofluorescence study with neurofilament and laminin antisera. In preparation.

Bignami, A., Chi, N.H., Dahl, D. (1984c). Early expression of laminin in peripheral nerve, cerebral blood vessels and skeletal muscle. Int. J. Dev. Neurosci. 2, 367–376.

Bignami, A., Delpech, B. (1985). Extracellular matrix glycoprotein (hyaluronectin) in early cerebral development. Int. J. Dev. Neurosci. 3, 301–307.

Bignami, A., Raju, T.R., Dahl, D. (1982). Localization of vimentin, the nonspecific intermediate filament protein, in embryonal glia and in early differentiating neurons. Dev. Biol. 91, 286–295.

Bignami, A., Ralston, H.J. (1969). The cellular reaction of Wallerian degeneration in the central nervous system of the cat. Brain Res. 13, 444–461.

Chi, N.H., Bignami, A., Bich, N.T., Dahl, D. (1980). Autologous sciatic nerve grafts to the rat spinal cord: Immunofluorescence studies with neurofilament and gliofilament (GFA) antisera. Exp. Neurol. 68, 568–580.

Chi, N.H., Dahl, D. (1983). Autologous peripheral nerve grafting into murine brain as a model for studies of regeneration in the central nervous system. Exp. Neurol. 79, 245–264.

Dahl, D. (1981). The vimentin-GFA protein transition in rat neuroglia cytoskeleton occurs at the time of myelination. J. Neurosci. Res. 6, 741–748.

Dahl, D., Bignami, A. (1983). The glial fibrillary acidic protein and astrocytic 10-nanometer filaments. In: Handbook of Neurochemistry, 5. Lajtha, A. (ed.). New York: Plenum, pp. 127–151.

Dahl, D., Bignami, A. (1985). Intermediate filaments in nervous tissue. In: Cell and Muscle Motility Vol. 6. Shay, J.W. (ed.). New York: Plenum, pp. 75–96.

Dahl, D., Rueger, D.C., Bignami, A., Weber, K., Osborn, M. (1981). Vimentin, the 57,000 dalton protein of fibroblast filaments, is the major cytoskeletal component in immature glia. Eur. J. Cell Biol. 24, 191–196.

Dahl, D., Strocchi, P., Bignami, A. (1982). Vimentin in the central nervous system. A study of the mesenchymal-type intermediate filament-protein in Wallerian degeneration and in postnatal rat development by two-dimensional gel electrophoresis. Differentiation 22, 185–190.

Delpech, B. (1982). Immunochemical characterization of the hyaluronic acid-hyaluronectin interaction. J. Neurochem. 38, 978–983.

Delpech, A., Girard, N., Delpech, B. (1982). Localization of hyaluronectin in the nervous system. Brain Res. 245, 251–257.

Delpech, B., Halavent, C. (1981). Characterization and purification from human brain of a hyaluronic acid-binding glycoprotein, hyaluronectin. J. Neurochem. 36, 855–859.

Delpech, B., Vidard, M.N., Delpech, A. (1976). Caracterisation immunochimique et immunohistologique d'une glycoproteine associée au système nerveux. Immunochemistry 13, 111–116.

Kalderon, N. (1982). Role of the plasmin-generating system in the developing nervous tissue. I. Proteolysis as a mitogenic signal for the glial cells. J. Neurosci. Res. 8, 509–522.

Kao, C.C., Chang, L.W., Bloodworth, J.M.B., Jr. (1977). Axonal regeneration across transected mammalian spinal cord: An electron microscopic study of delayed microsurgical nerve grafting. Exp. Neurol. 54, 591–615.

Krystosek, A., Seeds, N.W. (1981). Plasminogen activator secretion by granule neurons of developing cerebellum. Proc. Natl. Acad. Sci. USA 78, 7810–7814.

Liesi, P., Dahl, D., Vaheri, A. (1983). Laminin is produced by early rat astrocytes in primary culture. J. Cell Biol. 96, 920–924.

Manthorpe, E., Engvall, E., Ruoslahti, F., Longo, F.M., Davis, G.E., Varon, S. (1983). Laminin promotes neuritic regeneration from cultured peripheral and central neurons. J. Cell Biol. 97, 1882–1890.

Moonen, G., Grau-Wagemans, M.P., Selak, I. (1982). Plasminogen activator-plasmin system and neuronal migration. Nature 298, 753–755.

Reier, P.J., Stensaas, L.J., Guth, L. (1983). The astrocytic scar as an impediment to regeneration in the central nervous system. In: Spinal Cord Reconstruction. Kao, C.C., Bunge, R.P., Reier, P.J. (eds.). New York: Raven Press, pp. 163–191.

Richardson, P.M., Aguayo, A.J., McGuinness, V.M. (1983). The role of sheath cells in axonal regeneration. In: Spinal Cord Reconstruction. Kao, C.C., Bunge, R.P., Reier, P.J. (eds.). New York: Raven Press, pp. 293–304.

Schnitzer, J., Franke. W.W., Schachner, M. (1981). Immunocytochemical demonstration of vimentin in astrocytes and ependymal cells of developing and adult mouse nervous system. J. Cell Biol. 90, 435–447.

Soreq, H., Miskin, R. (1981). Plasminogen activator in brain. Brain Res. 216, 361–374.

Stensaas, L.J., Brugess, P.R., Horch, K.W. (1979). Regenerating dorsal root axons are blocked by spinal cord astrocytes. Soc. Neurosci. Abst. 5, 684.

Tapscott, S.J., Bennett, G.S., Toyama, E., Kleinbart, E., Holtzer, H. (1981). Intermediate filament proteins in the developing chick spinal cord. Dev. Biol. 86, 40–54.

Tello, F. (1911). La influencia del neurotropismo en la regeneración de los centros nerviosos. Trab. Lab. Invest. Biol. Univ. Madrid 9, 123–128.

Timpl, R., Rohde, H., Risteli, L., Oh, V., Gehron-Robey, P., Martin, G.R. (1980). Laminin. Methods Enzymol. 82, 831–838.

Yokoyama, K., Mori, H., Kurokawa, M. (1981). Astroglial filament and fibroblast intermediate filament proteins in cytoskeletal preparations from spinal cord and optic nerve. FEBS Lett. 135, 25–30.

Chapter 9

The Role of Schwann Cells in the Repair of Glial Cell Deficits in the Spinal Cord

SHIRLEY A. GILMORE* and TERRY J. SIMS†

General Background

The occurrence of Schwann cells in the central nervous system (CNS) of humans has been recognized for many years. These Schwann cells and peripheral-type myelin have been reported by some to represent regenerative processes (Klintworth 1964, Druckman 1955) to be associated with destructive lesions within the CNS (Payan and Levine 1965, Hughes and Brownell 1963, Bernstein et al. 1973) and to occur in the absence of any known lesion (DeMyer 1965, Adelman and Aronson 1972, Sung et al. 1981). Compression of the spinal cord owing to abnormalities of the vertebral column such as intervertebral disc protrusion (Druckman and Mair 1953, Mair and Druckman 1953) or to tumor (Druckman and Mair 1953) is also associated with intraspinal Schwann cells. Finally, axons myelinated by Schwann cells are often present in plaques in multiple sclerosis (Feigin and Popoff 1966, Feigin and Ogata 1971, Ghatak et al. 1973, Itoyama et al. 1983, Ogata and Feigin, 1975). The papers cited here are more selective than exhaustive in order to point out that in the human being the presence of Schwann cells within the CNS is a rather nonspecific response, as suggested by Koeppen and colleagues (1968), and may represent a reaction to both mechanical and metabolic injury (Adelman and Aronson 1972).

The nonspecific nature of the circumstances under which Schwann cells occur in the human nervous system is paralleled, to an extent, in the research laboratory. With respect to destructive lesions and possible regenerative processes, Schwann cells and Schwann cell myelin occur in the CNS following transection of the dorsal funiculi (Lampert and Cressman 1964) or of the entire spinal cord (Matthews et al. 1979) and in cases of cyanide intoxication or

* Department of Anatomy, University of Arkansas for Medical Sciences, Little Rock, Arkansas 72205 U.S.A.
† Department of Neurology, Stanford University and the VA Medical Center, Palo Alto, California 94304 U.S.A.

implantation of triethyltin (Hirano et al. 1969). Compression of the spinal cord by tumor transplanted into the vertebral canal or restriction of its circumferential growth by ligature is also accompanied by intraspinal Schwann cells and peripheral-type myelin (Duncan 1955). Remyelination following injection of diphtheria toxin (Harrison et al. 1972), 6-aminonicotinamide (Blakemore 1975), lysolecithin (Blakemore 1976, 1978, or ethidium bromide (Yajima and Suzuki 1979, Blakemore 1982) is accomplished, at least in part, by Schwann cells. These cells are also responsible for remyelinating CNS axons in cases of chronic experimental allergic encephalomyelitis (Raine et al. 1978, Snyder et al. 1975, Wisniewski and Madrid 1983). Finally, as in the human being, Schwann cells occur in the CNS of normal laboratory animals with no known lesions (Bellhorn et al. 1979, Büssow 1978, Raine 1976, Wyse 1980, Wyse and Spira 1981). In spite of the differing experimental circumstances under which Schwann cells develop in the CNS of laboratory animals, at least two observations are common to these studies. First, the Schwann cells are not pervasive in the CNS and form only limited foci. Second, the animals used for the studies (except for the growth restriction studies of Duncan (1955) were mature, so that the Schwann cells remyelinated axons, i.e., they myelinated axons previously myelinated by oligodendrocytes.

There is one experimental situation in which the development of intraspinal Schwann cells (ISC) and associated peripheral-type myelin is rather extensive, is predictable, and is different from all other experimental models in that it is a primary myelination of CNS axons and not a remyelination. This experimental situation is the induction of ISC by ionizing radiation in the immature rat, originally described by Gilmore and Ducan in 1968. This induction is predictable and has been substantiated by later studies in this laboratory (Gilmore 1971, Gilmore et al. 1982, 1983, Heard and Gilmore 1980, Sims and Gilmore 1983) and by others (Beal and Hall 1974, Blakemore and Patterson 1975). The fact that this phenomenon is predictable with respect to incidence, location, and extent of ISC development has made it possible to examine the circumstances under which ISC will or will not develop. These data should be helpful in our understanding of the conditions that will be supportive in attempts to graft peripheral nerve or to transplant components of peripheral nerve (e.g., Schwann cell cultures) into the CNS.

Techniques

The technique for inducing ISC is a relatively simple one in that the immature rat, usually 3 days old, is exposed to a beam of soft x-rays. During the exposure period, the animal is restrained by taping it to a synthetic sponge with adhesive tape. A strip across the shoulder area and another across the hindlimbs is usually sufficient to immobilize a rat of the age studied (from birth to 5 days of age). The animal is then covered with a lead shield containing an aperture measuring 5×10 mm, and the shield is oriented so that the aperture allows exposure of a 5-mm length of spinal cord.

The radiation beam is generated by a Philips Contact Therapy Apparatus operating under the following conditions: 50 kV(p), 2 mA, filter added, 0.25 mm Al. The target-skin-distance (TSD) is 8 cm, and the radiation is delivered at a rate of 722 R per minute. The half value layer (HVL) is 0.16 mm Al, which makes this beam fall into the category of "soft" x-rays. Although a beam of "soft" x-rays has been used consistently in studies in Gilmore's laboratory, this type of beam is not necessary, and Beal and Hall (1974) and Blakemore and Patterson (1975) have successfully induced ISC by using much "harder," more penetrating x-rays.

The use of "soft" x-rays in this laboratory has been preferred because most of these x-rays are absorbed within the first few millimeters of tissue. Therefore, with the beam passing from dorsal to ventral, the x-rays are absorbed for the most part by the vertebral column and related axial musculature, with the underlying viscera being exposed to a much reduced amount of radiation. In our experience, it is rare to lose an animal following this procedure. On the other hand, Blakemore and Patterson (1975) reported the loss of approximately 35% of the irradiated animals before 14 days of age (11 days post-irradiation). This significant loss could be due to damage to other viscera exposed to the more penetrating x-ray beam and also to the fact that they irradiated a much larger area of the animal.

Most observations have been made at the light microscopic level on spinal cords from animals perfused with 10% formalin via the abdominal aorta. Usually the spinal cords are embedded in paraffin and are serially sectioned (8 μm). At least 16 sections taken from specific sequential areas of these serially sectioned ribbons are mounted on slides. The procedure for mounting of the sections is carried out so that adjacent sections occur on consecutive slides. In this manner, one section from a given area can be stained with a general stain such as hematoxylin and eosin, the section next to it occurring on the next slide can be stained with a myelin stain such as luxol fast blue, and the next section on yet a third slide can be stained to demonstrate axis cylinders, etc. In this way, it is possible to determine the status of many constituents within a given region of the spinal cord. Of the many stains used in these studies, one of the most informative is the luxol fast blue-periodic acid Schiff (PAS) stain (Klüver and Barrera 1953). With this stain, it is possible to differentiate central (oligodendrocyte) myelin from peripheral (Schwann cell) myelin at the light microscopic level as pointed out by Feigin and Cravioto (1961). This permits a rather rapid evaluation of many sections for the presence, absence, location, etc., of peripheral-type myelin under varying experimental circumstances. Subsequently, the techniques of electron microscopy and immunocytochemistry can be reserved for more in-depth, detailed observations.

Some of the recent light microscopic observations have been made on material embedded in JB-4 embedding medium (Polysciences, Inc., Warrington, PA). This embedment can be sectioned on a rotary microtome with a steel knife and has an advantage in that it provides excellent routine sections that are thinner than those in paraffin. One disadvantage is that it is not easy to obtain ribbons to provide for serial sections. In general, however, the overall quality of the tissue is superior to that processed for paraffin embedment.

For ultrastructural examination the animals are anesthetized with chloral hydrate and perfused through the heart with a fixative containing 2% glutaraldehyde and 2% paraformaldehyde in 0.12 M Sorensen's phosphate buffer at pH 7.2 to 7.4. The fixative is delivered at room temperature via an adjustable speed roller pump, and flow is monitored with a drip chamber in the delivery line. Following perfusion for at least 10 minutes, the carcasses are stored at 4°C for 2 hours, and the lumbosacral region of the spinal cord is subsequently removed. The removed cord is cut into 2-mm segments and immersed in fixative overnight at 4°C. The following day the spinal segments are post-fixed in 2% OsO_4 in buffer for 2 hours at 4°C. These segments are then stained en block with uranyl acetate, dehydrated, infiltrated with Spurr plastic, and embedded in flat molds. Thick sections (1 μm) cut from hardened blocks are stained with toluidine blue. Thin sections are then cut, post-stained with uranyl acetate and lead citrate, and examined and photographed on a Siemens 101 electron microscope.

Light and Electron Microscopic Characteristics of ISC and Associated Peripheral-Type Myelin

One of the most prominent and characteristic features of the ISC-occupied areas in a section stained with a general cellular stain (hematoxylin and eosin, gallocyanin, toluidine blue, etc.) is the hypercellularity of these areas (Figure 9-1). The cell density is obviously much higher than in comparable areas of white or gray matter in the normal nervous system. Little cytoplasm is evident at the light microscopic level, and the nuclei appear to be either rounded or elongated, depending upon the plane of sectioning. Upon application of the luxol fast blue-PAS stain one finds that the myelin in these hypercellular areas is stained a darker, purplish-blue color in comparison with the more distinctly green color of normal CNS (oligodendrocyte) myelin (Figure 9-2). The coloration of the myelin in the ISC-occupied areas is the same as that in the nerve roots lying adjacent to the spinal cord in the same section, thus eliminating any question about the color differences being artifacts arising from the staining procedure per se. The designation of this intraspinal myelin as being that of the peripheral nervous system type is supported further by the recent use of an immunocytochemical technique to detect the presence of P_o protein, a major protein of myelin in peripheral nerve (Trapp et al. 1981). When the P_o protein antiserum is applied to sections of spinal cord containing Schwann cells, as identified on the basis of other staining characteristics, only the ISC-occupied areas and the adjacent spinal nerve roots are stained; myelin elsewhere in the spinal cord remains unstained. These same areas contain fine, argyrophilic fibers that are demonstrable by the Wilder stain for connective tissue fibers of the reticular type (Figure 9-3). Again, this is characteristic of peripheral nerve and not of the normal CNS.

Ultrastructurally, the majority of cells in these hypercellular areas contain irregular or ovoid nuclei. The cytoplasm is dense and contains numerous free ribosomes. Each cell is surrounded by a basal lamina (Figure 9-4). The sheaths

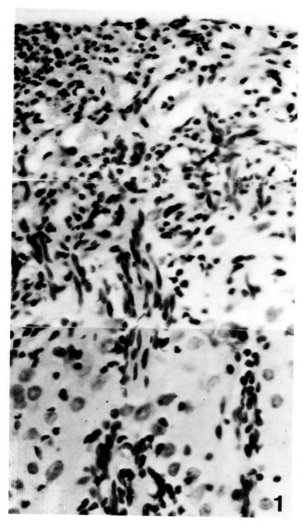

Figure 9-1. Montage showing area of ISC extending from the dorsal surface of the spinal cord through the dorsolateral portion of the dorsal funiculus and into the gray matter in an animal killed 45 days P-I (4000 R). Note the hypercellularity of the ISC-occupied area, in contrast to the normally less cellular area composed of CNS constituents. Note that the cells in the ISC-occupied area are darkly stained and that the nuclei appear to be either rounded or elongated, depending upon orientation within the section. Although this animal was injected with [³H]thymidine 1 hour prior to autopsy, cells in the ISC-occupied area are not labeled at this late post-irradiation interval. Hematoxylin and eosin stained autoradiograph. 428×.

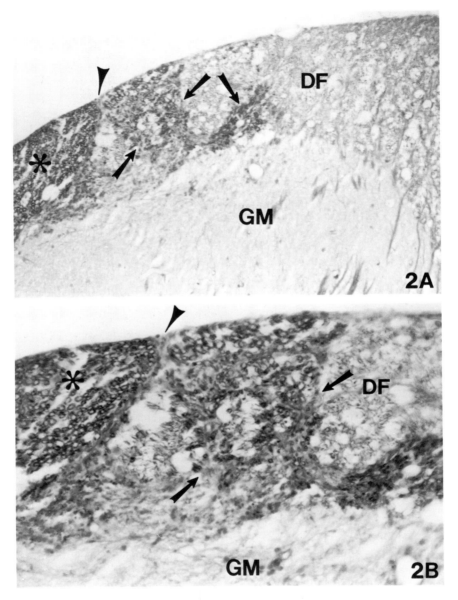

Figure 9-2. Luxol fast blue-PAS stained section photographed with two different objectives: A, 171×; B, 295×. This section was taken from an animal irradiated (2500 R) in the lumbosacral region and killed 60 days later. The dorsal root is indicated by the asterisk (*), and the boundary between the root and the spinal cord is indicated by the arrowhead. The myelin within the dorsal funiculus (DF) and extending into the dorsal gray matter (GM) is stained two different colors, which appear as two different intensities on these photographs. The darker staining myelin in the ISC-occupied regions of the spinal cord (arrows) resembles that in the dorsal root. The oligodendrocyte myelin in the remainder of the dorsal funiculus does not stain as darkly.

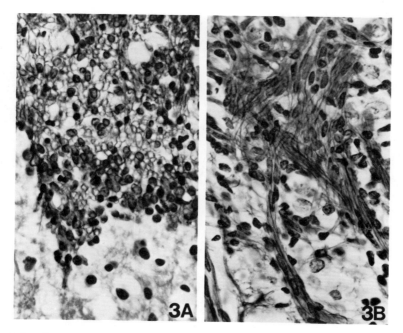

Figure 9-3. Photographs taken in two different regions of a well-developed area of ISC within the same spinal cord section stained with Wilder's reticular stain to demonstrate connective tissue fibers. This section was taken from a rat irradiated with 4000 R (lumbosacral area) and killed 60 days later. (A) The upper two-thirds of the photograph shows the hypercellular ISC-occupied region in which the argyrophilic connective tissue fibers are oriented such that they form a honeycomb arrangement, as one would see in a cross section of a peripheral nerve. (B) The fine, argyrophilic connective tissue fibers are oriented longitudinally along the long axis of the cells in the hypercellular ISC-occupied areas. Note the absence of these fibers from the lower portions of both illustrations occupied by normal CNS constituents. 485×.

of compact myelin are characteristic of those of peripheral nerve, with the periodicities of this intraspinal Schwann cell myelin being different from those of normal central myelin (Gilmore and Duncan 1968). Nodes of Ranvier with Schwann cell myelin on one side and oligodendrocyte myelin on the other are present within the depths of the spinal cord (Gilmore and Duncan 1968). Extracellular space is abundant in the ISC-occupied areas (Figure 9-4) in comparison with a similar area in control animals (Gilmore et al. 1982). Fibroblasts have not been observed in any of the material, in spite of the connective tissue fibers observed at the light microscopic level (Figure 9–3) and of the observation of a few collagen fibrils at the ultrastructural level (Figure 9-4; also Sims and Gilmore 1983). The presence of these connective tissue elements in the absence of fibroblasts is not totally unexpected, however, because of the observations that Schwann cells are capable of producing small-diameter (18 nm) collagenous fibrils, as well as basal lamina, *in vitro* in the presence of neurons (Bunge et al. 1980).

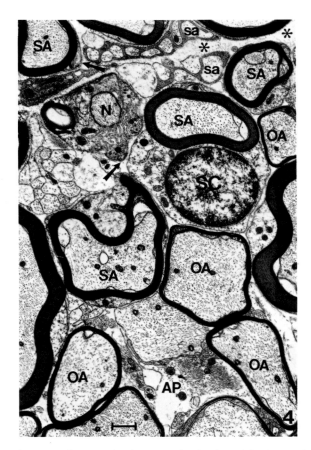

Figure 9-4. An electron micrograph of an area in the dorsal funiculus from a rat killed
90 days P-I. This figure represents a transition zone between Schwann cell-myelinated
axons and oligodendrocyte-myelinated axons deep within the funiculus. The Schwann
cells (SC) myelinate large axons (SA) and ensheath some of the smaller axons (sa).
Schwann cells and their processes are surrounded by a basal lamina (arrows). Intermingled with the peripheral-type myelinated axons are oligodendrocyte-myelinated axons
(OA). An astrocyte process (AP) is present; however, these processes are far less
numerous than in controls. The plane of section in this figure passes through the node of
a Schwann cell-myelineated axon (N). Collagenous fibrils are present in extracellular
spaces (*) and may be responsible for the connective tissue staining observed at the light
microscopic level (Figure 9-3; see text also). Bar = 1 μm.

Patterns of and Experimental Conditions Related to the Development of Intraspinal Schwann Cells

The original observations of radiation-induced ISC were made in animals irradiated when 3 days of age and killed 9 to 60 days post-irradiation (P-I) (Gilmore
and Duncan 1968). These animals received a single, total dose of 4000 R to a

5-mm length of the lumbosacral spinal cord. The hypercellular, ISC-occupied areas were present in the dorsum of the spinal cord, in both white and gray matter, and in some sections occupied almost the dorsal half of the cord. The elongated nuclei of these cells were often arranged in parallel with the bundles of axons that pass from the dorsal funiculi into the dorsal gray matter. These ISC-occupied areas occurred in all animals killed at 19 or more days P-I. In these rats, there was a predilection for these cell aggregates to occur in the caudal portion of the 5 mm long irradiated area and to be absent from the rostral portion.

Subsequently, Beal and Hall (1974) and Blakemore and Patterson (1975) carried out similar studies using the immature rat, 3 days of age. The actual irradiation procedure differed markedly from that of Gilmore and Duncan (1968) in that (1) a beam of "harder" x-rays was used, (2) different amounts of x-rays were delivered to the irradiated sites, and (3) larger areas of the animals were exposed to the x-ray beam. Beal and Hall (1974) used an exposure of 2000 R, and Blakemore and Patterson (1975) used a minimal dose of 2000 rad. The possible maximal dose was not reported by the latter investigators. In the study by Beal and Hall (1974), the animals were shielded so that the entire spinal cord from the mid-thoracic region caudally was exposed, whereas that portion caudal to the T_{12}/L_1 vertebral junction was exposed in the investigation by Blakemore and Patterson (1975). Areas occupied by ISC and resembling those described by Gilmore and Duncan (1968) were observed by both Beal and Hall (1974) and Blakemore and Patterson (1975). The ISC were concentrated in the dorsal portion of the irradiated area in the latter studies, as in the original one from this laboratory, in spite of the differences in the irradiation procedure. An interesting observation also common to all three studies was that irrespective of the length of spinal cord irradiated, the ISC development was most pronounced in the caudal portion of the irradiated area and was virtually absent from the most rostral regions. This observation was consistent, although Beal and Hall (1974) irradiated a portion of the thoracic spinal cord as well as the entire lumbosacral spinal cord, Blakemore and Patterson (1975) irradiated the entire lumbosacral spinal cord, and Gilmore and Duncan (1968) irradiated only a 5-mm length of lumbosacral spinal cord, leaving normal, unexposed areas both rostrally and caudally. These results then raised the question of whether or not there may be regional differences in the development of ISC.

Subsequently a study was undertaken in this laboratory (Heard and Gilmore 1980) in which two short (5 mm in length) but separate lengths of spinal cord, one in the mid-thoracic region and one in the lumbosacral region, were irradiated. The amount of radiation administered was 4000 R, as in the original study. This study included experimental groups of animals in which the mid-thoracic area alone or the lumbosacral area alone was irradiated. In a third group, both areas were irradiated leaving an unexposed intermediate area. Included in the objectives were: (1) a determination of whether ISC occurred predominantly at the caudal portion of the irradiated regions or if the ISC were distributed evenly throughout the irradiated region, and (2) an evaluation of whether or not the development of ISC was markedly different in the two areas. The results showed that ISC were absent from the most rostral portions of the irradiated areas in both the mid-thoracic region and the lumbosacral region. This pattern was present in all three irradiated groups. In addition, ISC development was much less extensive in the mid-thoracic region, where these cells and their associated peripheral-type myelin were limited to small, intermittent foci located near the dorsal root entry zone. In the lumbosacral region, on the other hand, the ISC formed a continuum rostrocaudally. The extent of development increased rostrocaudally, with these cells extending into the gray matter in the caudal portion of the irradiated areas. In general, the results indicated that the pattern of ISC development was quite different in the two regions of spinal cord studied (mid-thoracic versus lumbosacral) even though these two regions were separated by only a 5-mm length of spinal cord. Studies of these two regions in the normal 3-day-old are in progress in order to determine what, if any, differences in the developmental status of the animal at the time of irradiation may influence the subsequent development of ISC. The differences in the extent of ISC development between the mid-thoracic and the lumbosacral areas point out again the necessity of comparing similar regions of the spinal cord when studying immature animals, rather than considering one region of spinal cord as being representative of the spinal cord as a whole.

In view of the regional differences in ISC development reported by Heard and Gilmore (1980), a series of investigations, some of which are ongoing, were planned in order to elucidate factors related to the development of ISC. One of these studies examined the relationship between the amount of radiation administered and the pattern of ISC development in the lumbosacral spinal cord. Since the previous studies (Gilmore and Duncan 1968, Heard and Gilmore 1980) delineated the pattern of ISC development in the lumbosacral spinal cord following exposure to 4000 R at 3 days of age, this investigation examined ISC development after exposure to smaller amounts of radiation. Four groups of animals were used, and they were exposed to doses of 1000 R, 2000 R, 2500 R, or 3000 R when 3 days of age. The results showed in general that ISC development was less extensive with decreasing doses of radiation. Exposure to 1000 R resulted in a pattern of ISC development in the lumbosacral region that was very similar to that reported by Heard and Gilmore (1980) in the irradiated mid-thoracic region, i.e., ISC were restricted to small, intermittent foci adjacent to the dorsal root entry zone. Following exposure to 2000 R, ISC development was limited to the dorsal funiculi, whereas after exposure to 2500 R or 3000 R, ISC extended also in the dorsal gray matter. Although ISC developed in the gray matter in the two latter groups, the development was never as extensive as following exposure to 4000 R. An interesting and yet unexplained observation is that although the pattern of ISC development was the same in animals receiving 1000 R to the lumbosacral region and 4000 R to the mid-thoracic region, the incidence was quite different. Exposure of the mid-thoracic region to 4000 R resulted in the presence of ISC in all animals killed later than 2 weeks P-I (Heard and Gilmore 1980), whereas exposure of the lumbosacral region to 1000 R resulted in an incidence of only 33% (Gilmore et al. 1983). In the latter study an incidence of 86% or more was found in all other groups exposed to 2000 R or more.

Other ongoing studies of factors influencing the incidence and extent of ISC development have considered the factor of age. Since ISC development was so limited in the mid-thoracic area in animals exposed to 4000 R when 3 days of age (Heard and Gilmore 1980), would this development be more extensive in the mid-thoracic area if the animals were irradiated under the same conditions but at a younger age? The studies are incomplete, but the preliminary data indicate that the pattern of ISC development in the mid-thoracic region in animals irradiated at 1 and 2 days of age is similar to animals irradiated when 3 days of age (Heard and Gilmore 1980). All animals irradiated when 1 or 2 days old and examined to date showed ISC development limited to the dorsolateral portions of the dorsal funiculi, near the dorsal root entry zone. In no case has ISC developed more extensively, as following exposure of the lumbosacral region. Conversely, would the development be less extensive in the lumbosacral region if the animals were irradiated at later ages? To date, animals up to 5 days of age have been exposed to 4000 R, and the results show essentially the same pattern of ISC development as at 3 days of age. Further studies of older, larger animals have not been undertaken to date because of the need to consider certain technical problems. First, as the animal ages, it not only increases in size, but the vertebral arches overlying the spinal cord ossify and calcify. These factors of size and vertebral maturation would result in a decrease in the amount of x-rays reaching the spinal cord. In order to overcome this, a different x-ray source will have to be used. Second, as the animals mature, they cannot be restrained solely by taping them to the sponge, and the use of anesthetics may have to be employed. The latter are known to modify the effects of radiation and, thus, would introduce another variable into the study. Examination of the results, including the illustrations, from studies of adult animals in which the spinal cords were irradiated (Bradley et al. 1977, Innes and Carsten 1961, Kogel and Barendsen 1974, Kogel 1977, Mastaglia et al. 1976) reveals that although radiation-induced demyelination (as well as other degenerative changes) occurs, there is no evidence for the development of ISC in the mature rat. Therefore, the determination of the latest age at which ISC can be induced following exposure of ionizing radiation again could lead to a better understanding of the factors that hinder or facilitate the development of ISC.

The development of ISC in the dorsum of the spinal cord suggests that the dorsal roots may be the source of the ISC. This is supported (1) by the earliest observations of the ISC near the dorsal root entry zone and in the dorsolateral portions of the dorsal funiculi in animals receiving 4000 R to the lumbosacral area (Beal and Hall 1974, Gilmore and Duncan 1968, Heard and Gilmore 1980) and (2) by the restriction of the small foci of ISC to these same areas in animals receiving 1000 R to the lumbosacral area (Gilmore et al. 1983) or 4000 R to the mid-thoracic area (Heard and Gilmore 1980). In a few instances, areas of ISC, totally separated from those in the dorsum of the spinal cord, have been observed in the ventral regions of the irradiated lumbosacral spinal cord exposed to 4000 R (Figure 9-5). In these instances, it is rare to find the ISC in the ventral funiculus, particularly in the ventral root-spinal cord junctional zone as illustrated in Figure 9-3 in the original paper by Gilmore and Duncan (1968). More

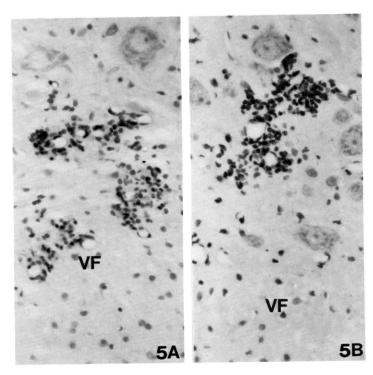

Figure 9-5. Portions of ventral gray matter and adjacent ventral funiculus (VF) from an animal irradiated with 4000 R (lumbosacral area and injected with [³H]thymidine 1 hour prior to sacrifice at 60 days P-I. (A) Small foci of ISC in gray matter and adjacent white matter in this section stained with gallocyanin-PAS. (B) Small area of ISC restricted to the gray matter. This autoradiograph stained with hematoxylin and eosin revealed no labeling of cells in the ISC-occupied areas at this time. Note in both sections that the ISC appear in part to be associated with blood vessels and that these ISC-occupied areas do not extend superficially to the spinal cord-ventral root transition zone. 248×.

commonly the ventral foci are limited to the ventral gray matter or to the junction of the ventral gray and ventral white matter, as shown in Figure 9-5. The conclusion that the areas of ISC in Figure 9-5 are not continuous (1) with the spinal cord-ventral root transition zone or (2) with ISC in the dorsum of the spinal cord is based on the fact that our observations are made on multiple serial sections as described in *Techniques* above. The ventrally located areas of ISC were noted in only a few instances in the earlier studies. However, such areas have been observed more frequently in recent studies in this laboratory. Since the region of spinal cord irradiated (lumbosacral), the amount of radiation (4000 R), and the conditions for the administration of the x-rays have been kept constant, some other factor then must account for the increased frequency of the ventrally located areas of ISC in more recent observations. After examination of all aspects of these studies, it became obvious that the ventrally located areas of ISC occurred in animals autopsied at intervals longer than 30 days P-I.

To date, 60 irradiated animals included in several studies have been evaluated, and ventrally located ISC were present in 8 of 19 rats killed at 30 or more days P-I and in only 1 of 41 animals killed prior to that time. Studies of additional animals autopsied through 60 days P-I are ongoing.

The consistent and predictable development of ISC in the dorsal funiculi (discussed above) supports the assumption that the Schwann cells in dorsal roots may be a source of the ISC. However, another observation not included in previous publications raises the need to consider an alternate source(s). This observation is the occasional association of foci of ISC with blood vessels, and the failure of examination of adjacent sections to demonstrate that these are in continuity with foci of ISC extending either to the spinal cord surface or to the root-cord transition zone. Figure 9-6 shows two of these foci, which are quite small and, consequently, could easily remain undetected on cursory examination. Both of these foci are well isolated from other areas of ISC. The isolation of these vessel-associated areas of ISC is especially pronounced in animals receiving the smaller amounts of x-rays and in which ISC development is not extensive (Gilmore et al. 1983). In such cases small areas of ISC were found underlying the dorsal median spinal vein. Further association of ISC and blood

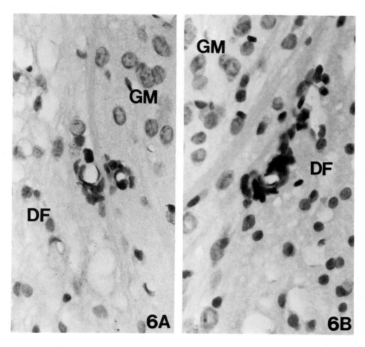

Figure 9-6. Both of these photographs show tiny aggregates of ISC in association with blood vessels and well separated from any other foci of ISC. In both, the blood vessels are located near the interface between the lateral border of the dorsal funiculus (DF) and the adjacent gray matter (GM). (A) From an animal killed 30 days P-I (4000 R, lumbosacral area). (B) From a rat killed 45 days P-I (4000 R, lumbosacral area). 456×.

vessels can be noted in the cases where ISC develop in the ventral aspect of the spinal cord (Figure 9-5). Schwann cells within the CNS have been considered to arise from a number of sources, including nerve roots (Raine et al. 1982), migration along blood vessels (Hirano et al. 1969, Raine et al. 1978, Snyder et al. 1975), multipotential cells of the mesenchymal type within the CNS (Feigin and Ogata 1971, Feigin and Popoff 1966), or division of the few Schwann cells normally found within the CNS (Itoyama et al. 1983), but the data and techniques to date do not provide direct evidence for any of these. An additional observation at the ultrastructural level in our laboratory is that many capillaries in the ISC-occupied regions lacked the complete astrocyte covering normally occurring in control animals (Sims and Gilmore 1983). Whether the same situation occurs on the isolated blood vessel surrounded by a few ISC, as shown in Figure 9-6, remains to be determined.

Proliferative Capacities of Intraspinal Schwann Cells (ISC) and Characteristics of Intraspinal Schwann Cell Myelin

In the original study by Gilmore and Duncan (1968), it was observed that the ISC were present initially in the dorsolateral portion of the white matter near the dorsal root entry zone. Subsequently, as the post-irradiation interval increased, these cells spread deeper into the spinal cord, occupying both dorsal gray and dorsal white matter. In view of this pattern of occurrence of ISC, a question arose as to (1) whether these cells arose in the dorsal roots and migrated into the spinal cord or (2) whether these cells, irrespective of their origin(s), were capable of dividing within the intraspinal environment. The answer to this question was sought by designing a light microscopic autoradiographic study to evaluate the pattern of [³H]thymidine uptake by these cells during the early stages of their development, i.e., through 3 weeks P-I (Gilmore 1971). Litters of 3-day-old rats were irradiated (4000 R) in the lumbosacral region. At 7, 11, and 15 days P-I, the rats received a single injection of [³H]thymidine. These groups were then subdivided to be autopsied at intervals from 4 hours to 7 days following injection of the isotope. The results showed that the ISC were capable of incorporating [³H]thymidine and that the ISC were heavily labeled in animals killed at the shortest post-injection intervals. If, however, the interval between injection and autopsy was increased to 3 or 7 days, the cells were only lightly labeled, indicating that cell division(s) occurred. Thus, these data clearly demonstrated that Schwann cells were capable of undergoing division within the spinal cord, an environment normally foreign to them.

Although the study just described (Gilmore 1971) demonstrated that the ISC are highly proliferative during the first few weeks following irradiation, other data indicated that a factor or factors within the spinal cord caused this proliferation to cease. This assumption is based on the observation in the studies by Gilmore and Duncan (1968) and Heard and Gilmore (1980) that the ISC occupy only specific regions within the irradiated area. Subsequently, a study was undertaken (1) to examine the pattern of labeling of ISC at intervals up to 2 months P-I by light microscopic autoradiography and (2) to correlate these findings, if possible, with a parallel ultrastructural study (Gilmore et al. 1982). All animals received 4000 R to a 5-mm length of lumbosacral spinal cord. The majority of these rats were used for light microscopic autoradiography and were perfused-fixed 1 hour following [³H]thymidine injection at intervals ranging from 15 to 90 days P-I. The remainder of the animals were prepared for electron microscopy. The ISC in animals in this study, as well as in other earlier studies from this laboratory, were confined to the dorsolateral portions of the dorsal funiculi at 15 and 20 days P-I and were heavily labeled. As the areas of ISC increased in size, i.e., as they extended ventrally into the spinal cord substance, it appeared that the majority of labeled cells occurred in the depths of the ISC, at its interface with the CNS constituents. This was particularly evident at 25 days P-I, when labeled cells were abundant at this interface but were much decreased in numbers dorsally where heavily labeled cells had been prominent earlier. Correlated with this finding was the observation that the peripheral-type (Schwann) myelin was more mature near the dorsal surface of the spinal cord than in the depths of the ISC-occupied regions where cell proliferation was still quite active. Dorsally, near the surface, myelin sheaths were compact and varied in thickness with the caliber of the axon, whereas in the depths of the ISC-occupied areas the state of myelination was less mature, characterized by loose spiralling of the mesaxon and the lack of major dense lines. By 30 and 45 days P-I, labeled cells were rare in the dorsal, superficial portions of the ISC-occupied regions. Only a few cells were labeled more deeply in the 30-day P-I group, and such cells were virtually absent from the 45-day P-I animals (Figure 9-1). A dorsal-ventral gradient in maturity of the myelin sheaths was still evident, however. By 60 and 90 days P-I, labeled cells were extremely rare in the ISC-occupied regions and mature, compact myelin was present throughout. These findings indicated that the mitogenic stimulus for the Schwann cells had essentially disappeared by 30 days P-I, thereby accounting for the restriction of ISC to certain areas within the irradiated length of spinal cord. Further aspects of the proliferative activities of ISC will be discussed in the next section.

Interrelationships and Interactions between Intraspinal Schwann Cells and Neuroglia

The observations made in the studies by Gilmore and associates suggest that the development of Schwann cells in the spinal cord and their subsequent involvement in myelination of intraspinal axons is related to the effects of radiation on the neuroglial population. In a light microscopic study in 1963, Gilmore demonstrated that exposure of the rat lumbosacral spinal cord to x-rays (4000 R or more) at 3 days of age resulted in a marked loss of neuroglia throughout the irradiated area as early as 2 days P-I (Gilmore 1963). As the animal aged, and particularly as it reached the second postnatal week, this loss of neuroglia was further evidenced by the fact that the irradiated white matter in all funiculi was hypomyelinated or even amyelinated. On the other hand, in the nonirradiated portion of spinal cord in the same animal or in appropriate control animals of this age, myelin was clearly evident in all funiculi by light microscopic techniques. Therefore, it was concluded that exposure of the spinal cord to this amount of x-rays at 3 days of age destroyed the neuroglia present in the white matter (as well as some in the gray matter), and perhaps some of their precursors, and consequently the pattern of myelinogenesis was altered. In the normal 3-day-old spinal cord very few axons are myelinated (Figures 9-7 and 9-8); therefore, the subsequent myelination of these axons by Schwann cells in the irradiated animal is a primary myelination and not a remyelination.

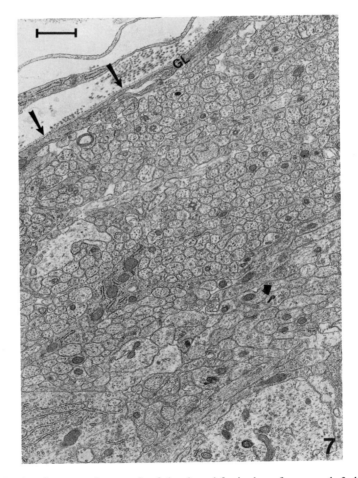

Figure 9-7. An electron micrograph of the dorsal funiculus of a normal, 3-day-old rat. The axons are generally of small diameter and are rarely myelinated at this time. A thin glia limitans (GL) is present at the surface of the spinal cord and is covered, in turn, by a basal lamina (arrows). Bar = 1 μm.

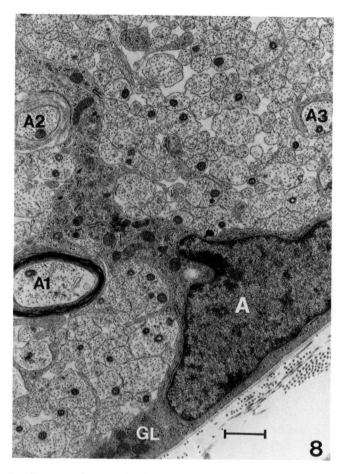

Figure 9-8. An electron micrograph of the ventral funiculus of a normal, 3-day-old rat. Most axons are unmyelinated at this age, but an occasional axon with compact myelin (A1) can be observed. Other axons (A2 and A3) appear to be in the early stages of myelination and are surrounded by spirals of oligodendrocyte cytoplasm. Sub-pial astrocytes (A) are seen more frequently than in the dorsal funiculus, and the glia limitans (GL) is generally thicker than its dorsal counterpart. Bar = 1 μm.

During the second post-irradiation week, when Schwann cells are first noted in the spinal cord, the oligodendrocyte population is markedly depleted, and the axons lack oligodendroglial myelin. Wood and Bunge (1975) have shown in tissue culture that sensory axons of the dorsal root ganglia have a mitogenic effect on Schwann cells, and a subsequent study (Salzer et al. 1980) demonstrated that this mitogenic stimulus is located on the neurite surface. Therefore, it is possible that the radiation-induced ISC that are in contact with the unensheathed central neurites receive their proliferative stimuli from these structures. Later, by approximately 1 month post-irradiation, when the neuroglial population is recovering and participating in its normal functions, the naked neurites become ensheathed by Schwann cells, by oligodendrocytes, or by astrocytes (to be discussed below), and the ISC cease proliferation. The ability of the oligodendrocytes to myelinate the intraspinal axons after a radiation-induced delay is evidenced by the presence of oligodendrocyte-myelinated axons adjacent to Schwann cell-myelinated axons and by the existence in the depths of the spinal cord of nodes of Ranvier at which the two types of myelin are apposed (Gilmore and Duncan 1968, Gilmore et al. 1982, Sims and Gilmore 1983). Areas in which axons myelinated by Schwann cells were intermixed with axons myelinated by oligodendrocytes were described also by Blakemore and Patterson (1975). Although the neuroglial population shows some degree of recovery in the dorsal funiculi, there is no evidence that this population ultimately attains primacy over the ISC, i.e., the ISC-myelinated areas are not eventually replaced by normal spinal cord constituents. This statement is based on the observation that areas of ISC persist for periods of 2 or more years following irradiation (Gilmore 1973).

The interactions of Schwann cells and oligodendrocytes at later post-irradiation intervals (60 and 90 days) suggest that the irradiated spinal cord of the immature rat may serve as an interesting model for studying the signals for myelination. As pointed out above, Schwann cell myelin, once established, becomes a stable component of the irradiated spinal cord. On the other hand, axons of small diameter that were initially ensheathed by ISC subsequently become myelinated by oligodendrocytes. These unpublished observations were made recently in spinal cords from rats killed at 60 and 90 days P-I in which an increased number of small (1 to 3 μm in diameter) axons myelinated by oligodendrocytes were found in ISC-occupied regions. In these situations, small axons located in the center of ISC-ensheathed axons profiles were observed to be in various stages of myelination by oligodendrocytes. One possible interpretation of these findings is that ISC, like their counterparts in the peripheral nervous system, do not myelinate axons less than 1.5 μm in diameter (Berthold 1978), whereas oligodendrocytes myelinate spinal cord axons as small as 0.2 μm in diameter (Chung and Coggeshall 1983). This implies that while some small-caliber axons possess a trophic signal to initiate myelination, the Schwann cell requires either a higher threshold signal (e.g., axons of larger diameter) or a different signal from that required by oligodendrocytes. Further aspects of this problem are under investigation.

The spinal cord of the rat irradiated prior to normal myelination of its axons by oligodendrocytes is proving to be an interesting model for studies that may be useful in understanding normal developmental events. It has already been established that irradiation at 3 days of age results in a rapid and marked loss of neuroglia in all funiculi (Beal and Hall 1974, Gilmore 1963, Rodgers 1965). In the ventral funiculus, the glial population is undergoing reconstitution at 25 days P-I, but ISC are not present at this time (see above). Ultrastructural examination of this region reveals foci in which axons possess myelin sheaths that are reduced in thickness in comparison with sheaths on similar-sized axons in adjacent regions of the same funiculus (Sims, unpublished data). This reduction in myelin thickness is likely to be due to the fact that the number of oligodendrocytes is reduced, thereby necessitating the myelination of more axons than normal by each oligodendrocyte. If this is the case, the oligodendrocyte may compensate for the increased demand for membrane formation by reducing the normal number of turns of myelin lamellae around each axon, thus reducing the thickness of the sheath. This suggests that the thickness of each axonal sheath is regulated in part by the total demand for membrane production and maintenance placed on a given oligodendrocyte. There is evidence also that myelin sheath thickness for each axon is regulated independently at a site close to the axon (Friedrich and Mugnaini 1983). Similar evidence for local regulation of sheath thickness has been observed recently in the ventral funiculi of rats irradiated in Gilmore's laboratory and killed 10 days P-I (Waxman and Sims, 1985). At this time the number of oligodendrocytes and myelin sheaths is markedly reduced in the irradiated (4000 R) lumbosacral area as compared to the controls, as discussed above (Beal and Hall 1974, Gilmore 1963, Rodgers 1965). Thus, the probability that the few myelinated axons clustered about a given oligodendrocyte derive their myelin sheath from that cell is certainly greatly increased within this background of non-myelinated axons. Most axons within a myelinated cluster are similar with respect to diameter and to myelin sheath thickness. However, in some clusters, myelinated axons having diameters only about one-half those of other axons have been observed (Waxman and Sims, 1985). These axons of small diameter have thinner myelin sheaths than the larger axons, suggesting that the oligodendrocyte adjusts local membrane production in accordance with the diameter of each axon it myelinates.

The presence of Schwann cells within the spinal cord suggests that the astrocyte population is not functioning in its normal capacity of delimiting the boundaries of the CNS (Reier et al. 1983). This role is particularly evident at the transition zone located on both cranial and spinal nerves, at which point the central and the peripheral nervous systems are in continuity but yet quite distinct from one another (Berthold and Carlstedt 1977a, b, Carlstedt 1981, Fraher 1978, Gamble 1976, Haller et al. 1972, Maxwell et al. 1969, Steer 1971). In this transition zone are found the nodes of Ranvier where the transition between oligodendrocyte myelin and Schwann cell myelin normally takes place. As pointed out above, such nodes occur also well within the depths of the spinal cord in areas occupied by ISC (Gilmore and Duncan 1968, Gilmore et al. 1982, Sims and Gilmore 1983).

In order to understand the role of the astrocyte population in the development of ISC, a recent study was carried out in which spinal cords of irradiated rats (4000 R, 3 days of age) were examined at intervals from 5 to 60 days P-I (Sims and Gilmore 1983). By studying these intervals, it is possible to evaluate the astrocyte population prior to, during, and following the establishment of ISC. The animals killed 5 days P-I in this study confirmed the earlier observations of a rapid, marked loss of neuroglia including sub-pial astrocytes. By 10 days P-I, interruptions appeared in the glia limitans, resulting in the presence of naked axons on the surface of the spinal cord underlying the intact basal lamina. It is about this time that ISC are found within the spinal cord. As the post-irradiation interval increases, the paucity of astrocytes in general becomes more marked, and this is particularly evidenced by the abundance of extracellular space in the ISC-occupied areas. Some of the astrocytes that were present had swollen processes. Such processes were not restricted to areas of ISC but occurred throughout the irradiated spinal cord. The rapid radiation-induced depletion of the astrocyte population, as well as the distribution within the irradiated spinal cord of astrocytes having swollen processes, is emphasized because Blakemore and Patterson (1975) also observed the absence of astrocytes from areas occupied by ISC and attributed this to a toxic interaction between the astrocytes and Schwann cells. Their conclusion was based on observations made in animals killed well after ISC were established in the spinal cord, and they failed to appreciate the earlier, radiation-induced changes in the astrocyte population. By 45 days P-I, after proliferation of ISC has essentially ceased (Gilmore et al. 1982), several variations were noted in the neuroglial-Schwann cell arrangements (Sims and Gilmore 1983). In one of these, Schwann cell-myelinated axons were apposed to areas where the neuroglial composition was essentially normal, as evidenced by the presence of oligodendrocyte-myelinated axons and normal astrocyte processes. In other areas, Schwann cell-myelinated and oligodendrocyte-myelinated axons intermingled, but astrocyte processes were absent (Figure 9-4). Finally, in some areas normal astrocyte processes distinctly separated groups of naked axons from adjacent bundles of Schwann cell-myelinated axons. This border was not effected by a multiplicity of astrocyte processes as would be present in a glial scar such as that occurring after direct physical disruption of the spinal cord (Berry 1979, Matthews et al. 1979, Puchala and Windle 1977). Instead, a single astrocyte process was sufficient to establish this boundary. As indicated above, the mitogenic stimulus for Schwann cells is located on the surface of the axon membrane (Salzer et al. 1980), and perhaps the ensheathment of bundles of unmyelinated axons by a single astrocyte process is sufficient to separate the ISC from their mitogenic stimuli and, thus, account for the rare uptake of [^{3}H]thymidine by ISC by this post-irradiation interval. As a result, the astrocyte population, although reduced in number, could serve as an effective barrier to the extension of Schwann cells within the spinal cord.

The interrelationships between ISC and neuroglia are suggested further from data obtained in other studies cited above of factors related to ISC development. In the study by Heard and Gilmore (1980) in which ISC development was shown to be restricted to small, isolated foci near the dorsal root entry zone of the irradiated mid-thoracic spinal cord (4000 R, 3 days of age), it was found also that the neuroglial population recovered quite rapidly (Heard 1981). As in the irradiated lumbosacral area, there was an obvious decrease in the neuroglial population of the white matter that was evident through 13 days P-I. Concurrently, the funiculi were hypomyelinated. By 19 days P-I, the number of neuroglia was obviously increased as was the intensity of the myelin staining, and by 25 days P-I the irradiated mid-thoracic area could not be distinguished from that in the controls. In contrast, at these post-irradiation intervals, the radiation-induced changes in neuroglia and myelin were clearly evident in the lumbosacral levels. Thus, although detailed autoradiographic and ultrastructural analyses have not yet been completed in the mid-thoracic area, the light microscopic evaluations indicate that the neuroglial population recovers much more quickly than in the lumbosacral area, thus perhaps obviating the development of ISC. Data yet unpublished from spinal cords included in the study of ISC development in the lumbosacral area following exposure to different amounts of x-rays (1000–3000 R) (Gilmore et al. 1983) indicate also that the lower doses induce less marked losses of neuroglia. It will be recalled from the discussion of that study above that exposure of the lumbosacral spinal cord to 1000 R results in the same restricted patterns of ISC development as observed in the mid-thoracic area after exposure to 4000 R. These data suggest again that the very limited ISC development is related to the recovery of the neuroglial population. Thus, it appears from the foregoing data that there is a competition between the ISC and neuroglia for axonal surfaces and that recovery of the neuroglial population influences the development of ISC. Further quantitative analyses of spinal cords from animals in the studies described above may be helpful in determining whether or not such a competition exists.

Summary

This chapter (1) describes an experimental model in which Schwann cells can be induced to populate the intraspinal environment and to myelinate intraspinal axons and (2) summarizes the studies to date utilizing this model. Since the development of ISC is predictable and can be rather extensive, this model is of value in determining the behavior and the potential of Schwann cells within the environment of the CNS. The definition of conditions under which Schwann cells will develop within the spinal cord provides the experimental framework for further elucidation of factors that either enhance or inhibit this phenomenon. In addition, this model presents an opportunity to examine aspects of oligodendrocyte myelination in a situation in which that process has been delayed. It is anticipated that data derived from studies carried out in this model will add to our understanding of repair processes in the CNS, of conditions necessary for transplantation into the spinal cord, and of normal development of that structure.

Acknowledgments. This work has been supported continuously and primarily by NIH grant NS 04761 from the National Institute of Neurological and Communicative Disorders and Stroke. Other recent sources of support include the Graduate Student Research Funds from the University of Arkansas for Medical Sciences and Grant NSF/ISP 8011447.

Dr. Bruce D. Trapp, Laboratory of Molecular Genetics, National Institute of Neurological and Communicative Disorders and Stroke, NIH, Bethesda, MD, is gratefully acknowledged for carrying out the immunostaining.

Mr. Napoleon Phillips is thanked for his capable technical assistance throughout these studies, and Mr. Ralph Nichols is thanked for his technical skills in the ultrastructural studies. Ms. Jane Leiting is acknowledged for her assistance in preparation of this manuscript, and Mrs. Yvonne Wingfield and Mrs. Nancy Stone are thanked for their secretarial assistance.

References

Adelman, L.S., Aronson, S.M. (1972). Intramedullary nerve fiber and Schwann cell proliferation within the spinal cord (schwannosis). Neurology 22, 726–731.

Beal, J.A., Hall, J.L. (1974). A light microscopic study of the effects of x-irradiation on the spinal cords of neonatal rats. J. Neuropathol. Exp. Neurol. 33, 128–143.

Bellhorn, R.W., Hirano, A., Henkind, P. (1979). Schwann cell proliferations mimicking medullated retinal nerve fibers. Am. J. Ophthal. 87, 469–473.

Bernstein, J.J., Collins, G.H., Bernstein, M.E. (1973). Ultrastructure of a human spinal neuroma. J. Neurol. Sci. 18, 489–492.

Berry, M. (1979). Regeneration in the central nervous system. In: Recent Advances in Neuropathology. Cavanaugh, J.B., Smith, W.T. (eds.). New York: Churchill Livingstone, pp. 67–111.

Berthold, C.H. (1978). Morphology of normal peripheral axons. In: Physiology and Pathobiology of Axons. Waxman, S.G. (ed.). New York: Raven Press, pp. 3–63.

Berthold, C.H., Carlstedt, T. (1977a). Observations on the morphology at the transition between the peripheral and the central nervous system in the cat. II. General organization of the transitional region in S_1 dorsal rootlets. Acta Physiol. Scand. Suppl. 446, 23–42.

Berthold, C.H., Carlstedt, T. (1977b). Observations on the morphology at the transition between the peripheral and the central nervous system in the cat. III. Myelinated fibers in S_1 dorsal rootlets. Acta Physiol. Scand. Suppl. 446, 43–60.

Blakemore, W.F. (1975). Remyelination by Schwann cells of axons demyelinated by intraspinal injection of 6-aminonicotinamide in the rat. J. Neurocytol. 4, 745–757.

Blakemore, W.F. (1976). Invasion of Schwann cells into the spinal cord of the rat following local injections of lysolecithin. Neuropathol. Appl. Neurobiol. 2, 21–39.

Blakemore, W.F. (1978). Observations on remyelination in the rabbit spinal cord following demyelination induced by lysolecithin. Neuropathol. Appl. Neurobiol. 4, 47–59.

Blakemore, W.F. (1982). Ethidium bromide induced demyelination in the spinal cord of the cat. Neuropathol. Appl. Neurobiol. 8, 365–375.

Blakemore, W.F., Patterson, R.C. (1975). Observations on the interactions of Schwann cells and astrocytes following x-irradiation of neonatal rat spinal cord. J. Neurocytol. 4, 573–585.

Bradley, W.G., Fewings, J.D., Cumming, W.J.K., Harrison, R.M., Faulds, A.J. (1977). Delayed myeloradiculopathy produced by spinal x-irradiation in the rat. J. Neurol. Sci. 31, 63–82.

Bunge, M.B., Williams, A.K., Wood, P.M., Uitto, J., Jeffrey, J.J. (1980). Comparison of nerve cell and nerve cell plus Schwann cell cultures, with particular emphasis on basal lamina and collagen formation. J. Cell Biol. 84, 184–202.

Büssow, H. (1978). Schwann cell myelin ensheathing C.N.S. axons in the nerve fibre layer of the cat retina. J. Neurocytol. 7, 207–214.

Carlstedt, T. (1981). An electron microscopical study of the developing transitional region in feline S_1 dorsal rootlets. J. Neurol. Sci. 50, 357–372.

Chung, K., Coggeshall, R.E. (1983). Propriospinal fibers in the rat. J. Comp. Neurol. 217, 47–53.

DeMyer, W. (1965). Aberrant peripheral nerve fibers in the medulla oblongata of man. J. Neurol. Neurosurg. Psychiat. 28, 121–123.

Druckman, R. (1955). Review of structural evidence of regeneration of nerve fibers in injury to the human spinal cord. In: Regeneration in the Central Nervous System. Windle, W.F. (ed.). Springfield, IL: C.C. Thomas, pp. 241–246.

Druckman, R., Mair, W.G.P. (1953). Aberrant regenerating nerve fibers in injury to the spinal cord. Brain 76, 448–454.

Duncan, D. (1955). Experimental compression of the spinal cord. In: Regeneration in the Central Nervous System. Windle, W.F. (ed.). Springfield, IL: C.C. Thomas, pp. 247–258.

Feigin, I., Cravioto, H. (1961). A histochemical study of myelin. A difference in the solubility of the glycolipid components in the central and peripheral nervous system. J. Neuropathol. Exp. Neurol. 20, 245–254.

Feigin, I., Ogata, J. (1971). Schwann cells and peripheral myelin within human central nervous tissues: The mesenchymal character of Schwann cells. J. Neuropathol. Exp. Neurol. 30, 603–612.

Feigin, I., Popoff, N. (1966). Regeneration of myelin in multiple sclerosis. The role of mesenchymal cells in such regeneration and in myelin formation in the peripheral nervous system. Neurology 16, 364–372.

Fraher, J.P. (1978). The maturation of the ventral root-spinal cord transition zone. An ultrastructural study. J. Neurol. Sci. 36, 427–449.

Friedrich, V.L., Mugnaini, E. (1983). Myelin sheath thickness in the CNS is regulated near the axon. Brain Res. 274, 329–331.

Gamble, H.J. (1976). Spinal and cranial nerve roots. In: The Peripheral Nerve. Landon, D.N. (ed.). New York: J. Wiley and Sons, Inc., pp. 330–354.

Ghatak, N.R., Hirano, A., Doron, Y., Zimmerman, H.M. (1973). Remyelination in multiple sclerosis with peripheral type myelin. Arch. Neurol. 29, 262–267.

Gilmore, S.A. (1963). The effects of x-irradiation on the spinal cords of neonatal rats. II. Histological observations. J. Neuropathol. Exp. Neurol. 22, 294–301.

Gilmore, S.A. (1971). Autoradiographic studies of intramedullary Schwann cells in irradiated spinal cords of immature rats. Anat. Rec. 171, 517–528.

Gilmore, S.A. (1973). Long-term effects of ionizing radiation on the rat spinal cord: Intramedullary connective tissue formation. Am. J. Anat. 137, 1–18.

Gilmore, S.A., Duncan, D. (1968). On the presence of peripheral-like nervous and connective tissue within irradiated spinal cord. Anat. Rec. 160, 675–690.

Gilmore, S.A., Heard, J.K., Leiting, J.E. (1983). Patterns of x-radiation-induced Schwann cell development in spinal cords of immature rats. Anat. Rec. 205, 313–319.

Gilmore, S.A., Sims, T.J., Heard, J.K. (1982). Autoradiographic and ultrastructural studies of areas of spinal cord occupied by Schwann cells and Schwann cell myelin. Brain Res. 239, 365–375.

Haller, F.R., Haller, A.C., Low, F.N. (1972). The fine structure of cellular layers and connective tissue space at spinal nerve root attachment in the rat. Am. J. Anat. 133, 109–124.

Harrison, B.M., McDonald, W.I., Ochoa, J. (1972). Remyelination in the central diphtheria toxin lesion. J. Neurol. Sci. 17, 293–302.

Heard, J.K. (1981). Changes induced by x-irradiation of the mid-thoracic and lumbosacral levels of neonatal rat spinal cord with special reference to the occurrence of

    intramedullary Schwann cells. Doctoral Dissertation, The University of Arkansas
    for Medical Sciences, Little Rock, AR.

Heard, J.K., Gilmore, S.A. (1980). Intramedullary Schwann cell development following
    x-irradiation of mid-thoracic and lumbosacral spinal cord levels in immature rats.
    Anat. Rec. 197, 85–93.

Hirano, A., Zimmerman, H.M., Levine, S. (1969). Electron microscopic observations
    of peripheral myelin in a central nervous system lesion. Acta Neuropathol. (Berlin)
    12, 348–365.

Hughes, J.T., Brownell, B. (1963). Aberrant nerve fibres within the spinal cord. J.
    Neurol. Neurosurg. Psychiat. 26, 528–534.

Innes, J.R.M., Carsten, A. (1961). Demyelinating or malacic myelopathy. A delayed
    effect of localized x-irradiation in experimental rats. Arch. Neurol. 4, 190–199.

Itoyama, Y., Webster, H.DeF., Richardson, Jr., E.P. Trapp, B.D. (1983). Schwann cell
    remyelination of demyelinated axons in spinal cord multiple sclerosis. Ann.
    Neurol. 14, 339–346.

Klintworth, G.K. (1964). Axonal regeneration in the human spinal cord with formation
    of neuromata. J. Neuropathol. Exp. Neurol. 23, 127–134.

Klüver, H., Barrera, E. (1953). A method for the combined staining of cells and fibers in
    the nervous system. J. Neuropathol. Exp. Neurol. 12, 400–403.

Koeppen, A.H., Ordinario, A.T., Barron, K.D. (1968). Aberrant intramedullary periph-
    eral nerve fibers. Arch. Neurol. 18, 567–573.

Kogel, A.J., van der. (1977). Radiation tolerance of the rat spinal cord: Time-dose
    relationships. Radiology 122, 505–509.

Kogel, A.J., van der, Barendsen, G.W. (1974). Late effects of spinal cord irradiation
    with 300KV x-rays and 15 MeV neutrons. Brit. J. Radiol. 47, 393–398.

Lampert, P., Cressman, M. (1964). Axonal regeneration in the dorsal columns of the
    spinal cord of adult rats. An electron microscopic study. Lab. Invest. 13, 825–839.

Mair, W.G.P., Druckman, R. (1953). The pathology of spinal cord lesions and their
    relation to the clinical features in protrusion of cervical intervertebral discs. Brain
    76, 70–91.

Mastaglia, F.L., McDonald, W.I., Watson, J.V., Yogendran, K. (1976). Effects of x-
    radiation on the spinal cord: An experimental study of the morphological changes
    in central nerve fibers. Brain 99, 101–122.

Matthews, M.A., St. Onge, M.F., Faciane, C.L., Gelderd, J.B. (1979). Axon sprouting
    into segments of rat spinal cord adjacent to the site of a previous transection.
    Neuropathol. Appl. Neurobiol. 5, 181–196.

Maxwell, D.S., Kruger, L., Pineda, A. (1969). The trigeminal nerve root with special
    reference to the central-peripheral transition zone—an electron microscopic study
    in the Macaque. Anat. Rec. 164, 113–126.

Ogata, J., Feigin, I. (1975). Schwann cells and regenerated peripheral myelin in multi-
    ple sclerosis: An ultrastructural study. Neurology 25, 713–716.

Payan, H., Levine, S. (1965). Focal axonal proliferation in pons (central neurinoma).
    Association with cystic encephalomalacia. Arch. Pathol. 79, 501–504.

Puchala, E., Windle, W.F. (1977). The possibility of structural and functional restitution
    after spinal cord injury. A review. Exp. Neurol. 55, 1–42.

Raine, C.S. (1976). On the occurrence of Schwann cells within the normal central
    nervous system. J. Neurocytol. 5, 371–380.

Raine, C.S., Brown, A.M., McFarlin, D.E. (1982). Heterotopic regeneration of periph-
    eral nerve fibers into the subarachnoid space. J. Neurocytol. 11, 109–118.

Raine, C.S., Traugott, U., Stone, S.H. (1978). Glial bridges and Schwann cell migration during chronic demyelination in the C.N.S. J. Neurocytol. 7, 541–553.

Reier, P.J., Stensaas, L.J., Guth, L. (1983). The astrocytic scar as an impediment to regeneration in the central nervous system. In: Spinal Cord Reconstruction. Kao, C.C., Bunge, R.P., Reier, P.J. (eds.). New York: Raven Press, pp. 163–196.

Rodgers, C.H. (1965). Alterations in spinal cords of neonatal rats following x-irradiation. Exp. Neurol. 11, 502–515.

Salzer, J.L., Bunge, R.P., Glaser, L. (1980). Studies of Schwann cell proliferation. III. Evidence for the surface localization of the neurite mitogen. J. Cell Biol. 84, 767–778.

Sims, T.J., Gilmore, S.A. (1983). Interactions between intraspinal Schwann cells and the cellular constituents normally occurring in the spinal cord: An ultrastructural study in the irradiated rat. Brain Res. 276, 17–30.

Snyder, D.H., Valsamis, M.P., Stone, S.H., Raine, C.S. (1975). Progressive demyelination and reparative phenomena in chronic experimental allergic encephalomyelitis. J. Neuropathol. Exp. Neurol. 34, 209–221.

Steer, J.M. (1971). Some observations on the fine structure of rat dorsal nerve roots. J. Anat. (London) 109, 467–485.

Sung, J.H., Mastri, A.R., Chen, K.T.K. (1981). Aberrant peripheral nerves and neuromas in normal and injured spinal cords. J. Neuropathol. Exp. Neurol. 40, 551–565.

Trapp, B.D., Itoyama, Y., Sternberger, N.H., Quarles, R.H., Webster, H.DeF. (1981). Immunocytochemical localization of P_o protein in Golgi complex membranes and myelin of developing rat Schwann cells. J. Cell Biol. 90, 1–6.

Waxman, S.G., Sims, T.J. 1985. Specificity in central myelination: Evidence for local regulation of myelin thickness. Brain Res. 292, 179–185.

Wisniewski, H.M., Madrid, R.E. (1983). Chronic progressive experimental allergic encephalomyelitis (EAE) in adult guinea pigs. J. Neuropathol. Exp. Neurol. 42, 243–255.

Wood, P.M., Bunge, R.P. (1975). Evidence that sensory axons are mitogenic for Schwann cells. Nature (London) 256, 662–664.

Wyse, J.P.H. (1980). Schwann cell myelination in the nerve fibre layer of the BW rat retina. J. Neurocytol. 9, 107–117.

Wyse, J.P.H., Spira, A.W. (1981). Ultrastructural evidence of a peripheral nervous system pattern of myelination in the avascular retina of the guinea pig. Acta Neuropathol. (Berlin) 54, 203–210.

Yajima, K., Suzuki, K. (1979). Demyelination and remyelination in the rat central nervous system following ethidium bromide injection. Lab. Invest. 41, 385–392.

Chapter 10

The Motoneuron and Its Microenvironment Responding to Axotomy

GEORG W. KREUTZBERG*

Grafting pieces of nervous tissue into the brain and expecting axons to grow out from the transplant implies that we are dealing with axotomized neurons and with regenerating neurons. In this context it might be useful to review the basic events that occur in neurons of the peripheral nervous system as a consequence of axotomy. In general, it is accepted that these events are somehow related to regeneration. However, as we will discuss later, this is questionable, since at least some of the retrograde changes can be suppressed without inhibiting regeneration (Carlsen et al. 1982). It should also be pointed out that changes occurring during regeneration may also take place in neurons exposed to other noxious stimuli such as hypoxia. An example for this is the increase of ornithine decarboxylase (ODC) (Kleihues et al. 1975).

This enzyme shows an early transient increase in activity in sympathetic neurons (Gilad and Gilad 1983), a finding we have recently been able to confirm also for motoneurons (Tetzlaff and Kreutzberg, 1985). As early as 2 hours after the cut, the activity was increased to 200% and by 10 hours a peak was reached of about 450% above control values. ODC is the rate-limiting enzyme in polyamine synthesis, and it is thought to play a potentially important role in regulating cellular growth and proliferation. However, when ODC induced by nerve crushing was inhibited irreversibly by α-difluoro-methylornithine, axonal growth occurred nevertheless, and the optic nerves of goldfish regenerated (Kohsaka et al. 1982).

One of the most consistently produced changes in axotomized neurons is the increase of activity in hexose monophosphate shunt enzymes (Kreutzberg 1963, Härkönen and Kauffman 1974). We have recently reinvestigated these changes quantitatively in the facial nucleus of rats following seventh nerve lesioning. After 7 days, glucose-6-phosphate dehydrogenase was 130% and 6-phosphogluconate dehydrogenase was 135% of control values (Tetzlaff and Kreutzberg 1984). Increased levels of these enzymes were observed for a dura-

---

* Max Planck Institute for Psychiatry, Munich, F.R.G.

tion of at least 4 weeks. The pathway is thought to serve the synthesis of ribose that could be necessary for the increased RNA metabolism in regenerating neurons. This most interesting aspect has been reviewed by Austin and Langford (1980). There appears to be more than just a general increase in RNA, as reflected in the ultrastructural changes of chromatolytic neurons with the augmentation of ribosomes and the dispersion of the Nissl bodies. Detailed analysis revealed changes in different RNA species at different times post-lesioning.

Such changes in template formation may well go along with the increased production of certain structural and matrix proteins such as tubulin, calmodu-lin, actin (Heacock and Agranoff 1976, Bisby 1979, Hall et al. 1978, Hoffman and Lasek 1980), but also with the appearance of new proteins. These so-called growth associated proteins (GAPs) were discovered by Skene and Willard (1981a,b). It might be of special interest to look for GAPs appearing not only in regenerating nerves but also in growing fiber tracts during neurogenesis. GAPs are, however, absent in systems not capable of regeneration or growth, such as the adult mammalian optic nerve. It would be interesting to see if neurons in transplants with successful axonal outgrowth contain GAPs. GAPs are trans-ported in the fast component of axonal transport. It seems that they are mem-brane constituents, and it is not unlikely that they play a role in the growth cones or sprouts (Willard and Skene 1982).

Increased glucose uptake as revealed by the [^{14}C]deoxyglucose method oc-curs also as an early response to axotomy (Singer and Mehler 1980, Kreutzberg and Emmert 1980). Only 24 hours after transection of the facial or hypoglossal nerves the motor nuclei show increased radioactivity. Contact autoradiographs taken from these areas do not allow for finer resolution, but it seems apparent that glucose consumption is high not only in the neuronal cell bodies but in the neuropil as well. The increase in glucose metabolism can be seen over a period of at least 4 weeks. It clearly does not require increased activities of oxidative enzymes, because succinic dehydrogenase, malate dehydrogenase, or cyto-chrom oxidase remain unchanged.

All the above-mentioned changes could be referred to as an increase in cell work, the metabolic counterparts of neuronal hypertrophy. A number of changes, however, point in another direction, namely that of reduced activity. This applies especially to neurotransmitter-related proteins such as receptors or enzymes involved in the biosynthesis or degradation of transmitters, e.g., muscarinic receptors (Rotter et al. 1979), dopamine-β-hydroxylase and tyro-sine hydroxylase (Ross et al. 1975). choline acetyl transferase, or acetyl cholin-esterase (Watson 1966, 1976), to mention a few examples. AChE probably is the best investigated representative of this group. It decreases to about 60% of normal activity in the rat N VII nucleus and stays at this value for about 4 weeks before it slowly recovers. Light microscopic and electron microscopic histochemistry shows enzyme activity disappearing quickly from the neuropil, i.e., the dendrites, while staining of perikarya is still visible. In the guinea pig facial nucleus, AChE seems to be increasingly secreted from the dendrites to the extracellular space leading to widespread enzyme deposits at the basal laminae of the local capillaries (Kreutzberg and Tóth 1974, Kreutzberg et al. 1975).

We have recently studied butyryl cholinesterase in the dorsal motor nucleus of the vagal nerve where this enzyme of unknown function is particularly strong (Kreutzberg et al. 1984). After the vagus is cut, the enzyme disappears from the neurons even faster than AChE. Thus, BuChE behaves similarly to other transmitter-related enzymes in regenerating neurons.

As an enzyme transported in dendrites, AChE distribution in axotomized neurons may tell us something of the dynamics of these cell processes during regeneration. A shrinkage of the total neuropil area can be seen in enzyme histochemical preparations (Tetzlaff and Kreutzberg 1984). Because dendrites contribute considerably to this area, a volume change of these processes could be suspected to be the basis for such a finding. Golgi preparations of regenerating motoneurons have indeed demonstrated that their dendritic field is diminished considerably (Sumner and Watson 1971, Sumner and Sutherland 1973). It has been thought that this change reflects retraction and reexpansion of the dendrites. We have seen similar changes when we investigated dendritic transport processes in spinal motoneurons of cats 3 weeks following ischiadectomy (Schubert and Kreutzberg, unpublished observations). When single motoneurons were injected intracellularly with [³H]glycine, the radioactive proteins synthesized thereafter became distributed in the complete dendritic arborization (Schubert et al. 1972). In regenerating neurons the spread of the dendritic field showed a deficit of 34%, and the mean length of labeled dendrites was diminished by 24%. In tissue culture of neuroblastoma cells, we have also observed some dynamic changes of neurites following the transection of the "axon" by a laser shot (Rieske and Kreutzberg 1978). Recently we were able to confirm this finding in a rather impressive way in motoneurons *in vitro* where we found retraction of most of the neurite processes after severing the presumably axonal process by laser microsurgery. It is tempting to interpret these findings in the sense that there occurs a rerouting of neuroplasmic material away from the dendrites into the axon. This change could temporarily supply the growing process with more material before the synthetic machinery of the perikaryon is able to feed all its processes adequately.

The changes in the dendrites are neuronal, and it remains to be discussed how far other elements of the brain tissue participate in the retrograde response. We have briefly mentioned the capillary system that becomes AChE-positive because of an enhanced extracellular secretion of this enzyme from dendrites. We have also seen that alkaline phosphatase of the endothelial cells increases strongly in the first week after nerve transection (Kreutzberg et al. 1974). A most interesting change can be observed in the perineuronal glia that is thought to be of microglial origin. These are cells with a rather dense ground cytoplasm and a small fusiform perikaryon from which rectangular processes derive. Within a few days (3–8) these cells are proliferating and then are seen covering most of the surface of the motoneurons, especially the cell bodies and the stem dendrites (Blinzinger and Kreutzberg 1968). This leads to a loss of the majority of normally inserted presynaptic terminals. The neurons appear deafferented. The synaptic stripping has consequences for the electrophysiology of the cells. They lose the spontaneous miniature EPSP's with a fast time rise to peak, whereas those with a slow time rise to peak representing the dendritic periphery become more prominent and remain (Lux and Schubert 1975).

We have seen in this brief review that retrograde changes are of a rather complex nature. They concern size, shape, finer morphology, metabolism, and electrophysiology of the axotomized neurons. They extend to the neuropil and involve glial cells and the local vasculature. Many of the changes can be viewed teleologically as fitting the concept of a neuron supplying its growing axon with the necessary materials. However, it must be honestly admitted that we do not really know what all the changes mean in terms of regeneration and whether they are really necessary to guarantee axonal growth. Many exceptions from the general rules we have sketched here do exist (Kreutzberg 1982). Variations with system, age, species, proximity of lesion, etc., make it difficult to decide what the prerequisites of axonal regeneration are.

References

Austin, I., Langford, C.J. (1980). Nerve regeneration: A biochemical view. Trends Neurosci. 3, 130–132.

Bisby, M.A. (1979). Changes in the composition of labeled protein transported in motor axons during their regeneration. J. Neurobiol. 11, 436–445.

Blinzinger, K., Kreutzberg, G.W. (1968). Displacement of synaptic terminal from regenerating motoneurons by microglial cells. Z. Zellforsch. 85, 145–157.

Carlsen, R.C., Kiff, J., Ryugo, K. (1982). Suppression of the cell body response in axotomized frog spinal neurons does not prevent initiation of nerve regeneration. Brain Res. 234, 11–25.

Gilad, G.M., Gilad, V.H. (1983). Early rapid and transient increase in ornithine decarboxylase activity within sympathetic neurons after axonal injury. Exp. Neurol. 81, 158–166.

Hall, M.E., Wilson, D.L., Stone, G.C. (1978). Changes in synthesis of specific proteins following axotomy: Detection with two-dimensional gel electrophoresis. J. Neurobiol. 9, 353–366.

Härkönen, M.H.A., Kauffman, F.C. (1974). Metabolic alterations in the axotomized superior cervical ganglion of the rat. II. The pentose phosphate pathway. Brain Res. 65, 141–157.

Heacock, A.M., Agranoff, B.W. (1976). Enhanced labeling of a retinal protein during regeneration of optic nerve in goldfish. Proc. Nat. Acad. Sci. USA 73, 828–832.

Hoffman, P.N., Lasek, R.J. (1980). Axonal transport of the cytoskeleton in regenerating motor neurons: Constancy and change. Brain Res. 202, 317–353.

Kleihues, P., Hossmann, K.A., Pegg, A.E., Kobayashi, K., Zimmermann, V. (1975). Resuscitation of the monkey brain after one hour complete ischemia. III. Indications of metabolic recovery. Brain Res. 95, 61–73.

Kohsaka, S., Heacock, A.M., Klinger, P.D., Porta, R., Agranoff, B.W. (1982). Dissociation of enhanced ornithine decarboxylase activity and optic nerve regeneration in goldfish. Devel. Brain Res. 4, 149–156.

Kreutzberg, G.W. (1963). Changes of coenzyme (TPN) diaphorase and TPN-linked dehydrogenase during axonal reaction of the nerve cell. Nature 199, 393–394.

Kreutzberg, G.W. (1982). Acute neural reaction to injury. In: Repair and Regeneration of the Nervous System. Dahlem Konferenzen 1982. Nicholl, J.G. (ed.). Berlin/ Heidelberg/New York: Springer-Verlag, pp. 57–69.

Kreutzberg, G.W., Emmert, H. (1980). Glucose utilization of motor nuclei during regeneration: A ^{14}C 2-deoxyglucose study. Exp. Neurol. 70, 712–716.

Kreutzberg, G.W., Tetzlaff, W., Tóth, L. (1984). Cytochemical changes of cholinesterases in motor neurons during regeneration. In: Cholinesterases—Fundamental and Applied Aspects. Brzin, M., Kiauta, T., Barnard, E.A. (eds.). Berlin: Walter de Gruyter & Co. pp. 273–288.

Kreutzberg, G.W., Tóth, L. (1974). Dendritic secretion: A way for the neuron to communicate with the vasculature. Naturwissenschaften 61, 37.

Kreutzberg, G.W. Tóth, L., Kaiya, H. (1975). Acetylcholinesterase as a marker for dendritic transport and dendritic secretion. In: Physiology and Pathology of Dendrites. Kreutzberg, G.W. (ed.). Advances in Neurology, Vol. 12, New York: Raven Press, pp. 269–281.

Kreutzberg, G.W. Tóth, L., Weikert, M., Schubert, P. (1974). Changes in perineuronal capillaries accompanying chromatolysis of motoneurons. In: Pathology of Cerebral Microcirculation. Cérvos-Navarro, J. (ed.). Berlin: Walter de Gruyter Verlag, pp. 282–287.

Lux, H.D. Schubert, P. (1975). Some aspects of the electroanatomy of dendrites. In: Physiology and Pathology of Dendrites. Kreutzberg, G.W. (ed.). Advances in Neurology, Vol. 12. New York: Raven Press, pp. 29–44.

Rieske, E., Kreutzberg, G.W. (1978). Neurite regeneration after cell surgery with laser microbeam irradiation. Brain Res. 148, 478–483.

Ross, R.A., Joh, G.H., Reis, D.J. (1975). Reversible changes in the accumulation and activities of tyrosine hydroxylase and dopamine-β-hydroxylase in neurons of nucleus locus coeruleus during the retrograde reaction. Brain Res. 92, 57–72.

Rotter, A., Birdsall, N.J.M., Burgen, A.S.V., Field, P.M., Smolen, A., Raisman, G. (1979). Muscarinic receptors in the central nervous system of the rat. IV. A comparison of the effects of axotomy and deafferentation on the binding of [^{3}H]probylbenzilylcholine mustard and associated synaptic changes in the hypoglossal and pontine nuclei. Brain Res. Rev. 1, 207–224.

Schubert, P., Kreutzberg, G.W., Lux, H.D. (1972). Neuroplasmic transport in dendrites: Effect of colchicine on morphology and physiology of motoneurons in the cat. Brain Res. 47, 331–343.

Singer, P., Mehler, S. (1980). 2-Deoxy[^{14}C]glucose uptake in the rat hypoglossal nucleus after nerve transection. Exp. Neurol. 69, 617–626.

Skene, J.H.P., Willard, M. (1981a). Axonally transported proteins associated with axon growth in rabbit central and peripheral nervous systems. J. Cell Biol. 89, 96–103.

Skene, J.H.P., Willard, M. (1981b). Characteristics of growth-associated proteins (GAPs) in regenerating toad retinal ganglion cells. J. Neurosci. 1, 419–426.

Sumner, B.E.H., Sutherland, E.I. (1973). Quantitative electron microscopy on the injured hypoglossal nucleus in the rat. J. Neurocytol. 2, 315–328.

Sumner, B.E.H., Watson, W.E. (1971). Retraction and expansion of the dendritic tree of motor neurones of adult rats induced in vivo. Nature 233, 273–275.

Tetzlaff, W., Kreutzberg, G.W. (1984). Enzyme changes in the rat facial nucleus following a conditioning lesion. Exp. Neurol. 85, 547–564.

Tetzlaff, W., Kreutzberg, G.W. (1985). Ornithine decarboxylase in motoneurons during
regeneration. 4 Exp. Neurol. 89, 679–688.

Watson, W.E. (1966). Quantitative observations upon acetylcholine hydrolase activity
of nerve cells after axotomy. J. Neurochem. 13, 1549–1550.

Watson, W.E. (1976). Cell Biology of Brain. London: Chapman and Hall.

Willard, M., Skene, J.H.P. (1982). Molecular events in axonal regeneration. In: Repair
and Regeneration of the Nervous System. Dahlem Konferenzen 1982. Nicholls,
J.G. (ed.). Berlin/Heidelberg/New York: Springer-Verlag, pp. 71–89.

Chapter 11

Cellular Interactions between Transplanted Autonomic Ganglia and the Developing Brain

Jeffrey M. Rosenstein* and Milton W. Brightman†

Introduction and Rationale

Within the past few years, attempts to restructure damaged or deficient circuitry within the central nervous system (CNS) have involved the use of fetal CNS tissue transplants as specific replacements (Lund and Hauschka 1976, Perlow et al. 1979, Gash et al. 1980). Necessarily, the placement of grafts in these systems involves damage to the host brain. Experimental methods entail either direct insertion into the parenchyma or the establishment of a resection cavity for subsequent graft placement (Das and Altman 1972, Stenevi et al. 1976, Björklund and Stenevi 1979). Either means, although successful in terms of connectivity, may produce not only an extensive astroglial reaction but the ensuing brain wound violates the blood–brain barrier (BBB) and thus serves to liberate systemically derived macrophages (see Imamoto and LeBlond 1977).

Our approach to neural transplantation studies is a different one than those in which the brain is injured. In utilizing the fourth ventricle as a transplantation site, we can assess the mutual interactions of foreign, transplanted neurons and the adjacent undamaged brain. Tissue grafted within the fourth ventricle rests upon the internal (ependyma) or external (glial) surfaces of the brain, and the underlying parenchyma remains undisturbed (for detailed methodology see Rosenstein and Brightman 1978, 1979). In this system of minimal disturbance, cellular events and changes are uncomplicated by excessive scar formation, inflammation, or edema. The relatively accessible fourth ventricle makes it possible to examine neurons, glia, and blood vessels from the peripheral (autonomic) nervous system and the central nervous system. Autonomic ganglion tissues regenerate briskly in its new cerebrospinal fluid (CSF) environment.

* Department of Anatomy, George Washington University. Medical Center, N.W., Washington, D.C. 20037 U.S.A.
† Laboratory of Neurobiology, NINCDS, National Institutes of Health, Bethesda, Maryland 20205 U.S.A.

Fetal CNS tissue is particularly useful to study both cellular development in isolation and angiogenesis and neovascularization, presently one of our active areas of study.

In addition to the study of cellular alterations, another motivating reason for using the CSF compartment as a graft site is that the CSF freely communicates with the extracellular fluid of the brain. This humoral communication could influence interactions between various cerebral regions and the transplant by the dissemination of neuroactive agents secreted by the transplanted tissue. Our recent experiments indicate that transplanted neural tissue can markedly affect the integrity of the host BBB. Moreover, our hypothesis that peripheral nervous tissue which contains fenestrated, permeable vessels might provide a direct link into the CNS from the systemic vasculature has been borne out (Rosenstein and Brightman 1983, 1984). This transplantation system provides a model whereby grafted neural tissue could serve as a portal for systemically administered substances to enter the CNS (see below). This approach has a distinct advantage over the more accessible anterior chamber of the eye as a transplantation site: it enables one to follow the mutual interaction between graft and relatively undisturbed central nervous tissue. By the same token, for the study of neuronal development, the anterior eye chamber is most advantageous because the grafted tissue can be observed directly and is accessible to microelectrodes so that its functional state can be readily determined.

Growth of autonomic ganglion tissue, particularly the superior cervical ganglion (SCG), has been well characterized in tissue culture (Mains and Patterson 1973, Rees and Bunge 1974). Morphological changes in the SCG after axotomy *in situ* have also been studied (Hendry 1975). One of our original intentions was to follow the cellular changes and regeneration of the SCG, divorced from neural or vascular connections, as an *in vivo* organ culture within the CSF compartment. We felt it might be possible for regenerating neurites, from a completely foreign source, to enter the undamaged host brain because the surface is comprised of but a few thin astroglial slips or ependymal cells. While the host brain proves remarkably accommodative for the survival of the graft, movement of any of the myriad regenerating neurites into the host is very meager. Thus, a disadvantage of our system is that it appears that only after mechanical lesions can transplanted axons enter the host. The slight but inevitable disruption at the time of graft placement might provide conditions necessary for successful grafting: Neuritic ingrowth after damage to host brain has been demonstrated repeatedly in grafted autonomic and CNS tissue but few have illustrated the nature of the wound site. Ramon y Cajal (1928) proposed the presence of "alluring substances," possibly neuronal, at a lesion site. These substances may well be needed for successful ingress of foreign axons, yet the growth-promoting characteristics of non-neuronal cells, i.e., macrophages, at brain wound sites must not be overlooked (Imamoto and LeBlond 1977).

An interesting aspect that has arisen during the course of our investigations of neural transplantation concerns marked differences in the developmental or regenerative properties between peripheral and central nervous tissue. Discussion of these differences appears in previous papers (Rosenstein and Brightman 1979, 1984). Briefly, we have found that neural tissue from the periphery, autonomic ganglia (Rosenstein and Brightman 1978, 1979), dorsal root ganglion, and adrenal medulla (unpublished observations) must be *mature* to flourish after transplantation. Ganglion tissue, in order to survive *in vitro*, must be taken from fetal or neonatal donors, whereas the same tissue will not survive transplantation to the *in vivo* site, the brain (Rosenstein and Brightman 1978, 1979). Conversely, central nervous tissue, in order to survive *in vivo* after transplantation to the brain, must be derived from fetal sources: The younger the fetal tissue, the better the prospects of survival within the brain. Such profound differences between fetal CNS nerve cells and those nerve cells derived from the neural crest may provide further information on the requisites for neuronal development.

Results and Implications

In this review we will attempt to depict the neural, glial, and vascular changes brought about by grafted autonomic ganglia. The major thrust of our studies is to demonstrate the cellular alterations that take place within the host brain and its capacity to conform to the presence of a graft.

Regeneration

A mature SCG allograft undergoes a predictable course of regeneration. There is an initial period of degeneration when many neurons die, but others only chromatolyze and sprout numerous neurites. Within 1–2 weeks after transplantation, surviving ganglion cells have a normal appearance (Figure 11-1) al-

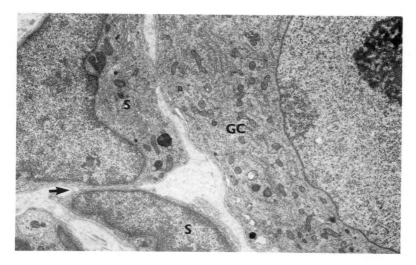

Figure 11-1. A regenerated grafted SCG ganglion cell (GC) rest, near two satellite cells (S) that share a basal lamina (arrow). Six weeks postoperative.

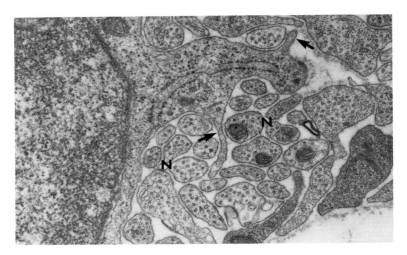

Figure 11-2. A Schwann cell (S) emits newly formed processes (arrows) that sequester groups of neurites (N). One week postoperative.

though SIF cells, according to electron microscopic data, do not recover (Rosenstein and Brightman 1979). Growth cones are recognizable and are present for at least 6 months. Schwann cells proliferate and undergo changes to accommodate the massive growth of regenerated neurites (Figure 11-2). Over time, as neuronal tissue gradually diminishes, Schwann cells will envelop individual axons as in the mature state. This suggests that, after transplantation, an SCG allograft regresses to an immature state composed of neurites and growth cones and eventually redevelops into a mature, stable ganglion albeit with fewer nerve cells. This may be considered an adaptative response owing to the fact that in its transplantation site there are fewer targets.

Allografts of SCG appear to survive indefinitely, at least 30 months in rats. There is, however, gradual loss of neurons over time, resulting not from immunological rejection but from a lack of appropriate targets (Rosenstein and Brightman 1979, 1984). If an SCG is allografted to a recipient animal that has been bilaterally ganglionectomized, nearly four times as many neurons survive at 1 month postoperative and seven times as many neurons at 6 months when compared to recipients with intact SCG (Rosenstein and Brightman 1984). Removal of the SCG caused afferent terminals on blood vessels of the pia and choroid plexus to degenerate and thus become available to the regenerating axons of the graft.

Tropic Effects

The survival of grafted autonomic ganglion is determined, in part, not only by the availability of target tissue but by its revascularization. Even after the removal of its capsule, the grafted ganglion cells and their processes are separated from the CSF by layers of Schwann cells and fibroblastic sheaths. What nutrients there are in the CSF must diffuse through these layers to reach the neurons. A more effective and certain means of sustaining the neurons is the invasion of its graft by endothelial sprouts from the surrounding subarachnoid, choroid plexus, and parenchymal blood vessels extrinsic to the graft. This sprouting would be accompanied, presumably, by a regeneration of vessels intrinsic to the graft.

Within 9 hours after transplantation, anastomoses between intrinsic and extrinsic vessels are formed in a few animals, as judged by the entry of India ink-gelatin into graft vessels after the mixture is injected into the heart of an aldehyde-fixed recipient (Tsubaki and Brightman, unpublished observations). By 18 hours, the graft vessels of all the hosts examined had anastomosed with extrinsic vessels (Figure 11-3). Thus, a powerful *angiotropic effect* is exerted by the graft on the surrounding vessels. The degree of vascularity, determined by measuring the total length of blood vessels in a given volume of the graft, reaches a peak at about 1 week after transplantation. It is presumed that some of the extrinsic vessels, subarachnoid and choroidal, had been damaged during insertion of the graft and that the new vessel sprouts arose from these vessels. Preliminary data employing tritiated thymidine indicate that grafted fetal cerebral tissue is vascularized within 24 hours (Krum and Rosenstein, unpublished observations).

The permeability of the vessels within the graft, whether it is inserted into the parenchyma of the cerebellum or upon its pial surface, is the same. The permeability of graft vessels to a small neutral amino acid, alpha-amino isobutyric acid labeled with ^{14}C, has been measured by quantitative autoradiography. The transfer rate across the grafts' vessels is considerably higher than that

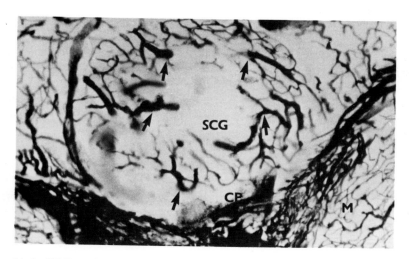

Figure 11-3. SCG graft (SCG) contains numerous India ink-gelatin containing vessels (arrows) as it rests on the medulla (M) and choroid plexus (CP). Twenty-four hours postoperative.

across parenchymal vessels with their blood–brain barrier. It would appear that the permeability of the grafts' vessels to macromolecules such as horseradish peroxidase is retained (Rosenstein and Brightman 1983) as is the permeability to an amino acid. However, our measurements reveal that the transfer rate of the isobutyrate in the grafts is never as high as that of the undisturbed, *in situ* ganglion. Further, the permeability to the amino acid diminishes with the age of the graft, perhaps because of a decrement in the area of fenestrated vasculature. The blood flow, as measured with ^{14}C-labeled antipyrine, is consistently greater in the vessels of grafts that have anastomosed with pial vessels than with parenchymal vessels (Tsubaki et al., unpublished observations). It is conceivable, therefore, that pial and choroidal vessels may provide a more effective source of blood to a graft than do parenchymal vessels.

Placement of an SCG allograft on the surface of the cerebellum has a marked *neurotropic* influence. In the rat, cells of the external granule layer, the outermost mantle of the neonatal cerebellum, begin inward migration toward the Purkinje neurons around postnatal day 7. They complete their journey, forming the internal granule layer, by day 24 (Heinsen 1977) leaving the newly formed molecular layer free of granule cells. When the SCG graft is adjacent to the cerebellum, whole laminae or clusters (Figure 11-4) of granule neurons remain permanently arrested at their superficial point of origin, at the cerebellar surface. This phenomenon does not occur in adjacent folia. Not only are granule neurons arrested, but many of these undergo a post-mitotic anomalous migration out of the confines of the brain in a tissue bridge composed of both granule neurons and glia to enter the foreign graft (Rosenstein and Brightman 1981). In addition, these bridges contain parallel fibers and mossy fibers as the central element of a glomerulus. The ectopic position of glomeruli suggests that the incoming mossy fiber probed the environment in a tropic manner, seeking

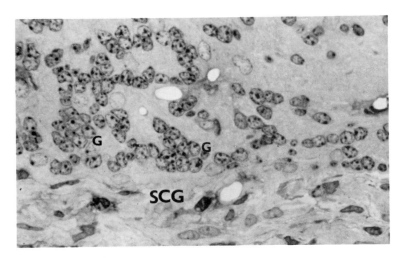

Figure 11-4. Laminae of granular cells (G) are arrested at the surface of the cerebellum contiguous with the SCG graft (SCG). Five months postoperative.

specific groups of granule neurons. Alternatively, the growing mossy fiber was passively entrained by anomalous moving granule cells to which it was synaptically bound.

It has recently been demonstrated that transplanted fetal CNS tissue can produce a similar ectopia in the neonatal cerebellum (Jaeger and Lund 1982). It seems that both the regenerating (PNS) and developing (CNS) tissue can alter the "programmed" neuronal migratory patterns in the cerebellum by, presumably, the secretion of a tropic substance. Based on our previous experiments the substance may well be neuronal as opposed to non-neuronal. When we grafted pieces of fresh and predegenerated sciatic nerve, the latter containing only viable Schwann cells and fibroblasts, there was no neuronal arrest (Rosenstein and Brightman 1981). Moreover, mechanical destruction or inert objects on the cerebellar surface produced no morphological changes. Further characterization of the agents that dramatically affect changes in neuronal migration could be useful in future neural transplantation experiments where rearrangements of neural circuitry are considered.

The presence of a ganglion graft on the undamaged brain surfaces produces changes in both ependyma and astroglia. When a graft is placed in the ventricle, the polarity of some ependymal cells may be altered; the ciliated surfaces turn inward and the basal surface, which now borders the ventricle, extends processes covered by basal lamina over the graft (Rosenstein and Brightman 1979). The entire ependymal lining responds to the graft by altering its normal conformation and forms a bridge extending to meet it (Figure 11–5).

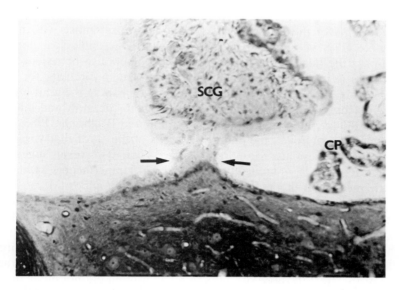

Figure 11-5. A bridge of ependymal and glial (between arrows) extend to meet the SCG graft (SCG) within the fourth ventricle. Choroid plexus (CP). 4-μ section. Six weeks postoperative.

The astroglia adjacent to the SCG graft participate in a subtle gliosis forming numerous thin parallel sheets (Rosenstein and Brightman 1979, Anders and Brightman 1980). It would appear that this gliotic elaboration of the untraumatized brain surface might effectively limit penetration of the regenerating neurites. On the other hand, according to histofluorescence studies, axons from autografted SCG can pass through glial scar tissue after appropriate trauma to enter the parenchyma (Björklund and Stenevi 1977).

After a few weeks post-transplantation, the SCG grafts exert a *gliotropic* effect on the host brain. There is a directed gliosis in which a few astrocytic cell bodies and their processes migrate from the host into the SCG graft. This transposition is determined by immunocytochemistry with anti-sera to glial fibrillary acidic proteins (GFAP) that stains for glial filaments. An advantage here is that GFAP is not found in autonomic ganglia (Jessen and Mirsky 1980), and their presence within the autonomic graft indicates that they have migrated from the undamaged brain (Rosenstein and Brightman 1984). This glial migration occurs from both the medullary and cerebellar surfaces where astroglia form a major part of the tissue bridge. There is still little information on the role played by astroglia in the establishment of cellular domains within transplants and host tissues.

The Blood–Brain Barrier

An intriguing consequence of transplanting peripheral ganglia to the undamaged brain surfaces is the effect on the host BBB. Since the blood vessels of the SCG are mostly fenestrated and permeable to protein (Jacobs 1977), we believed that some of these intrinsic vessels would anastomose with normally impermeable CNS vessels and produce a permanent, biological portal that could by-pass the host BBB. To test this idea horseradish peroxidase (HRP) (m.w. 40,000) is infused systemically and permitted to circulate for 1 to 60 minutes. Within 1 minute HRP reaction product appears in the graft but not in the subjacent brain. Only after 15 minutes are both the graft and underlying brain inundated by the glycoprotein (Rosenstein and Brightman 1983). At the electron microscopic level, the endothelial cells of the cerebellar vessels contain more pits and vesicles than normal (Figure 11-6). This result suggests that the SCG graft might have induced the nearby CNS impermeable capillaries to become permeable. If this is the case then perhaps the imposition of the graft mimics those central endothelial wall linings seen in experimental models by hyperosmolarity (Brightman et al. 1973) or even tumor induction (Groothius et al. 1982). A more likely explanation for the circumvention of the BBB is that, since the HRP was first exuded from SCG vessels and required time in order to reach the interstitial fluid of the brain, the HRP has flowed from the extracellular clefts of the graft to those of the brain. The protein did not enter the brain parenchyma from its blood vessels but rather from the extracellular clefts of the graft (Rosenstein and Brightman 1983). These results reveal an aspect of neural

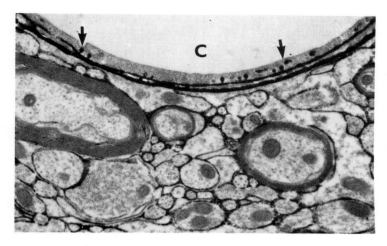

Figure 11-6. Intercellular spaces of the brain parenchyma underlying the SCG graft are filled with HRP 30 minutes after intravascular infusion. Endothelial cell lining a capillary (C) contains many HRP-containing vesicles (arrows). Three months postoperative.

transplantation that heretofore has not been addressed. A significant interaction between host and graft is the confluence of their extracellular compartments; blood-borne substances have access to the host via extracellular clefts of the graft. Future studies on this work will be expanded to include both CNS tissue and adrenal medulla. Not only can a neural graft make axonal connections with its host, but it can also establish extracellular connections. Our observations have broadened the term "connectivity" to include not only neural interconnections but also extracellular ones as well. It is along the interstitial connection that bioactive peptides, amines, and hormones could be exchanged between graft and host.

Acknowledgments. This study was supported in part by NIH grant NS-17468 to J.M.R.

References

Anders, J.J., Brightman, M.W. (1980). Assemblies of particles in the cell membranes of developing, mature and reactive astrocytes. J. Neurocytol. 8, 777–795.

Björklund, A. Stenevi, U. (1977). Experimental reinnervation of the rat hippocampus by grafted sympathetic ganglia. I. Axonal regeneration along the hippocampal fimbria. Brain Res. 138, 259–270.

Björklund, A., Stenevi, U. (1979). Reconstruction of the nigrostriatal dopamine pathway by intercerebral implants. Brain Res. 177, 555–560.

Brightman, M.W., Hori, M., Rappoport, S., Reese, T.S., Westergaard, E. (1973). Osmotic opening of tight junctions in cerebral endothelium. J. Comp. Neurol. 152, 317–326.

Das, G.D., Altman, J. (1972). Studies on the transplantation of developing neural tissue in the mammalian brain. I. Transplantation of cerebellar slabs into the cerebellum of neonate rats. Brain Res. 38, 233–249.

Gash, D., Sladek, C.D., Sladek, J.R. (1980). A model system for analysing functional development of transplanted peptidergic neurons. Peptides Suppl. 1, 125–134.

Groothius, D.R., Fischer, J.M., Lapin, G., Bigner, D.D., Vick, N.A. (1982). Permeability of different experimental brain tumor models to horseradish peroxidase. J. Neuropath. Exp. Neurol. 41, 164–185.

Heinsen, H. (1977). Quantitative anatomical studies of the postnatal development of the cerebellum of the albino rat. Anat. Embryol. 151, 201–218.

Hendry, I.A. (1975). The response of adrenergic neurons to axotomy and nerve growth factor. Brain Res. 94, 87–97.

Imamoto, K., LeBlond, C.P. (1977). Presence of labeled monocytes, macrophages and microglia in a stab wound of the brain following an injection of bone marrow cells labeled with ^{3}H-uridine into rats. J. Comp. Neurol. 174, 255–280.

Jacobs, J.M. (1977). Penetration of systematically injected horseradish peroxidase into ganglia and nerves of the autonomic nervous system. J. Neurocytol. 61, 607–618.

Jaeger, C.B., Lund, R.D. (1982). Influence of grafted glial cells and host mossy fibers on anomalously migrated host granule cells surviving in cortical transplants. Neuroscience 7, 3069–3076.

Jessen, K.R., Mirsky, R. (1980). Glial cells in the enteric nervous system contain glial fibrillary acidic proteins. Nature (London) 286, 736–737.

Lund, R.D., Hauschka, S.D. (1976). Transplanted neural tissue develops connections with host brain. Science 193, 582–584.

Mains, R.E., Patterson, P.H. (1973). Primary cultures of dissociated sympathetic neurons. I. Establishment of long term growth in cultures and studies of differentiated properties. J. Cell Biol. 59, 329–345.

Perlow, M.J., Freed, W.J., Hoffer, B.J., Seiger, A., Olson, L., Wyatt, R. (1979). Brain grafts reduce motor abnormalities produced by destruction of nigrostriatal dopamine system. Science 204, 643–647.

Ramon y Cajal, S. (1928). Degeneration and Regeneration of the Nervous System, Vol. 1. May, R. (trans. and ed.). London: Oxford Press.

Rees, R.P., Bunge, R. (1974). Morphological and cytochemical study of synapses formed in culture between isolated superior cervical ganglion neurons. J. Comp. Neurol. 157, 1–12.

Rosenstein, J.M., Brightman, M.W. (1978). Intact cerebral ventricle as a site for tissue transplantation. Nature (London) 275, 83–85.

Rosenstein, J.M., Brightman, M.W. (1979). Regeneration and myelination in autonomic ganglia transplanted to intact brain surfaces. J. Neurocytol. 8, 359–379.

Rosenstein, J.M., Brightman, M.W. (1981). Anomalous migration of central nervous tissue to transplanted autonomic ganglia. J. Neurocytol. 10, 387–409.

Rosenstein, J.M., Brightman, M.W. (1983). Circumventing the blood-brain barrier with autonomic ganglion transplants. Science 221, 879–881.

Rosenstein, J.M., Brightman, M.W. (1984). Some consequences of grafting autonomic ganglia to brain surfaces. In: Neural Transplants: Development and Function. Sladek, J., Gash, D. (eds.). New York: Plenum Press.

Stenevi, U., Björklund, A., Svendgaard, N. A. (1976). Transplantation of central and peripheral monoamine neurons to the adult rat brain: Techniques and conditions for survival. Brain Res. 114, 1–20.

Chapter 12

A Behavioral and Histological Examination of Young Rats Receiving Homotopic Embryonic Neural Transplants in Motor Cortex

JEFFREY HARNSBERGER and ROBERT B. WALLACE*

General Information

Neural transplantation is a field extensively researched from as early as the beginning of the twentieth century. Studies have been conducted with three broadly defined objectives and have evolved chronologically as follows: (1) the use of transplants (both neuronal and extraneuronal) simply to assess the viability of "nerve grafts," and as a tool for studying regeneration in the central nervous system; (2) studies centering on neural transplantation as a method for elucidating the phenomena of neuronal migration and specificity and the relationship of these events to the ordering of the CNS during embryogenesis; and (3) neural transplantation from the standpoint of a technically viable and specialized field of research, with emphasis on the anatomical, functional, and physiological nature of the transplants. It has been in the context of this latter domain that the clinical implications of transplantation work have recently received considerable attention. A review of the primary studies carried out in these three general subgroups follows.

Early Transplantation Studies with Mammals

Regenerative Capacity of the Central Nervous System

After extensive investigations by Ramon y Cajal and numerous other researchers into the anatomical nature of the mammalian brain, attention began to turn towards the nature of the functional characteristics and capacities of that organ. Early physiological and anatomical studies in general were often directed toward the capabilities of an organ system to recover from injury or disease—the brain, being "the seat of the soul," was not excluded from extensive re-

* University of Hartford, Departments of Psychology and Biology, West Hartford, Connecticut 06117 U.S.A.

search in this area. With the development of the silver-based histological techniques by Ramon y Cajal and Bielschowsky in the early 1900s, investigations into regeneration and repair in the CNS began.

Early research on regenerative events in the central nervous system following insult yielded equivocal results. Ramon y Cajal (1928) summed up a large body of experimental research on central regeneration. His results confirmed earlier findings demonstrating signs of axonal sprouting following both peripheral and central damage. He concluded, however, that such restorative events were extremely limited in the CNS and that extensive regeneration was not accomplished and, in fact, was largely aborted. Extensive studies since then have pointed unequivocally to the fact that the mammalian CNS is quite restricted in terms of its regenerative capacity. For an overview of much of the early work done on regeneration in the central nervous system, the reader is referred to Glees (1955).

Extraneuronal and Peripheral Nervous System Transplants

Early research took a somewhat different tack to study aspects of CNS regeneration in response to events other than trauma. This work involved examining the neuronal events that occurred subsequent to the implantation of viable tissue into the central nervous system. Ranson (1914) and Tidd (1932) transplanted spinal ganglion cells into the cerebral cortex of rats and found that they survived for up to 99 days. Sprouting from these implants, however, reached only the host/donor tissue border. LeGros Clark (1942, 1943), using rabbits, inserted spinal ganglia, sciatic nerve segments, or the stump of cut facial or occipital nerves (posterior primary ramus of the second nerve) into the brain substance. Results showed little if any fiber ingrowth from the host brain, and only limited outgrowth of fibers was seen emanating from the implants that survived. From these studies, LeGros Clark concluded (somewhat erroneously) that there was no regenerative capacity of the intrinsic fibers of the rabbit's brain.

Considerably more success was obtained by Glees (1955), and in his earlier works he pointed out that while LeGros Clark had used homografts (grafts taken from a different animal of the same species), he used autografts (one animal as both donor and host). To test what trophic influences (if any) end organs might have on central regeneration, Glees inserted grafts of Pacinian bodies, temporal muscle, and ectodermal skin (since this has the same embryonic ancestor as neuroectoderm) into the brain of rabbits. While muscle grafts did not survive and did not prompt growth of new cerebral fibers, Pacinian bodies did become revascularized but again showed minimal interconnections with the host brain. Skin grafts into hippocampus and brain stem did, however, give evidence of regenerative attempts on the part of the host brain. These consisted of fairly extensive ingrowths of nerve fibers from the host brain directly into the graft. Additionally, these grafts continued to develop extensively (exhibiting hair follicles, etc.) in the host.

From the above studies, it becomes apparent that although the CNS had very limited intrinsic regenerative capacity, it could act as a culture medium for growth and survival of certain tissue types that had been removed from their original environment. However, peripheral nervous and ectodermal tissue had long been known to have regenerative capacities far superior to that of the central nervous system, and thus viability of such tissue after transplantation would not be unexpected. To look at CNS regenerative phenomena from a slightly different viewpoint, studies examining the fate of central (rather than peripheral) nervous system tissue transplanted to a host brain were undertaken by several researchers.

Central Nervous System Transplants

As early as the 1900s, Ranson (1903) and Saltykow (1905) took neural tissue from the cerebral cortex of rats and transplanted it to the neocortex of adult animals. Although these transplants did not become an integral part of the host brain, they did survive for varying lengths of time and developed sprouting processes. Dunn (1917) utilized neonatal neural tissue and observed fairly extensive fiber outgrowths from cortical slabs transplanted to age-matched hosts, provided a piece of choroid plexus was attached to the donor tissue. Additionally, cortical neurons survived within the transplant and showed growth characteristics quite similar to those in normal cortex; however, their morphology was somewhat different.

In later studies, Greene and Hildegarde (1945) utilized the anterior chamber of the eye of rabbits as a host site for homologous embryonic neocortical donor tissue. Additionally, both human and rabbit embryonic cortical tissues were used as donor tissue in transplants to the guinea pig anterior chamber. All such transplants (including the use of tumor and meninges as donor material) were successful in terms of the growth and survival of the transplants. Adult donor tissue, however, was found not to survive transplantation to the same site.

Both LeGros Clark (1940) and Glees (1955) transplanted fetal neural tissue from rabbits to the brain of adult hosts. In both instances, mature cortical neurons were seen to have differentiated from the primitive neuroblasts and extensive neurofibrillar outgrowths were seen growing out of the transplants.

It should be pointed out that in the latter studies cited, concern was no longer merely with regeneration of the central nervous system *per se*. Rather, the research was beginning to be carried out to assess specifically the inherent capabilities of primitive neural tissue to grow, differentiate, and survive in a site devoid of its original neuroembryological influences. Although no clear-cut conclusions were drawn from these early studies, when viewed collectively, two main points become evident: (1) Anatomical regeneration in the central nervous system in terms of actual neural repair and replacement is negligible, and (2) despite its limited intrinsic regenerative capacity, the CNS does seem to have some capability to accept and integrate with donor neural tissue, especially of fetal origin. After numerous although somewhat equivocal early demonstrations of the transplantability of neural tissue, renewed interest in its applicability to CNS study came with advances in neurohistological techniques (e.g., autoradiography, horseradish perioxidase, and Fink-Heimer staining) that allowed visualization of neuronal pathways of connectivity.

Modern Applications of Neural Transplants

The early investigations of neural transplantation in mammals led to varying degrees of success in terms of growth and differentiation of transplants in the host brain. It did become clear, however, that the most promising results occurred when immature or even fetal brain regions were utilized as donor tissue (LeGros Clark 1940, Greene and Hildegarde 1945, Glees 1955). After this time period, however, transplantation research nevertheless went through a relatively quiescent 15- or 20-year interval before renewed interest in its applicability to the study of embryogenesis of the nervous system arose in the early 1970s. When viewed in retrospect, one realizes that a prime reason for the resurgence of transplantation research was the technological gains that had been made since the 1950s. Tremendous advances in microscopy, neurohistological procedures, and even understanding of the mammalian central nervous system allowed researchers not only to perfect the methods for achieving successful transplants, but also to study in fine detail their development and effect on the host neural environment.

The modern era of transplantation research really began with a series of studies published by G.D. Das and co-workers in the early 1970s. Although previous transplantation had been achieved with varying degrees of success, the research done by Das was the first truly systematic and methodological approach to the study of neural transplantation.

Studies Elucidating the Phenomena of Neuronal Migration and Specificity

In the first study published, Das and Altman (1971) used rats as host and donor animals, both 7 days of age. To allow accurate identification of the transplanted neural tissue, donor animals were injected with [^{3}H]thymidine, thus labeling mitotic cells. Slabs of cerebellar cortex largely containing proliferating cells of the external granular layer were taken from the donors and gently embedded into a surgical incision in the host cerebellum. Host rats were then sacrificed at various times after tranplantation, and the fate of the transplanted tissue followed by processing the brains for autoradiography.

The results of Das and Altman's original study, as well as those from a similar one confirming the first (Das and Altman 1972), indicated that both the transplants and the host brains did undergo fairly substantial degenerative changes: however, this did not seem to produce any chronic pathologic changes in the cerebella. Furthermore, a few days following transplantation, large numbers of labeled spindle-shaped cells could be seen streaming from the external layer of the transplants into the cortex of the host cerebellum. In animals that were allowed to survive for 10 to 16 days, labeled cells were seen to have migrated to the internal and molecular layers of the host. It is interesting to note that this migration occurred even amidst the degenerative and regenerative events that were occurring subsequent to the initial trauma. By examining the labeled cells, it was found that these were granule, basket, and stellate cells, indicating that the donor neuronal precursors had differentiated in the host cerebellum. To insure that these results were not merely species specific, a similiar study was conducted with rabbits and the same pattern of results was seen (Das 1973).

The relevance of these studies to neurogenesis is apparent. For example, were the transplanted neural elements predetermined to become granule, basket, and stellate cells, or did the host neural environment influence in some way the differentiation of these immature neurons? Such questions of pluripotency and specified development had long been researched, and neural tranplantation appeared to be a new method whereby these questions could be further explored.

In 1974, Das published an extensive study (Das 1974) in which a new technique for transplantation in rats was presented, technical details and comments of which were expanded upon in a later work (Das 1979). Additionally, utilizing the techniques of autoradiography and cresyl-violet staining, Das presented in this study the first detailed elaboration of the applicability of neural transplants specifically to studies of neurogenesis.

The techniques that Das (1974, 1979) developed had several advantages over previous methods: (1) There was decreased trauma to the host neural tissue, thus reducing the necrotic changes that were often seen subsequent to the transplantation procedure; (2) specific neural structures (e.g., cerebellum, inferior colliculus, diencephalon, brain stem, etc.) were able to be isolated, obtained, and transplanted selectively; and (3) it utilized embryonic neural tissue, specifically neuroblasts (post-mitotic, undifferentiated neurons), and thus there were no dendritic or axonal processes that would be dismembered from the neurons through actual physical manipulation during the transplant procedure. These advances greatly improved the success rate for transplantation such that growth, survival, and integration of the transplants could be achieved in nearly all cases.

In terms of neuroembryogenesis, Das (1974) was able to demonstrate several points from this study: (1) Neuroblasts from 18-day-old donor embryos are specified to differentiate into neurons defined by their source of origin; i.e., the fate of the donor neuroblasts was largely predetermined and not influenced by the host neural environment; (2) homotopic transplants appeared continuous or blended with, while heterotopic transplants were distinct from, the host neural tissue—this indicating some sort of affinity between cells of similar embryonic origin; (3) the cytoarchitectural and topographic organization achieved by the differentiated transplant reflected specification of the neuroblastic tissue according to its site of origin—e.g., transplanted embryonic cerebellar tissue in general maintained its typical trilaminar appearance after differentiation, while nuclear structures (brain stem, diencephalon) displayed characteristic nuclear appearance even after being transplanted to cerebellum; and (4) the developing transplant did not affect the normal cytoarchitectural or morphological embryogenesis of the host brain.

Lastly, in this study Das emphasized that neural transplantation could not, as in the past, be defined merely by the fact that transplants survive and grow, for this could be achieved in tissue cultures. Das continued that, in addition, there must necessarily be anatomical integration of the transplanted tissue with the host, either in terms of sharing a common neuropil or the exchange of axons and dendrites between the two (transplant and host). This definition would therefore exclude many of the previous studies (e.g., transplants enveloped by pia mater, transplants to the anterior chamber of the eye, etc.) as being true neural transplants, and appropriately so if conclusions are to be made with regard to neuroembryogenesis and any possible functional or physiological aspects of the transplants.

In what would be the first of several extensive and important studies in the field of transplantation research, Lund and Hauschka (1976) made the first in-depth analysis of the pathways of connectivity between transplant and host neural tissue. Utilizing rats and a transplantation technique similar to that developed by Das (1979), superior collicular fragments of 15- and 16-day-old donor embryos were transplanted into homologous sites of newborn hosts. In the hope of identifying fiber projections ramifying between transplant and host, the Fink-Heimer method for staining degenerating axons, a neurofibrillar stain, and autoradiography were employed.

Results from the Fink-Heimer technique provided evidence that the transplanted superior collicular tissue was able to receive afferents from host structures that would normally innervate it, e.g., retina and visual cortex. Additionally, neurofibrillar staining demonstrated numerous fiber bundles coursing into and out of the transplant; these were presumed to be afferent and efferent axons. Data from this study also indicated that the transplant was innvervated by host afferents in a specific manner. This was presumed to be due to the fact that the transplant was not innervated totally by host visual afferents, even if placed in a region normally receiving many such afferents. From this, it was suggested that only those regions of the transplants that would normally receive visual afferents possess specific affinities for these visual inputs. Conversely, the areas of the transplant that possessed no such affinity did not have the capacity to influence the host afferents.

These relatively early studies by Das and Lund and Hauschka were the first comprehensive analyses of the techniques, applicability, and ramifications of neural transplants. The utility of applying neural transplantation to questions concerning the embryogenesis of the nervous system had become apparent. It is important, however, to note at this point that the mechanisms (biochemical or otherwise) underlying these observations were not being studied by these investigators. Rather, novel phenomenological and anatomical discoveries were being made to give other researchers possible approaches to the problem of solving questions of the mechanics of neurogenesis, e.g., genetic preprogramming, cell–cell interactions, tissue specificities, etc.

Systematic transplantation research was, however, only in its infancey, and detailed studies utilizing modern microscopy and neuroanatomical tracing techniques could proceed now that many of the technical and methodological difficulties had been conquered. After several quiet years, many studies began to appear in the late 1970s that carried these earlier transplantation investigations several steps further.

The Effects of Existing Neuronal Substrate on Developing Nerve Fibers

To evaluate in more detail the untrastructure of neural tissue transplanted into cerebellum, Das (1975, 1976) used Golgi–Cox preparations as well as electron microscopy. Results indicated that in both homo- and heterotopic transplants, the basic pattern of dendritic arborization was specified by the site of tissue origin. However, host influences were for the first time demonstrated because both the course and length of dendritic branches were altered. This suggested that the general dendritic pattern that neuroblasts differentiate into is predetermined: however, the extent of this growth is influenced in some way (possibly trophic influences, effect of host afferents, etc.) by the host neural tissue. Additionally, utilizing electron microscopic analysis, differentiated neuroblasts were found to have synapses on their somata and dendrites, suggesting that the transplants may have been physiologically active.

Further confirmation of these results was published later by Das (1979) in a more extensive study utilizing embryonic heterotopic transplants from spinal cord, brain stem, thalamus, hypothalamus, hippocampus, cerebral cortex, and basal ganglia into cerebellum. Again, the neuroblasts had developed dendritic patterns nearly identical to those that would have developed had they remained in their original location. Additionally, dendritic and axonal projections could be seen extending between the host neural tissue and transplant. Golgi studies demonstrating results nearly identical to these were later reported by Jaeger and Lund (1981) utilizing cortical transplants into the tectum of neonatal rats.

Examining Ordering of CNS Connections During Neuroembyrogenesis

To elucidate the patterns of connectivity in heterotopic cerebellar transplants, Das and co-workers utilized some of the methods used earlier by Lund and Hauschka (Hallas et al. 1980b, Oblinger et al 1980). In these studies, both host afferents and transplant efferents were identified using Fink-Heimer, Bodian, and HRP staining techniques.

Afferents included projections from contralateral inferior olivary nuclei, pontine nuclei, ipsilateral spinal cord, and lateral reticular nuclei. Efferents were observed to project to the deep cerebellar nuclei, reticular formation, and medullary cerebellar regions; additionally, fibers were identified ramifying within the transplant itself. Both afferents and efferents were concluded to be nonspecific in that it appeared to be the topographic availability of fibers that determined which connections would or would not be made. For example, transplanted tissue in cerebellum seemed to project to sites that would normally be innervated by fibers from that region of the host cerebellum. Similarly, cerebral cortex transplanted to cerebellum did not receive distant afferents, for example, from thalamus, as it normally would.

In an extension of these studies on connectivity of the transplants, Oblinger and Das (1981) examined the effect of host age on afferent innervation of the transplant. In this work, it was found that transplants in more immature animals received a greater proportion of afferents, presumably reflecting a more plastic state of the younger host brain.

Later in the 1970s and early 1980s, Jaeger and Lund extended in several respects the work of Lund and Hauschka (1976). Utilizing embryonic neural tissue from the dorsal telencephalic vesicle of rats as donor tissue, transplants were made into either tectum or occipital cortex of newborn hosts (Jaeger and Lund 1978). Neurofibrillar staining demonstrated successful transplantation in terms of fiber connections coursing both between host and donor tissue, as well as within the transplant itself.

Autoradiography indicated that the transplanted cortical tissue continued normal cell histogenesis despite its new environment within the host tectum or cerebral cortex (Jaeger and Lund 1980a). The differentiated transplants did display, however, an abnormal distribution, e.g., patchy distribution rather than laminar organization. This it was hypothesized, was due either to an actual physical disturbance of the tissue during transplantation or to the absence of normal extrinsic fiber projections to the cortical tissue. Demonstrating successful transplantation into this neuroanatomical system, quite different embryologically from the cerebellum utilized by Das et al., lent itself well to in-depth studies of connectivity within this framework.

In a series of more extensive studies, Jaeger and Lund (1979a,b, 1980b) examined the morphology and efferent and afferent connections of occipital cortex transplants situated in the tectum of host rats. Utilizing a combination of Golgi impregnation, autoradiography, horseradish peroxidase (HRP) tracing, Fink-Heimer, and neurofibrillar procedures, a detailed evaluation of the nature of these transplants was achieved.

In the mature transplants, the three cell types typical of occipital cortex were identified using the Golgi method, namely, pyramidal cells and spiney and smooth stellate cells (Jaeger and Lund 1980b, 1981). Generally, these cortical transplants had a structural morphology quite similar to that of their original anatomical location without the normally well-defined degree of lamination. Additionally, the transplants had a high degree of internal fiber ramification. The extent of these host/donor fiber interactions was next researched.

In examinations of host afferents, numerous axonal projections were seen coursing to the transplant. These included those from occipital, somatosensory, and cingulate cortices, superior colliculus, pretectal areas, and various brain stem regions (central gray, raphe nuclei, hypothalamus). None, however, were seen from retina, lateral geniculate nucleus (LGN), or dorsal thalamus. In general, it was found that these afferent connections were fairly specific; for example, nearby neurons might fail to innervate the transplant, while distant sites sent fibers to the transplant. Clearly, however, some unexpected connections were made, while some expected ones were not observed, e.g., from LGN. These results were suggested to indicate that both topographical (Jaeger and Lund 1979a) as well as neuron-specific type influences (Jaeger and Lund 1980b) were directing the host afferents.

Transplant efferents tended to show a more variable pattern, but in general, projections were to superior colliculus and pretectal regions (Jaeger and Lund 1979b, 1980b). The collicular projections were expected of occipital cortex; however, the fibers to central gray were atypical. Again, transplant fibers did not merely innervate local host regions. From these results, further work was proposed to establish more clearly whether it is inherent properties of the donor tissue or host influences that determine the extent and specificity of connections.

Studies focusing on patterns of connectivity were conducted by McLoon and Lund (1979, 1980) in which embryonic retinal tissue was transplanted to superior colliculus of newborn rats. Fully differentiated transplants showed relatively normal cell and plexiform layers; however, some minor abnormalities were seen in terms of the layering of the different retinal cell types as well as underdevelopment of the outer photoreceptor segments.

Neurofibrillar, HRP, and Fink-Heimer procedures revealed various transplant projections. These consisted mainly of efferents to optic tract and nuclei that are normally retino-recipient, e.g., superior colliculus, pretectum, and lateral geniculate nucleus. Those regions closest to the transplant efferents received the heaviest fiber distribution, while those most distant received a lighter innervation. Interestingly, early unilateral enucleation contralateral to the site of the transplant caused a more extensive efferent fiber projection from the transplant; a lack of host afferent competition at potential synaptic sites was offered as a possible explanation. This research tended to suggest a more special affinity of retinal efferents for visual structures, this not being the case, as shown earlier, with cortical transplants to the same region (Jaeger and Lund 1980).

Most recently, Harvey and Lund (1981) have transplanted embryonic tectal tissue into the tectum of newborn rats. As with earlier transplantation of retinal and cortical tissue to the same region, tectal transplants developed a cytoarchitecture quite similar to a normally differentiated tectum. Using retrograde HRP tracing techniques, labeled cells were identified in nearly 50 host regions. Most dense afferent connections were from occipital cortex; however, other projections were seen from pretectum, parabigeminal nucleus, and superior and inferior colliculi. In the first study of this system (Lund and Harvey 1981), retinal afferents were identified using anterograde tracing techniques; this was not found to be the case, however, in the second study, which utilized retrograde labeling. These discrepancies were most likely due to the fact that the retina projects to very discrete regions of the transplants, these regions being infrequently labeled when retrograde techniques are used.

Results from these studies suggested that despite their abnormal position and the donor/host age differences, transplanted tectum could grow and differentiate to make fairly normal fiber connections. The fact that afferents did not simply innervate the transplant as a result of local proximity and that, in general, only projections from structures that would normally innervate the tectum were seen coursing into the transplant again tend to suggest some sort of host/transplant selectivity of connections (Harvey and Lund 1981). The fiber connections demonstrated in the tectum-tectum transplant model also were quite clearly different from cortical-tectum and retinal-tectum transplants, further supporting the concept of unique cytoarchitectural and embryological specificities of each system.

When viewed collectively, these studies point to the fact that neural transplantation is possible at several different levels and can be utilized in studies of neurogenesis. There remains, however, another aspect of transplantation research that has in recent years received considerable attention. This aspect applies to studies that have as their goal simply elucidating and expanding the field of neural transplantation as a specialized area of scientific inquiry. It is within this realm that the more functional and physiological aspects of transplant/host interaction are examined.

Neural Transplantation as a Specialized Field of Research

Studies on the Nature of Neural Transplants

One of the primary limitations of much of the transplant research has been the restriction of its use to young host animals. Embryonic neural tissue had clearly been shown to be the optimal donor tissue; however, even this tissue did not seem to grow or survive in adult hosts (Das 1974). In fact, much of the early transplantation research was likely labeled a failure owing to the use of mature donor as well as host neural tissue. The major problem, however, with the use of adult hosts may not have been simply an inherent inability of the mature brain to accept transplants, but rather may have reflected a technological level not sophisticated enough to achieve successful transplantations in adult hosts.

In studies addressing this issue, Stenevi, et al. (1976) and Svengaard (1977) were able to demonstrate successful transplantation of embryonic and newborn CNS neural tissue containing the neurotransmitters norepinephrine, dopamine, and 5-HT and pieces of superior cervical ganglion into the choroidal fissure of adult rat brains. Success in this location was found to be due largely to the immediate presence of a rich vascular bed; this was confirmed from demonstrations of successful transplantation using an artificial vascular bed of iris tissue. Success, however, was not achieved with similar intracerebral transplants. Although intriguing in terms of success of neural transplantation into the adult brain, the restricted location and conditions for transplant viability limited the generalizability and applicability of these results.

After advancing significantly the technique of neural transplantation, Das (1977) and Das and Hallas (1978) were able to demonstrate unequivocally successful transplantation into forebrain and cerebellum of host rats of various ages. Animals ranged in age from 3 to 12 months and all transplants were seen to be fully integrated with the host neuropil. In the most systematic study of transplant histogenesis, Das et al. (1980) compared the growth characteristics of embryonic donor tissue ranging in age from 15 to 21 gestational days. Futhermore, Hallas et al. (1980a) also examined in detail the volumetric growth of transplants in host animals 5 to 180 days of age.

Though successful in all respects in terms of cytoarchitectural differentiation and integration with host neuropil, transplants in younger hosts and from more immature embryos were found to afford the greatest growth potential. In terms of host age, growth was presumed to be restricted owing to the space-limiting effect of the more ossified cranium in older hosts. Donor tissue from 15-day-old embryos yielded a larger transplant in any age host than did any older embryonic tissue. This was due to the relatively higher proportion of actively mitotic neuroepithelial cells in the younger embryos. Such success in adult hosts was quite important in extending the realm of significance of future transplantation research.

In an effort to look specifically at the nature and course of various stages of transplant growth in rats, Das (1978) sacrificed host animals after having received cortical transplants into cerebellum as neonates at 2 and 4 hours, and at various times between 1 and 60 days. Although degenerative changes were seen initially (reaching a maximum by 12–24 hours), both transplants and host brain subsequently grew and differentiated normally, indicating some sort of mutual as well as independent regenerative capacity of both host and transplant neural tissue.

Transplants of neural tissue into the adult rat brain have also produced surprising results in terms of the mitotic activity and fiber outgrowth from the mature host neural tissue. Lundberg and Mollgard (1979) demonstrated a 3-mm zone of increased mitotic activity in occipital cortex, hippocampus, and brain stem following implantation of fetal CNS tissue. Weinberg and Raine (1980) have demonstrated extensive axonal sprouting from local CNS tissue into peripheral nerve segments implanted into rat midbrain. Additionally, myelinization of these segments seemed to be enhanced. Kromer (1980) has also shown that hippocampal transplants actually prevented typical astrocytic reactions and reduced the formation of glial scar at the interface between host brain and transplant.

These three studies again point to the possibility of some factor or influence from neural transplants on the host brain. Although the nature of these influences is unknown, the transplants appear to induce some form of regenerative activity on the part of even the adult host brain. The clinical implications of these findings, although premature and requiring further study, are obvious.

Physiological and Functional Properties of Neural Transplants

Several studies have been conducted to test more directly the functional and physiological properties of neural transplants in various brain regions. In research by Kimura et al. (1980), the striata of rats with an animal "model" of Huntington's disease were used as a host site. Four to 6 weeks following kanic acid lesioning of the striatum, neonatal striatal tissue was injected into the lesioned area. Analysis showed that the transplanted tissue grew, differentiated, formed fiber connections, and was metabolically active. Within this clinical model, a determination of the functional and physiological properties of the transplant was proposed.

In a study aimed specifically at analyzing the functional nature of neural transplants, Björklund and Stenevi (1979) transplanted embryonic substantia nigral tissue into adult rats that had several weeks earlier received unilateral 6-hydroxydopamine-lesioning of dopaminergic neurons of the substantia nigra. Long-term transplant survival was demonstrated, as well as fiber projections to regions normally receiving dopaminergic innervation in a majority of host brains. More interestingly, however, was the correlation of attenuation of amphetamine-induced ipsilateral turning with the magnitude of transplant dopamine-containing fiber ingrowth to the denervated striatum that occured over time. Perlow et al. (1979), utilizing this same anatomical system and the rotating rat model of Parkinson's disease, demonstrated promising results very similar to those of Björklund and Stenevi even up to 9 months post-surgery. These studies suggest this work as a possible method for studying functional recovery in human diseases involving this neuroanatomical substrate such as in Parkinson's disease.

Other evidence of the more physiological capacity of neural transplants was presented by Gash et al. (1975), utilizing hypophysectomized female rats. Embryonic Rathke's pouch tissue was transplanted into the hypothalamus of these rats and assays for LH and FSH were performed 4 weeks later. Stimulation of target organs by LH and FSH was detected in the host females indicating the possibility of a physiologically active transplant. Further study by Gash et al. (1979) demonstrated similar results using supraoptic neural transplants into adult rats congenitally lacking vasopressin-producing neurons. In both cases, however, there was considerable question as to the growth characteristics of these transplants in terms of host/donor integration. Additionally, transplants in the first study were found, in many cases, to be neoplastic in nature.

Electrophysiological Studies of the Transplants

Probably the first systematic electrophysiological work done on neural transplants was that by Björklund et al. (1979). Embryonic neural tissue from the area of locus coeruleus was transplanted into the hippocampus of rats in which adrenergic input has been removed by 6-hydroxydopamine and sympathectomy. In general, fairly specific anatomical reinnervation and integration by the transplant with hippocampus could be demonstrated. Electrophysiologic examinations showed spontaneous firing of transplant cells and an increased rate when aspartate was applied. Stimulation of the transplant also inhibited the electrical activity of the hippocampal cells (the hippocampus normally receives inhibitory innervation from the locus coeruleus), and this inhibition was reduced significantly by beta-receptor antagonists. This demonstration of the physiological activity and functional host/donor interactions is an extremely important step in assessing possibilities for the functional applicability of neural transplants.

Behavioral Examinations of Animals Receiving Neural Transplants

In the first studies looking specifically at the behavioral correlates of intercerebral transplants, Wallace and Das (1982) examined the effects of heterotopic transplants into the cerebella of neonatal rats. Animals receiving transplants were compared to those receiving cerebellar lesions and normal controls on a series of behavioral tests designed to assess motor functioning. While controls and transplants showed virtually no behavioral deficits, the lesioned animals were quite impaired. Because the transplant had caused during its growth and differentiation nearly an 80% compressive lesion of the host brain, it was posited that the transplant had in fact assumed some functional role.

Clinical Implications of Neural Transplants

As one reviews the literature on the physiological and functional properties of neural transplants, it is difficult to escape allusions to the clinical possibilities for such work. In fact, the studies by Kimura et al. (1980), Björklund and Stenevi (1979), and Perlow et al. (1979) specifically mention application of their research to investigations of neurological disorders such as Parkinson's disease.

In order for transplantation research to move in the direction of practical clinical application, an important first step would be, as in the case of any organ transplantation, having donor tissue available for immediate use. Attempts to culture and store viable embryonic neural tissue have thus been attempted.

Recently, McLoon et al. (1981) have been successful in culturing 14-day-old embryonic rat retinal explants for 2 to 14 days prior to transplantation to host superior colliculus. The normal lamination pattern was observed in the transplanted retinae as well as many of the fiber projections previously described (McLoon and Lund 1980).

In a more striking demonstration of the viability of stored neural tissue, Houle and Das (1980a,b) transplanted embryonic cortical tissue that had been kept frozen for 6 hours, 7 days, and 130 days. This procedure involved the use of an ultra-freeze and a specific sequence for the freezing and subsequent thawing of the neural tissue before transplantation. Deviation from this sequence resulted in donor tissue that was not viable.

Analysis of the differentiated transplants derived from the frozen neural tissue revealed cytoarchitecture and morphology nearly identical to that of normal transplants (Das 1975). These results were actually quite important in terms of hopes for transplantation in higher mammals, where storage of donor tissue might be required until conditions of optimal host age, etc., could be met. Additionally, this is an extremely important first step if clinical applications for neural transplants are to be realistically considered.

An anatomical location that would lend itself well to studies of the clinical application of neural transplants would be the spinal cord. Das (1981) has demonstrated that neural transplantation can even be successfully performed in the spinal cord of adult rats. The transplants became fully integrated with the host spinal cord and displayed morphology similar to their site of origin. Demonstrating successful transplants of this type in higher mammals would greatly advance the realm of clinical significance for neural transplants.

It should be emphasized that the clinical possibilities for neural transplants are presently only intriguing at best. The practical and technical difficulties of extending the transplantation procedure to higher mammals are immense. One must therefore keep in mind that at this point, speculation made from current research on the clinical future of neural transplants is just that—purely speculation.

Motor Cortex of the Rat: Its Applicability to Transplantation Studies

Reviewing the literature on neural transplantation leaves little doubt that it is an extremely relevant and expanding field of research in terms of examining neural mechanisms. However, to examine further the applicability (clinical and otherwise) of such research, new neuroanatomical locations need to be utilized as host sites; additionally, the functional implications of neural transplants require continued investigation. The motor cortex of rats appears to satisfy both of these prerequisites and thus will be discussed in terms of its anatomy, behavioral correlates, and potential as a host site for neural transplantation.

Cerebral Cortex as a Host Site for Neural Transplants

In the past, the cerebral cortex of rats has been used with limited success as a host structure for neural transplants (Ranson 1903, Saltykow 1905, Dunn 1917). Of these studies, Dunn appeared to have the most success, utilizing neonatal donors as well as hosts. More recently, Wenzel and Barlehner (1969) used slabs of adult cortex of mice as donor tissue and achieved marginal success in transplanting these to animals with extirpated sections of cerebral cortex. Success in terms of transplantation, it should be recalled, is defined not only as growth and differentiation of the transplant, but also anatomical integration of the donor tissue with the host neuropil. Implicit in this definition is the exchange of axonal fiber projections between the donor and host parenchyma. Most recently, Jaeger and Lund (1980a) have had considerable success in transplanting embryonic occipital cortex into the homologous location of rats. These studies indicate that cerebral cortex may be well suited as a recipient site for homotopic transplants. Presumably, any cortical region, such as motor cortex, would serve as an equally good host site.

Before delving directly into the possibilities for motor cortex in studies of neural transplantation, a brief discussion of this neuroanatomical entity, specifically in terms of the rat, is warranted.

Topographical Anatomy of the Rat Motor Cortex

Krieg (1946a,b) amassed a tremendous volume of data in the first systematic study of the topography and structure of the cerebral cortex of the rat. Utilizing earlier work by Lashley (1921) on "stimulable area" and effects on the control of locomotor activity, Krieg described a well-delineated region of the anterolateral cerebral cortex simply as "frontal cortex." Krieg further classified individual areas within this region by number, much like the system developed by Brodmann for the human brain. Later Settlage et al. (1949) after more extended studies labeled this same region as motor cortex, this corresponding to Krieg's areas 4, 6, 10, and 8.

More recently, Hall and Lindholm (1974) mapped the motor and somatosensory cortices of rats utilizing electrophysiological techniques. The area delineated by these researchers extended approximately 3 mm posterior and 5 mm anterior to bregma and extended 4 mm laterally from close to the sagittal suture. Of course, this description refers to the cortex underlying the cranial landmarks and is thus not exact and uniform for each animal. Generally, the cortical areas involved with control of the trunk centered on an area about 2 mm lateral to bregma, areas of forelimb control were located anterior to the trunk area, and cortical areas for hindlimb movement were posterior to the trunk region. Areas concerned with movement of vibrissae, rhinarium, jaw, lips, tongue, eyes, and eyelids generally were located more medial and rostral to the trunk and limb areas. This remains the most accurate, complete, and detailed analysis of the anatomical and functional properties of the rat motor cortex available.

Behavioral Correlates of Motor Cortex Function in the Rat

Analyses of motor cortex in terms of the behavioral manifestations of neuronal mechanisms have come largely from ablation studies. Lashley (1921) ascribed the function of cortical motor regions to be one primarily involved with regulation of postural reflexes. More recent research has yielded fairly dichotomous results depending on the region and extent of motor cortex lesioned.

In one set of studies, Castro (1972) and Spiliotis and Thompson (1973) lesioned the more frontal regions of motor cortex. From these works, it was concluded that damage to this area resulted in deficits on tasks that required precise use of the forepaw for manipulation and grasping. Price and Fowler (1981) have confirmed these results using a computerized analysis of force and rate of discrete forepaw responses. Quite different results, however, were seen when Maier (1935) lesioned more caudal areas of rat motor cortex. Damage here resulted in severe impairment of rats' ability to traverse a narrow elevated walkay. These results have been largely confirmed in more recent work by Gentile, et al. (1978) utilizing cinematographic analysis of locomotion on a walkway.

Utilizing irradiation, D'Amato and Hicks (1980) have produced more generalized cortical damage in rats. Behavioral results have demonstrated both difficulties in paw placement and locomotion resulting from corticospinal neuron depopulation in both the anterior and posterior motor areas.

Rationale for Utilizing Motor Cortex in Transplantation Research

Although not by any means exhaustive of the research carried out on the motor cortex of rats, the cited literature gives an overview of some of the more relevant studies. Particularly interesting is the fact that rats do in fact have at least a rough equivalent of the primate motor cortex; thus, the rationale for utilizing the rat to obtain applicable and relevant information on the function as well as dysfunction of this cortical region.

Extending the methods of neural transplantation to the motor cortex of rats appears technically feasible, although such research with this anatomical substrate is relatively sparse. As is apparent from the literature reviewed, several studies have successfully demonstrated methods for assessing motor cortex deficits. Thus, behavioral manifestations of motor cortex integrity should be apparent and quantifiable utilizing various experimental paradigms. Comparisons of animals receiving homotopic neural transplants into motor cortex to animals sustaining lesions to the same region are expected to yield needed information with respect to the possible functional characteristics of host-transplant neural interactions.

Methods

Subjects

Twenty-three Long-Evans hooded rats (obtained commercially from Blue Spruce Farms, Inc.), approximately 1 month of age on arrival in the Developmental Psychobiology Laboratories at the University of Hartford, served as subjects for this study. Ten of these animals received homotopic neural transplants, eight sustained cortical aspiration lesions, and five underwent sham operations and served as controls.

Apparatus

The apparati used in this study are described below under two separate subheadings. The first will consist of the major materials that were incorporated into the surgical procedures, and the second is a general description of the various items of behavioral test equipment that were used to evaluate the subjects.

Surgical Set-Up

The animal surgery room at the University of Hartford was utilized to perform all surgical procedures. Instrumental to these surgeries was the use of an Olympus OME surgical microscope to perform both the transplantation and lesioning. A stereotaxic apparatus was used to maintain the animals' heads in proper position during the drilling of burr holes in performing craniectomies on animals that were to receive lesions. Drilling of burr holes in the rat crania was performed with an Emesco dental drill.

Sodium pentobarbital (Nembutal) was used to induce deep anethesia in animals prior to each surgery. Various sterilized microsurgical and standard surgical instruments, especially important being microdissecting forceps, were used during both the transplantation and lesioning procedures. Serrefine clamps were available for temporarily closing surgical incisions so that batches of animals could be prepared to undergo experimental manipulations. Sterile lactated Ringer's solution was used for dissection and temporary storing of the embryonic neural tissue and for irrigation during all surgeries. Sterile gauze pads and glass petri dishes were on hand to use during dissection of the embryos. Gelfoam (Upjohn Co.) and sterile gauze pads were utilized to achieve hemostasis and sterile 5-0 twisted silk sutures were used in the closure of all surgical wounds. Topical antibacterial spray and injections of pennicillin (Wyeth Bicillin) were used to minimize the chances of postoperative wound or systemic infection.

To effect the actual transplantation of neural tissue, a glass tuberculin microsyringe with a 0.05-cc capacity was utilized. Attached to the syringe with epoxy cement was a thin-walled glass capillary tube 3 cm long, 0.8 mm in outer diameter, and 0.6 mm in inner diameter. Before mounting, the capillary tube was ground at one end to an oblique, sharp point (about 45°); subsequently, the opposite end was cemented into the neck of the glass syringe. For a more detailed description of the specifics of the syringe used for transplantation, the reader is referred to Das *et al.* (1979).

The lesioning procedure, which first required access to the brain substance, was achieved by making burr holes with a dental drill followed by chipping away the desired section of cranium using microrongeurs. Aspiration lesions were made using blunted 15-, 18-, and 20-guage syringe needles angled to allow easy access to the cortex. These were then connected through a suction cannula adapter to an electrical suction unit (Air Shield-Dia Pump). Suction pressure could be regulated with this apparatus as well as by using the thumb-hole in the suction cannula adapter.

Behavioral Tests

The battery of behavioral tests used in this study included: (1) neurological examination; (2) an open field test; (3) activity measurement in activity wheels; and (4) an elevated walkway task. The neurological exam utilized several approaches to assess the integrity of various CNS levels. Materials required for this test included: forceps, thin metal wire, several pads of foam rubber, a wire-mesh platform, a 1-inch diameter dowel, red safe-light filter, white noise source, a magnifying glass, a 30 c × 30 cm piece of plexiglass, a short length of rubber tubing, a stop watch, and a clean table on which the testing could be conducted.

The open field apparatus consisted of a 61 c × 61 c × 46 cm open box with plexiglass sides and a floor demarcated into 10 c × 10 cm squares. A red safe-light filter was used throughout the testing, and electrical counters were employed to tabulate the various behaviors. Various objects were also placed in the bottom of the box to provide manipulanda for the animals while being observed. The whole open field unit was elevated onto a table to allow easy observation of the animal. Seventy percent ethyl alcohol was used to quickly swab out the inside of the apparatus between each animal to eliminate possible olfactory cues from previously tested subjects.

Standard commercially available activity wheels (Lafayette Instrument Co.) that measure activity by digitally counting wheel revolutions were used to quantify animal movements.

The elevated walkway apparatus consisted of a piece of smooth wood 1.53 m long and 2.9 cm wide. The length was marked off in 8-cm intervals to allow calculation of the total distance traversed in a single test session. The entire apparatus was elevated 80 cm off the ground during the experimental sessions.

Surgical Techniques and Methods

The surgical procedures involved two distinct aspects, the transplantation of neural tissue and making the aspiration lesions. The sequence of events for the transplantation is dealt with first and consists of a general overview of the procedure; for a more detailed description of the procedure, the reader is referred to Das *et al.* (1979).

Transplantation Procedures

Care was taken to insure that before either of the two surgeries was begun, the surgery room had been thoroughly disinfected and that sufficient quantities and types of sterilized surgical instruments and supplies were available. Sterile surgical gloves and clean lab attire were worn by all personnel directly involved with the surgeries.

Subjects were 2 months of age on the day of surgery. Atropine was given one-half hour prior to surgery (1 mg/kg body weight), and subsequently deep anesthesia was induced using sodium pentobarbital (35 mg/kg body weight) prior to beginning any surgical procedures.

Before the transplantation of neural tissue could take place, viable donor embryos of 17 gestational days had to be obtained from a pregnant female rat. To accomplish this, female rats were placed with a proven male stud overnight, and sperm tests were performed the next morning on the females. Any females showing sperm-positive tests as determined by $400\times$ microscopic examination of vaginal smears were separated from the male and housed individually; this was designated as day 1 of gestation.

On day 17 of gestation, the donor embryos were removed from the mother via caesarian section. With the female deeply anesthetized and kept warm on a heating pad, the abdomen was shaved and prepped with betadine and a longitudinal abdominal incision 4 cm long was made. The uterine horns were gently exposed to check for viable embryos; with the number of such embryos determined, they were replaced into the abdominal cavity. A gauze pad moistened with sterile lactated Ringer's solution was used to pack the surgical wound. As donor embryos were needed, they were gently dissected out of the musculature of the uterus using fine forceps; at this point, the amniotic sac was not punctured. An embryo was then placed on a sterile gauze pad moistened with Ringer's lactate in a sterile petri dish.

Dissection of the embryo was then begun and carried out under the surgical microscope. The amniotic sac was punctured and the embryo exposed; viability was checked by looking for a heartbeat and reflexive movements of the limbs. Using fine-tipped microdissecting forceps, the integument and osteoid cranium were dissected away. The meningeal membranes were then gently teased away, thus exposing the brain *in situ*. In a modification of Das' original technique (Das *et al.* 1979) curved (nearly 90°) fine dissecting forceps were gently positioned under the brain in the base of the skull. By gently lifting the brain and at the same time slightly opening and closing the forceps to tear away any connective tissue and cranial nerve attachments, the entire intact brain at the level of the brain stem could be lifted from the open cranium. The brain was transferred (still positioned cradlelike in the curved tips of the forceps) to a sterile glass petri dish containing 2 ml of lactated Ringer's solution where further dissection was carried out.

At this point it should be mentioned that all dissection was carried out as rapidly as could be achieved skillfully, allowing the brain to be exposed to the air for as little time as possible. Dissection in the glass petri dish was carried out with the brain totally immersed in the Ringer's solution. Using the microdissecting forceps, the desired area of the brain (in this case cerebral cortex) was dissected away from the other structures. Mesenchymal tissue and vasculature were then meticulously teased away from the actual neural tissue, leaving in theory only embryonic neuroblasts. This tissue was then carefully drawn up into the tip of the 0.5-cc glass microsyringe so that only the 3-cm length of the specially fitted capillary tubing was filled; this allowed transplantation of approximately 5 mm³ of neural tissue. Care was exercised at this point not to inadvertantly introduce air bubbles into the donor neural tissue because this is not conducive to transplant growth. Likewise, any mesenchymal tissue left adherent to the donor tissue causes the transplant to be nonviable owing to the disproportinately rapid growth of mesenchymal tissue encapsulating the transplanted neural tissue.

At this stage, the donor neural tissue was ready to be transplanted to the host site. While the dissection of the donor embryos was taking place, the host animals were likewise prepared by an assistant so that the donor tissue could be immediately transplanted; the preparation of the host was as follows: Animals were first deeply anesthetized, the scalp shaved and scrubbed with betadine, and subjects then placed properly and securely in the stereotaxic apparatus. The scalp was incised at the rostral-most extent of the frontal bone and the incision extended caudally about 2 cm to allow adequate exposure of the cranium. The scalp was then retracted using mosquito clamps or small retractors, and the surface of the skull scraped clear of overlying connective tissue with a scalpel and thoroughly dried. A 1.5-mm diameter burr hole was then made unilaterally in the cranium using a dental drill. The coordinates for this were either 1 mm caudal to bregma and 2 mm lateral to the sagittal suture, or 1 mm rostral to bregma and 2 mm lateral to the sagittal suture; the rostral or caudal positions were counterbalanced as well as the position on either the right or left side of the sagittal suture. At this point a scalpel with a number 11 blade was gently inserted into the burr hole and the underlying dura incised; this resulted in a slight backflow of cerebrospinal fluid. In pilot studies, it was found that preparing host animals in batches of two or three ensured having hosts prepared to receive fresh neural tissue; this method was thus employed in this study. It was found, however, that several host animal could be kept waiting for transplants provided they were adequately anesthetized and the scalp incisions were kept moistened and clamped with Serrefine clamps.

As donor tissue began to be drawn into the microsyringe, a prepared host animal was transferred to the operating field. The sharp oblique tip of the syringe was then inserted through the burr hole at an angle approximately 45° to the surface of the cranium and about 1–2 mm directly into the cerebral cortex. The neural tissue was then slowly ejected from the syringe using very gentle pressure on the plunger. This part of the procedure was very tedious and had to be done carefully, since inserting the glass needle too deep would result in a subcortical transplant, while not plunging the tip deep enough would result in an extraparenchymal transplant and failure of neuronal integration (Das 1982). When injecting neural tissue via the caudally placed burr hole, the tip of the needle was inserted in a rostral orientation; when injecting via the rostrally placed burr hole, the tip of the needle was inserted in a caudal direction. Both of these approaches resulted in the neural tissue being injected almost directly under the coronal suture about 2 mm lateral to the sagittal suture, this being the central region of the rat motor cortex (Hall and Lindholm 1974).

After the neural tissue was injected, the syringe was rotated around its axis and gently withdrawn over a 20-second time period. After removing the glass needle, the scalp was immediately repositioned and pressure applied for 30 seconds on the transplant site. The cranial incision was then sutured with 5-0 silk sutures, topical antibacterial spray applied, and finally the surgical site sprayed with Aeroplast (Parke-Davis Co.) sterile spray bandage. A prophylactic dose of 60,000 units of penicillin was then given before the animals were placed in postoperative recovery cages. After surgical recovery, animals were returned to their original cages and continued to receive food and water *ad libitum*.

Lesioning Procedure

For the lesioning procedure, the surgical set-up and equipment were nearly identical to that used for the transplantation. Subjects were 3 months of age on the day of surgery. With the animals deeply anesthetized, they were placed securely in the stereotaxic instrument. A midline incision was made in the scalp overlying the rostral extent of the frontal bone and extended caudally 2 cm. The cranium was again scraped and dried and a burr hole made unilaterally on each side of the coronal suture (but very close to it) and 1 mm from the sagittal suture. Using microrongeurs, a craniectomy was made by chipping away bone outward from the edges of the burr holes. The craniectomy was extended 3 mm posterior and anterior from the coronal suture and laterally to 4 mm from the sagittal suture. The opening thus achieved was approximately 18 mm² in area and corresponded to the forelimb trunk, and hindlimb motor cortical areas as electrophysiologically mapped by Hall and Lindholm (1974).

Using metal suction cannulae (15, 18, and 20 gauge) attached to an electrical suctioning unit, the cortex exposed by craniectomy was aspirated completely as well as a small amount of cortex under the edges of the exposed cranium. Care was taken not to aspirate any of the underlying white matter in the process. The surgical wound was irrigated with sterile Ringer's, and Gelfoam was then cut to the appropriate size and packed into the resected brain cavity. The cranial incision was then closed with 5-0 silk sutures. Postoperative care was identical to that received by the animals receiving transplants.

At just over 3 months of age (6 days after the actual lesions were made), animals serving as controls for this study sustained midline cranial incisions identical to those of the animals receiving the transplants and lesions. The underlying cranial bone was likewise scraped with a scalpel and the incision then simply closed with continuous 5-0 silk sutures. The pre- and postoperative procedures were identical to those already mentioned.

Behavioral Evaluations

Animals receiving transplants into motor cortex were behaviorally tested beginning 6 weeks postoperatively; this allowed adequate time for the transplants to grow and differentiate. Animals sustaining motor cortex lesions and sham operations were behaviorally tested 1 1/2 weeks and 5 days, respectively, post-surgery; this allowed optimal opportunity to observe any motor deficits.

Each behavioral test used in this study was designed to assess a particular aspect of motor functioning and, when viewed collectively, gave a relatively comprehensive overview of the integrity of several neuroanatomical systems. The tests used and their methodologies are discussed separately below.

Neurological Examination

The neurological exam was utilized to assess the integrity of several levels of CNS function. The methodology for this was taken from the procedures developed by Bures et al. (1976), and the applicability and usefulness of the exam has been demonstrated by Tupper and Wallace (1980). The procedure in short consisted of several separately presented test situations with two observers noting the animal's response to these tests. Scoring consisted of placing a ''1'' on the score sheet for a correct response; inappropriate responding or no response received a rating of 0. The test was administered over 2 consecutive days.

Each of the separate subtests, a brief procedure for administering them, and the appropriate responses that would be observed in a normal animal are as follows: *Flexion Reflex:* the animal is picked up by the tail and toes are pinched with forceps; the pinched paw is moved away. *Grasping Reflex:* holding the rat by the tail, the forepaw is touched with a wire; the touched paw grips the wire. *Righting Reflex:* (a) the rat is turned over onto its back on a flat surface; it immediately rights itself; (b) the animal is held around the lower back and rear limbs and turned in either a clockwise or counterclockwise direction in the air; the head moves in the direction opposite the turning; (c) the rat is held upside-down (with its back facing the ground), 40 cm above a padded surface, and then dropped; it turns in the air to land on its feet. *Placing Reactions:* (a) the rat is held by the tail and brought toward the edge of the table; as the front paws approach the edge, it reaches for the table; (b) the same procedure as in (a), except as the chin nears the table edge, both paws are placed on the table; (c) the rat is restrained near the edge of the table; when one leg is forced over the edge, it is immediately placed back on the table; (d) the animal is held by the tail and brought toward the edge of the table its vibrissae are touching; the paws reach for the table; (e) same procedure as in (d) except that the whiskers are not allowed to touch the table; by sight the animal reaches for the edge. *Equilibrium Tests:* (a) the rat is placed facing down a wire platform elevated to 30 to 60°, it turns around to fall upward; (b) the animal is placed on a 2-cm wooden dowel wrapped with cloth tape; it should be able to stay on the bar for 3 minutes; (c) same procedure as in (b) but the dowel is rotated at 1 revolution/10 seconds; the rat should be able to maintain balance and stay on. *Corneal Reflex:* the cornea is touched with a whisp of cotton; the rat blinks its eye; *Pupillary Reflex:* the pupil is allowed to dilate under red light as observed with a magnifying glass; a white light source is shined in the eye and the pupil constricts. *Auditory Startle:* when the rat is standing quietly, hands are clapped loudly over its head; the animal extends its limbs and looks startled; *Toe Spreading:* the rat is placed on a piece of plexiglass that is then titlted; through the underside of the plexiglass, the toes are observed to spread. *Head shaking:* a puff of air is blown into the rat's ears through a rubber tube; the animal shakes its head. For a detailed description of the neuroanatomical level examined by each test, the reader is referred to Tupper and Wallace (1980).

Open Field

By employing the open field apparatus, it was possible to observe general activity of the animal as well as any general locomotor dysfunction. A counting device tabulated the number of blocks crossed (all four paws passing through a block), normal and abnormal rears, frequency of dysmetria and ataxia, and frequency of urination and defecation. Continuous records were also kept of general manipulative ability. The test was conducted over 4 consecutive days, each test session consisting of five consecutive 1-minute observation periods. Two observers were used to count the various behaviors.

Activity Measurement

Rats were placed in activity wheels for 23 consecutive hours with continuous access to water. After 23 hours, the animals were removed from the wheels for 1 hour and allowed free access to food. During this period, the number of revolutions was recorded and the units recalibrated according to the procedure of Lacey (1944). The activity measurements were made on 3 consecutive days.

Elevated Walkway

Two 45-mg Noyes pellets were placed at each end of the runway and the animal placed in the center (facing a randomly chosen end). Five 1-minute trials were used duing each test session. As the animal traversed the walkway, the numbers of falls, footfaults, and total number of intervals crossed were counted during each trial. General behavior and locomotor ability were also observed and continuously recorded. Two observers were used on each of the 2 consecutive days of testing.

Histology

Following behavioral testing, animals were sacrificed with an overdose of sodium pentobarbital and perfused transcardially using 10% buffered formalin. Macrophotography of representative brains was done before blocking. Following embedding in parablast, brains were cut in the coronal plane at 8 μm. For brains sustaining lesions, as well as controls, every seventh section was saved. Brains receiving embryonic neural tissue implants were cut similarly, and every fourth or in some cases serial sections were saved through the extent of the differentiated transplant. All tissue was subsequently stained using the Kluver–Barrera method for myelin and cell bodies (Kluver and Barrera 1953). Finally, the material was subjected to qualitative analysis and photomicrographs of representative brains were taken.

Results

Behavioral Data: Quantitative

Since previous research involving transplantation into cerebellum (Wallace and Das 1982) has shown that behaviorally, control and transplant animals are significantly different from lesioned animals, though not from one another, in the present investigation a series of t-tests (two-tailed) for independent samples was performed on the mean data for transplants versus lesions, transplants verus controls, and controls verus lesions (see Table 12–1). In some cases where t-tests yielded results that were close to though not significant at the .05 level, a nonparametric statistical procedure (Kruskal–Wallis one-way analysis of variance) was employed in an attempt to obtain some type of information with respesct to the directionality of the group data (Table 12–2).

Neurological Exam

All three groups of animals exhibited essentially the same number of appropriate responses (100%) on all subtests of the neurological exam except for the equilibrium test performed using the 2-cm wooden dowel.

Since the data collected (the specified behavior classified as either appropri-

Table 12-1. Summary of T-Test Data

Behavioral test	Transplant vs. lesion	Transplant vs. control	Control vs. lesion
Elevated walkway			
1. Blocks traversed	t = 4.91; p < 0.001[a]	t = 3.37; p < 0.01[a]	t = −1.12; p = 0.30
2. Hindleg misplacements	t = 0.71; p = 0.49	t = 5.62; p < 0.001[a]	t = 4.12; p < 0.005
3. Falls	t = −2.14; p = 0.07[b]	t = −0.72; p = 0.48[b]	t = 2.04; p = 0.08[b]
4. Turns	t = 2.47; p < 0.05[a]	t = 0.38; p = 0.72	t = 1.40; p = 0.21[b]
Open field			
1. Blocks crossed	t = 2.74; p < 0.05[a]	t = 2.61; p < 0.05[a]	t = −0.54; p = 0.60
2. Normal rears	t = 5.74; p < 0.001[a]	t = 3.29; p < 0.02[a]	t = −2.08; p = 0.06[b]
Activity wheel	t = 0.28; p = 0.79	t = −0.18; p = 0.86	t = −0.35; p = 0.74

[a] Indicates significance at the 0.05 level or less.
[b] See Kruskal–Wallis analysis of variance, Table 12-2.

Table 12-2. Kruskal–Wallis One-Way Analysis of Variance

Elevated walkway			
1. Falls	$H = 8.60; p < 0.01$[a]	$H = 0.45; p < 0.50$	$H = 4.82; p < 0.05$[a]
2. Turns	—	—	$H = 1.55; p < 0.20$
Open field			
1. Normal rears	—	—	$H = 4.20; p < 0.05$[a]

[a] Indicates significance at the 0.05 level or less.

ate or inappropriate) was actually nominal in nature, the Fisher exact probability test (a nonparametric procedure) was employed. Both control ($p < 0.025$) and transplant ($p < 0.005$) animals were found to differ significantly from lesioned animals using a one-tailed test (since directionality was presumed). Transplant and control groups, however, were not significantly different from one another.

Open Field

Of the various subtests utilized in the open field testing, the only truly quantifiable differences that could be examined between groups were number of blocks crossed and number of normal rears. Animals of the three groups performed essentially the same on the other quantitative aspects of the open field exam in that their scores on such items as incidents of intention and resting tremor, ataxia, dysmetria, and number of abnormal rears had a mean value of very close to zero. Further elaboration of such aspects of this test appears under the qualitative behavioral results.

1. Blocks crossed (Figure 12–1a): Animals receiving transplants showed a significantly greater mean number of blocks crossed per test session that either lesion ($t = 2.74$; $P < 0.05$) or control animals ($t = 2.61$; $p < 0.05$). Using the t-test as well as Kruskal–Wallis analysis of variance, control animals were found not to be significantly different from lesion animals on this subtest.

2. Normal rears: On this subtest, transplant animals showed significantly more activity than either lesion ($t = 5.74$; $p < 0.001$) or control ($t = 3.29$; $P < 0.02$) groups. The results indicate (Figure 12–1b), however, that transplantation and control groups had a greater number of normal rears than did the lesion group and in fact, using the t-test, a significant difference was nearly seen between control and lesion animals ($t = -2.08$; $p = 0.064$). Utilizing the Kruskal–Wallis nonparametric statistic, however, a significant difference was seen between lesion and control groups ($H = 4.2$; $p < 0.05$).

Activity Wheel

Significant differences between the three groups were not found utilizing t-tests; additionally, a one-way analysis of variance run on the data suggested no significant differences among the groups. The data are presented in Figure 12–2: however, differences between groups must be viewed tentatively because both the standard deviation and within-group variability were large.

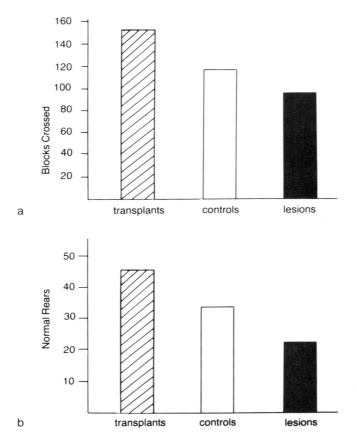

Figure 12-1. Results of open field tests. (a) Mean number of blocks crossed per test session. (b) Mean number of normal rears per test session.

Elevated Walkway

1. Blocks traversed: Animals in the transplant group showed the highest mean number of blocks traversed per test session (Figure 12–3a). T-tests showed values for the transplant group to be significantly greater than either lesion (t = 4.91; p < 0.001) or control (t = 3.37; p < 0.01) groups. Control animals did not differ significantly from lesion animals on this measure.

2. Falls: Significant differences utilizing t-tests between groups on mean number of falls per test session were not found at the 0.05 level. It should be noted, however, that mean number of falls for both control and transplant groups was much lower than the values for the lesioned animals (Figure 12–3b). The direction of this difference is actually borne out by the results of the t-tests, with transplants being significantly different from lesions at the 0.07 level, controls were significantly different only at 0.48 level. Further analysis utilizing the Kruskal–Wallis one-way analysis of variance showed transplants

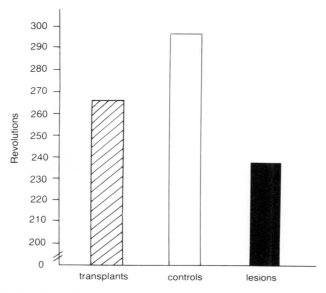

Figure 12-2. Results of activity wheel tests. Mean number of revolutions per day.

(H = 8/6; p < 0.01) and controls (H = 4.82; p < 0.50) to be significantly different from lesioned animals, yet not significantly different from one another (H = 0.45; p < 0.50).

3. Turns on the walkway: Transplant animals showed significantly more turns per test session than did lesions (t = 2.47; p < 0.05). Likewise, control animals showed a higher number of turns per test session than did lesions (Figure 12–3c); however, the significance of this difference reached only the 0.2 level utilizing both the t-test and the nonparametric Kruskal–Wallis test. Lack of a significant difference between transplants and controls is evident from the t-value (t = 0.377; p < 0.72).

4. Hindleg misplacements: Both lesion (t = 4.11; p < 0.01) and transplant (t = 5.62; p < 0.001) groups showed a significantly greater number of hindleg misplacements than controls. However, as Figure 12–4 indicates, for both control and transplant groups, the mean number of hindleg misplacemets per test session decreased, while the mean increased on subsequent test sessions for the lesion group. T-tests on the differences in mean number of hindleg misplacements per test session between days 1 and 2, 2 and 3, and 1 and 3 revealed no significant differences between transplants and controls. However, lesioned animals were found to differ significantly from both transplants and controls on this measure (with the exception of the difference between day 1 and 2 for lesions versus controls). Table 12–3 gives a summary of these results and along with Figure 12–4 indicates that while control and transplant animals showed approximately the same decrease in hindleg misplacements on succes- sive days, lesioned animals showed no such decrease and in fact were signifi-

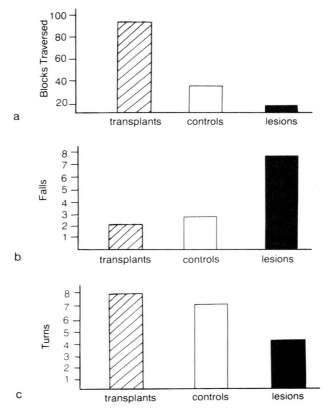

Figure 12-3. Results of elevated walkway tests. (a) Mean blocks traversed per test session. (b) Mean number of falls per session. (c) Mean number of turns on walkway per session.

Table 12-3. Summary of T-Tests on Differences in Hindleg Misplacements per Test Session between Specified Days of Testing

Comparison	Day 1–2	Day 2–3	Day 1–3
Transplants vs. lesions	t = 3.48; p < 0.005[a]	t = 2.75; p < 0.02[a]	t = 5.40; p < 0.001[a]
Transplants vs. controls	t = 1.71; p = 0.13	t = -0.65; p = 0.53	t = 1.78; p = 0.10
Controls vs. lesions	t = -1.02; p = 0.34	t = 2.74; p < 0.05[a]	t = 4.53; p < 0.001[a]

[a] Indicates significance at the 0.05 level or less.

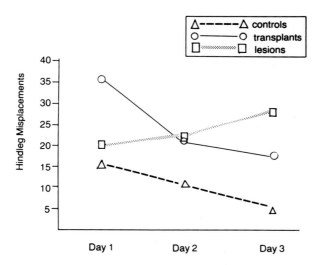

Figure 12-4. Results of elevated walkway tests. Hindleg misplacements per day for the three experimental groups.

cantly different in almost all cases from these two groups, showing an increase in this behavior on successive days.

Behavioral Data: Qualitative

Several general statements may be made regarding the overall motor capacities of the three groups of animals. Unilateral limb deficits contralateral to the side of the lesion were perhaps the most striking characteristics of the lesion group, being most apparent during equilibrium testing on the neurological exam and on the elevated walkway. Comprising such motor difficulties were a lack of limb control and coordination as manifested in an inability to properly grasp with and place the paws. On these two tests, hindlimb deficits were generally seen to be most profound, although forelimb deficits were also observed.

Although not quantifiable, it appeared that the lack of coordination seemed to be exacerbated by an apparent decrease in strength in the affected limbs. This was reflected in an animal's inability to maintain a grasp or posture during one of the tests.

Unilateral deficits were likewise quite apparent upon observing a lesioned animal's locomotor ability in the open field apparatus. Animals were frequently described as having a unilateral "hop" or "gimp" in their gait, and limb positioning was frequently abnormal both at rest and while locomoting (e.g., forelimb abducted or adducted). General coordinative ability was usually noted as "poor" as seen by difficulty in initiating turns to one side, crossing or aberrant placement of a limb, and occasional problems with the synchronous movement of limbs unilaterally. Such features were rarely, if ever, observed with transplant or control animals, most of the activity for these animals being described as symmetrical, smooth, or grossly normal.

Included in the various subtests of the open field evaluation related to motor ability (other than those mentioned previously under quantitative behavioral data) were incidents of ataxia, dysmetria, tremor at rest, intention tremor, number of abnormal rears, and qualitative judgement of manipulative ability. On these subtests, the three groups of animals performed essentially the same; i.e., nearly all animals had a mean score of zero or very close to it, suggesting that only on certain of the previously mentioned subtests were animals significantly different. It should be noted that at the gross observational level, lesioned animals did not appear to be markedly inferior to the other groups in terms of manipulative ability.

In summary of the qualitative data, then, deficits in the motor abilities of the lesioned animals did not appear to be simply generalized and nondescript; rather these deficits appeared to be related to those tasks that required the coordinated ability and strength to place and grasp with the extremities in order to maintain balance, or to synchronicity and controlled limb movements during locomotion.

Histological Data: Qualitative

Macroscopic

1. Transplants: Of the ten animals that recieved homotopic neural transplants, only two of these showed evidence of extensive transplant growth on macroscopic examination. In each of these cases, the transplant occupied an area of approximately 10 mm^2 and was found to be fairly well embedded into the host cortex. It should be noted, however, that even upon gross inspection, the transplant was seen to actually grow into the host cortical tissue at only one discrete region, the rest of the transplant simply displacing the host neuropil and remaining extraparenchymal. Six of the other brains receiving embryonic neural tissue showed as evidence of transplant growth only a small tuft of neural tissue approximately 1 mm^2 projecting from the cortical surface. In such cases it was not possible to establish macroscopically the extent of transplant growth that occured in the deeper cortical layers. Two of the ten brains showed no evidence of transplant growth upon gross inspection of the cortical surface.

2. Lesions: Figure 12–5 shows the approximate size and location of lesions in six of the lesioned brains. In the case of all lesioned brains, the desired area of cortex was adequately aspirated. In some cases, small areas of aspiration lesion extended beyond the cortex into the white matter (chiefly corpus collosum), underlying hippocampal structures to a minor degree, and in two cases as deep as the lateral ventricle on the side of the aspiration. In these latter two cases, fibers of the internal capsule and possible striatal structures may have been involved.

3. Controls: All of the brains from the control animals appeared grossly normal with no evidence of pathological changes.

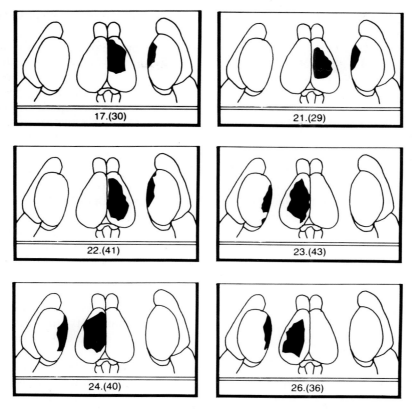

Figure 12-5. Drawings of the unilateral cortical lesions sustained at approximately 3 months of age; 10 days prior to behavioral testing. The first number below each specimen represents the identity of the animal; numbers within parentheses indicate estimated area of neocortex ablated in mm².

Microscopic

1. Transplants: In the case of the two large cortical transplants (10 mm²), microscopic analyses confirmed the initial observations of a fairly large region of the transplant displacing the host tissue, yet remaining extraparenchymal. At the point where the transplant was firmly embedded in the host neocortex, higher power magnification revealed continuity of host and donor neuropil as well as evidence of fiber projections coursing between the transplant and host neural tissue. This arrangement could be compared conveniently to the morphology of a mushroom, with its large "head" projecting above the cortical surface partially displacing it (i.e., extraparenchymally), and its "stalk" coursing down into the host neuropil establishing connectivity. In addition to this single "stalk" of neural tissue becoming integrated with the host brain, another discrete region of transplant growth was seen in both cases in the deeper cortical regions. These smaller regions were fully integrated with the host

tissue in terms of sharing a common neuropil, and in one of these cases, fibers were seen coursing between transplant and corpus callosum.

In the case of the other brains in which prior to processing for histology the tuft of neural tissue was seen projecting from the cortex, microscopic analyses revealed well-developed transplants just below the surface of the cortex extending down to the corpus callosum and in most cases actually embedding among its fibers. Notable massive growth of the transplant was seen in two cases, one in which the transplant had grown into the lateral ventricle and another in which contra- and ipsilateral hippocampal structures were invaded. Of all the brains examined microscopically, only one was found to show no evidence of transplant growth.

In terms of the transplant morphology, it was seen that this entity represented neural tissue that had become fully integrated with the host neuropil in that no pial or glial barrier separated the host/transplant interface. Additionally, perfectly normal-looking pyramidal cells were seen scattered throughout the transplant, yet the laminar character typical of neocortex was not observed. It thus should be emphasized that although the transplants did share a common neuropil with the host brain, their morphology was in fact quite distinctly different from the neural tissue with which they had become integrated.

Fiber projections coursing within the transplant as well as between host and donor tissue were also observed in the case of all transplants. In many cases these were represented by large bundles of axons from the corpus callosum plunging deep into the substance of the transplant as well as smaller callosal fibers extending into the more peripheral regions. In no instances were fiber projections seen to be "blocked" from integrating with the transplant by any type of glial or pial limiting membrane or substrate.

2. Lesions: After microscopic examination of the lesioned brains, two brains were in fact seen to have involvement of not only neocortex, but also extension of the lesion into the lateral ventricle, part of the internal capsule, and superficial hippocampal and striatal structures as well. All of the other lesioned brains showed at least minor involvement of callosal fibers in addition to neocortex, but lesions did not extend further than the deepest extent of this structure. In only one case was extensive enlargement of the lateral ventricles evident, and even in this case, there was not marked displacement of adjacent or contralateral structures.

3. Controls: The five control brains examined under magnifications up to $400 \times$ showed no cortical or subcortical abnormalities. The cortex was seen to have its normal laminar appearance, and there was no evidence of any subcortical nuclear pathology or ventricular enlargement.

Discussion

A discussion of the results of the present study will begin with a consideration of the data obtained on the various behavioral tests. Subsequently the histological findings will be explained, and, finally, conclusions from the study and suggestions for future research will be proposed.

With regard to the behavioral data, it can be said with some certainty at both the quantitatve and qualitative level that lesioned animals did in fact show deficits reflective of motor cortical damage that were not exhibited by either the transplant or control animals. This was perhaps most evident on the equilibrium subtest of the neurological exam utilizing the wooden dowel. Both transplants and control animals displayed no inappropriate responses on this test, whereas six of eight lesioned animals were seen to have some degree of difficulty maintaining balance and/or posture on the bar. These differences were borne out as significant utilizing the nonparametric Fisher test.

Similar results were also indicated from both the parametric and nonparametric statistical analysis of mean number of falls on the elevated walkway. The parametric t-tests, although not significant at the 0.05 level, nevertheless pointed clearly in the direction of transplant and control animals being less impaired than lesion animals on the elevated walkway in terms of number of falls. Nonparametric tests showed transplants and controls as in fact performing significantly better than lesions on this subtest at the 0.05 level or less. These data are in agreement with similar studies of motor cortex integrity (Maier 1935, Gentile et al. 1978).

In examining the data for an animal's hindleg misplacements on the elevated walkway, it is evident that the control animals performed significantly better than either transplant or lesion animals. At first glance, these data do not seem to support the contention that control and transplant groups should exhibit similar behavior. However, both control and transplant animals were seen to exhibit an improvement in performance with each successive day of testing; such was not the case for the lesioned animals; in fact, these animals showed an increase in hindleg misplacements each day. Again, such results for the lesioned and control animals reflect earlier work by Maier (1935) and Gentile et al. (1978); however, differences between transplant and control animals are difficult to speculate upon. The fact that both the control and transplant groups seemed to improve their performance on successive days does suggest that in fact the lesioned animals were more impaired than either of these two groups.

In considering the data from the remaining behavioral tests, such definitive statements cannot be made with regard to differences between the three groups. For example, it was found that on tests in which some level of activity was being recorded (e.g., blocks traversed on the elevated walkway and number of rears and blocks crossed as counted in the open field apparatus), transplant animals showed a significantly higher quantity of the measured behavior than either control or lesion animals. Although not significant at the 0.05 level for differences between transplants and control animals, this same pattern was seen as well on counts of turns on the elevated walkway. Although such a pattern was unexpected, still more baffling was the finding that except in the case of normal rears (open field), the lesion and control animals were not found to be significantly different from one another on these measures. Results similar to these have not appeared in literature, and thus one can only speculate as to the reasons for such results. At this point, one must logically look toward possible differences in the populations sampled; such possibilities will be considered in more detail later in the discussion.

Finally, it should be mentioned that little weight was placed on the results of the activity wheels. The reasons for this are severalfold: (1) No significant differences were found between any of the groups; (2) despite differences between the groups, there was a large standard deviation within groups; (3) nothing has appeared in the literature on motor cortex function that would suggest that there should be differences on this measure; and (4) there is some question as to the reliability of the data obtained from these measuring devices.

Before drawing conclusions from this study, a few statements may be made in consideration of the histological data. It should first be pointed out that the transplantation procedure utilized in this study resulted in successful transplants in nearly all cases. A successful and viable transplant was one that met at least one of the two major criteria established by Das (1974). These are integration with the host brain either by the sharing of a common neuropil or by the interchange of axons between transplant and host neural tissue. Thus, a successful neural transplant was not simply one that grew in any region of the brain; for example, a transplant may grow extensively in one of the cerebral ventricles if it receives a blood supply from the choroid plexus. Yet such a transplant could not be considered to be an anatomically integrated entity within the host brain for no pathways of neuronal connectivity could exist. Hence, functionality of the transplant in terms of synaptic transmission would not be possible; however, it might be capable of manifesting some type of hormonal influence if it possessed neurons that were secretory in nature.

In most of the recent transplantation studies mentioned earlier, areas of the host brain that proved well suited for transplant growth and integration were generally areas that were somewhat deep into the brain substance. The present study is unique in that a cortical region served as a host site for the transplant. The histological results showed that in fact neural transplants could be made into neural structures as superficial as neocortex and anatomical integration of the transplant with the host brain would occur. In transplanting into this site, however, growth of the neural tissue into the surrounding structures (corpus callosum, hippocampus, and lateral ventricles) does present a problem in that the transplant does not remain exclusively cortical. The depth of the rat neocortex simply is not great enough to accommodate the entire transplant, and any attempt to implant the neural tissue more superficially in the cortex results in a transplant that is largely extraparenchymal (as described in the "mushroom analogy"). A delicate balance therefore exists between a transplant that will end up as an extraprenchymal entity and a transplant that is implanted too deeply, thus invading adjacent structures during its growth.

Implications and Conclusions of this Study

Before any statements are made about the differences in the motor behavior of the animals in this study, the implications and effects of an animal receiving a neural transplant should be addressed. As mentioned previously, the histological findings of this study indicated that in virtually every case, the transplants appeared to be fully integrated with the host brain in a strictly defined sense. Although it cannot be proven unequivocally, there is no reason to assume that these transplants were not physiologically or at least metabolically normal neural tissue, for after all, they did grow and differentiate into a neural substrate quite normal in appearance.

Although clear proof of the functionality of the transplants would require electrophysiological methods, speculation from the present study can be made in light of past research. As was previously described, evidence has shown that neural transplants are both physiologically and electrophysiologically functional in several neuroanatomical systems (Gash et al. 1975, Björklund and Stenevi 1979; Björklund et al. 1979, Gash et al. 1979, Perlow et al. 1979, Kimura et al. 1980).

In support of the neurophysiological functionality of neural transplants are the many studies that have demonstrated unequivocally that neural transplants in several neuroanatomical systems quite specifically receive host afferents and send out efferent fibers. These studies include research on transplantation into sensory, nuclear, and relay systems (Lund and Hauschka 1976, Jaeger and Lund 1979a,b, 1980b, McLoon and Lund 1979, 1980, Harvey and Lund 1981), and similar work involving a motor system, namely cerebellum (Hallas et al. 1980b, Oblinger et al. 1980). Furthermore, Das (1975) has shown, utilizing electron microscopy, that transplants receiving afferents do indeed have synapses on their somata, although the functionality of these (e.g., the capacity for synaptic transmission) has not been established. The very fact that such pathways of connectivity become established (and sometimes over relatively long distances), suggests that the transplant/host interaction is indeed a very dynamic one. In addition, these studies have demonstrated that the patterns of connectivity are not simply random but rather are quite specific.

If one thus assumes that the neural tissue transplants in this and other studies did in fact perform some functional role, the logical next question to address is how might they have affected an animal's behavior? In research by Wallace and Das (1982) on behavioral analyses of animals receiving heterotopic neural transplants into cerebellum, the growing transplant was found to have displaced a substantial portion of the host brain. In that similar tissue loss effected by lesions of the cerebellum was seen to cause marked motor deficits, yet normal controls and the animals receiving transplants displayed no significant impairment, the contention was made that perhaps the transplants had indeed taken over the function of the displaced cerebellar tissue.

More recently, however, speculation has been made with respect to the possibility of the transplant in some way influencing the functioning of the cerebellar cortical tissue that remained subsequent to the compression lesion caused by the growing transplant. This hypothesis was put forward in light of the fact that the neocortical tissue used for transplantation would have neuroanatomical and physiological properties quite different from the cerebellar tissue into which it was transplanted. Although the nature of the influence of the transplant on the host neural tissue is not known, trophic factors would seem to be one such possibility.

In the present study, normal-looking neurons were seen scattered throughout the transplant; additionally, fiber bundles were seen projecting between host and transplant via a common neuropil, suggesting a possible route for neuronal interactions and connections to be made. Thus, although functionality (in terms of neurophysiological properties) of the transplants in the present study was not established, the morphological characteristics of these transplants and the findings of the mentioned studies suggest that they might at least have the potential to be functional.

In contrast to the study by Wallace and Das (1982), however, the present work did not yield such clear-cut behavioral results and transplant growth was not nearly as extensive. In fact, animals with transplants in many cases performed at significantly higher levels of activity than did controls on several behavioral tests. From such results, it is argued that the transplant at least had no deleterious effects on the host brain; beyond this, it is not possible to put forward supportable statements.

In light of current speculation, it could also be possible in the present study for the transplants to have exerted some trophic influence on the cortical tissue that had not been displaced by growth of the transplants. In support of such a possibility is the previously cited research by Lundberg and Mollgard (1979). Weinberg and Raine (1980), and Kromer (1980), in which neural transplants were seen to enhance regenerative events in the host brain.

Further mention should be made of the fact that in this study, transplant animals were actually more active on several of the behavioral tests (elevated walkway and open field). It is quite difficult to speculate and ascribe actual physiological causes to such differences. These results were likely to have been due to the small control group size affecting the numerical outcome of the statistical procedures that were utilized. Additionally, it is possible that the control group was in fact simply not a good population sample in terms of homogeneity of variance.

Another discrepancy in this study when contrasted to past work (Wallace and Das 1982) was also evident in comparisons between control and lesioned animals. Significant differences between these two groups were not found in all cases in which they were expected. It should be noted, however, that such results were on tests which measured a level of some activity (e.g., number of blocks traversed) and not on tests which reflected motor cortex deficits (e.g., hindleg misplacements on the walkway and equilibrium testing). Such differences thus could again have been due simply to sample size of the control group and variation within it.

In conclusion, it should be recognized that the behavioral tests used in this study were able to detect gross motor cortical deficits as represented in comparisons between lesioned and control animals. These included measures of hindleg misplacements, falls on the elevated walkway, and equilibrium testing. Additionally, animals receiving transplants did not perform any worse than controls on these subtests. This study thus appears to have been successful in at least supporting in direction the results of previous behavioral examinations of transplants into a motor system (Wallace and Das 1982).

In summarizing the results of the surgical procedures (lesioning and transplantation), it should be emphasized that this study dealt with a relatively new site for transplantation of neural tissue.

References

Bures, J., Burresova, D., Huston, J. (1976). Techniques and Basic Experiments for the Study of Brain and Behavior. Amsterdam: Elsevier Scientific Publishing Co.

Björklund, A., Segal, M., Stenevi, U. (1979). Functional reinnervation of rat hippocampus by locus coeruleus implants. Brain Res. 170, (pt 3) 409–426.

Björklund, A., Stenevi, U. (1979). Reconstruction of the nigrostriatal dopamine pathway by intracerebral nigral transplants. Brain Res. 177, 555–560.

Castro, A. (1972). The effects of cortical ablations on digital usage in the rat. Brain Res. 37, 173–185.

D'Amato, C., Hicks, S. (1980). Development of the motor system: Effects of radiation on developing corticospinal neurons and locomotor function. Exp. Neurol. 70, 1–23.

Das, G.D. (1973). Transplantation of cerebellar tissue in the cerebellum of neonate rabbits. Brain Res. 50, 170–173.

Das, G.D. (1974). Transplantation of embryonic neural tissue in the mammalian brain. I. Growth and differentiation of neuroblasts from various regions of the embryonic brain in the cerebellum of neonate rats. TIT J. Life Sci. 4, 93–124.

Das, G.D. (1975). Differentiation of dendrites in the transplanted neuroblasts in the mammalian brain. In: Advances in Neurology, Vol. 12. Kreutzberg, G.W. (ed.). New York: Raven Press.

Das, G.D. (1976). Transplantation of neuroblasts in the brain of rat: Dendritic differentiation. Anat. Rec. 184, 388.

Das, G.D. (1977). Transplantation of embryonic neural tissue in the brain of the adult rats. Anat. Rec. 187, 563.

Das, G.D. (1978). Neural transplants in the brain of the rat: Nature of degenerative changes in the host brain and the transplant. Anat. Rec. 193, 517.

Das, G.D. (1981). Neural transplants in the spinal cord of the adult rat. Anat. Rec. 199, 64A.

Das, G.D. (1982). Extraparenchymal neural transplants: Their cytology and survivability. Brain Res. 241, 182–186.

Das, G.D., Altman, J. (1971). Transplanted precursors of nerve cells: Their fate in the cerebellums of young rats. Science 173, 637–638.

Das, G.D., Altman, J. (1972). Studies on the transplantation of developing neural tissue in the mammalian brain. I. Transplantation of cerebellar slabs into cerebellum of neonate rats. Brain Res. 38, 233–249.

Das, G.D., Hallas, B. (1978). Transplantation of brain tissue in the brain of adult rats. Experientia, 34, 1304–1306.

Das, G.D., Hallas, B., Das, K. (1979). Transplantation of neural tissue in the brains of laboratory mammals: Technical details and comments. Experientia, 35, 143–153.

Das, G.D., Hallas, B., Das, K. (1980). Transplantation of brain tissue in the brain of rat. I. Growth characteristics of neocortical transplants from embryos of different ages. Am. J. Anat. 158, 135–146.

Dunn, E. (1917). Primary and secondary findings in a series of attempts to transplant cerebral cortex in the albino rat. J. Comp. Neurol. 27, 565–582.

Gash, D., Roos, T., Chambers, W. (1975). Development of Rathke's pouch tissue transplanted into adult hypophysectomized female rats. Neuroendocrinology 19, 214–226.

Gash, D., Sladek, J., Sladek, C. (1979). Development of normal fetal supraoptic neurons grafted into adult rats with a congenital lack of vasopressin producing neurons. Soc. Neurosci. Abst. 5, 445.

Gentile, A.M., Green, S., Nieburgs, A., Schmelzer, W., Stein, D.G. (1978). Disruption and recovery of locomotor and manipulatory behavior following cortical lesions in rats. Behav. Bio. 22, 417–455.

Glees, P. (1955). Studies on cortical regeneration with special reference to cerebral implants. In: Regeneration in the Central Nervous System. Windle, W.F. (ed.). Springfield, IL: C.C. Thomas.

Hall, R., Lindholm, E. (1974). Organization of motor and somatosensory neocortex in the albino rat. Brain Res. 66, 23–38.

Hallas, B., Das, G.D., Das, K. (1980a). Transplantation of brain tissue in the brain of rat. II. Growth characteristics of neocortical transplants in hosts of different ages. Am. J. Anat. 158, 147–159.

Hallas, B., Oblinger, M., Das, G. (1980b). Heterotopic neural transplants in the cerebellum of the rat: Their afferents. Brain Res. 196, 242–246.

Harvey, A., Lund, R. (1981). Transplantation of tectal tissue in rats. II. Distribution of host neurons which project to transplants. J. Comp. Neurol. 201, 505–520.

Houle, J., Das, G.D. (1980a). Freezing and transplantation of brain tissue in rats. Experientia 30, 1114–1115.

Houle, J., Das, G.D. (1980b). Freezing of embryonic neural tissue and its transplantation in the rat brain. Brain Res. 192, 570–574.

Jaeger, C., Lund, R. (1978). Development of cerebral cortex transplanted to cerebral cortex or tectum of newborn rat hosts. Soc. Neurosci. Abst. 4, 116.

Jaeger, C., Lund, R. (1979a). Connections between cerebral cortex transplants and rat host brain. Soc. Neurosci. Abst. 5, 628.

Jaeger, C., Lund, R. (1979b). Efferent fibers from transplanted cerebral cortex of rats. Brain Res. 165, 338–342.

Jaeger, C., Lund, R. (1980a). Transplantation of embryonic occipital cortex to the brain of newborn rats. An autoradiographic study of transplant histogenesis. Exp. Brain Res. 40, 265–272.

Jaeger, C., Lund, R. (1980b). Transplantation of occipital cortex to the tectal region of newborn rats: A light microscopic study of organization and connectivity of the transplants. J. Comp. Neurol. 194, 571–598.

Jaeger, C., Lund, R. (1981). Transplantation of embryonic occipital cortex to the brain of newborn rats: A Golgi study of mature and developing transplants. J. Comp. Neurol. 200, 213–230.

Kimura, H., McGeer, P., Noda, Y., McGeer, E. (1980). Brain transplants in an animal "model" of Huntington's disease. Soc. Neurosci. Abst. 6, 688.

Kluver, H., Barrera, E. (1953). A method for the combined staining of cells and fibers in the nervous system. J. Neuropath. Exp. Neurol. 12, 400–403.

Krieg, W. (1946a). Connections of the cerebral cortex. I. The albino rat. A. Topography of the cortical areas. J. Comp. Neurol. 84, 221–275.

Krieg, W. (1946b). Connections of the cerebral cortex. I. The albino rat. B. Structure of the cortical areas. J. Comp. Neurol. 84, 277–324.

Kromer, L. (1980). Glial scar formation in the brain of adult rats is inhibited by implants of embryonic CNS tissue. Soc. Neurosci. Abst. 6, 688.

Lacey, D. (1944). A revised procedure for the calibration of the activity wheel. Am. J. Psych. 57, 411.

Lashley, K. (1921). Studies of cerebral function in learning. No. III. The motor area. Brain 44, 255–285.

Le Gros Clark, W.E. (1940). Neuronal differentiation in implanted foetal cortical tissue. J. Neurol. Psych. (London) 3, 263–272.

Le Gros Clark, W.E. (1942). The problem of neuronal regeneration in the central nervous system. I. The influence of spinal ganglia and nerve fragments grafted in the brain. J. Anat. 77, 20–48.

Le Gros Clark, W.E. (1943). The problem of neuronal regeneration in the central nervous system. II. The insertion of peripheral nerve stumps into the brain. J. Anat. 77, 251–258.

Lund, R., Harvey, A. (1981). Transplantation of tectal tissue in rats. I. Organization of transplants and pattern distribution of host afferents within them. J. Comp. Neurol. 201, 191–209.

Lund, R., Hauschka, S. (1976). Transplanted neural tissue develops connections with host rat brain. Science 193, 582–584.

Lundberg, J., Mollgard, K. (1979). Mitotic activity in adult rat brain induced by implantation of pieces of fetal rat brain and liver. Neurosci. Lett. 13, 265–270.

Maier, N. (1935). The cortical area concerned with coordinated walking in the rat. J. Comp. Neurol. 61, 395–405.

McLoon, S., Lund, R. (1979). Development of retina transplanted to the tectum of neonatal rats. Soc. Neurosci. Abst. 5, 631.

McLoon, S., Lund, R. (1980). Specific projections of retina transplanted to rat brain. Exp. Brain Res. 40, 273–282.

McLoon, L., McLoon, S., Lund, R. (1981). Cultured embryonic retinae transplanted to rat brain: Differentiation and formation of projections to host superior colliculus. Brain Res. 226, 15–31.

Oblinger, M., Das, G.D. (1981). Age of host as an influencing factor on the growth and connectivity of neural transplants in the cerebellar hemisphere of the rat. Anat. Rec. 199, 185A–186A.

Oblinger, M., Hallas, B., Das, G.D. (1980). Neocortical transplants in the cerebellum of the rat: Their afferents and efferents. Brain Res. 189, 228–232.

Perlow, M., Freed, W., Karoum, D., Hoffer, B., Seiger, A., Olson, L., Wyatt, R. (1979). Substantia nigra grafts reduce motor abnormalities produced by destruction of negro-striatal dopamine system. Soc. Neurosci. Abst. 5, 681.

Price, A., Fowler, S. (1981). Deficits in contralateral and ipsilateral forepaw motor control following unilateral motor cortical ablations in rats. Brain Res. 205, 81–90.

Ramon y Cajal, S. (1928). Degeneration and Regeneration of the Nervous System, Vols. 1 and 2. May, R.M. (trans. and ed.). London: Oxford University Press.

Ranson, S. (1903). On the medullated nerve fibers crossing the site of lesions in the brain of the white rat. Comp. Neurol. 13, 185–207.

Ranson, S. (1914). Transplantation of the spinal ganglion, with observations on the significance of complex types of spinal ganglion cells. J. Comp. Neurol. 24, 547–558.

Saltykow, S. (1905). Versuche uber Gehirnplantation, zugleich ein Beitrag zur Kenntniss der Vorgange an den Zelligen Gehirnelementen. Arch. Psych. (Berlin) 40, 329–388.

Settlage, P., Bingham, W., Suckle, H., Borge, A., Woolsey, C. (1949). The pattern of localization in the motor cortex of rat. Fed. Proc. 8, 114.

Spiliotis, P., Thompson, R. (1973). The "manipulative response memory system" in the white rat. Physiol. Psych. 1, 101–114.

Stenevi, U., Björklund, A., Svendgaard, N. (1976). Transplantation of central and peripheral monamine neurons to the adult rat brain: Techniques and conditions for survival. Brain Res. 114, 1–20.

Svendgaard, N. (1977). Transplantation of monoaminergic neurons to the adult rat brain: Conditions for survival and mode of growth. Acta Neurochir. 37, 302.

Tidd, C.W. (1932). The transplantation of spinal ganglion of the white rat. A study of the morphological changes in surviving cells. J. Comp. Neurol. 55, 531–543.

Tupper, D., Wallace, R. (1980). Utility of the neurological examination in rats. Acta Neurobiol. Exp. 40, 999–1003.

Wallace, R., Das, G.D. (1982). Behavioral effects of CNS transplants in the rat. Brain Res. 243, 133–139.

Weinberg, E., Raine, C. (1980). Reinnervation of peripheral nerve segments implanted into the rat central nervous system. Brain Res. 198, 1–11.

Wenzel, J., Barlehner, F. (1969). Zur regeneration des Cortex cerebri bei *Mus masculus*. II. Morphologische Befunde regenerativer Vorgange nach Replantation eines Cortexabschnittes. Z. Mikroskop. Forsch. 81, 32–70.

Index